Intervention in Mental Health–Substance Use

MENTAL HEALTH–SUBSTANCE USE

Intervention in Mental Health–Substance Use

Edited by

DAVID B COOPER

Sigma Theta Tau International: The Honor Society of Nursing Award
Outstanding Contribution to Nursing Award
Editor-in-Chief, Mental Health and Substance Use
Author/Writer/Editor

Radcliffe Publishing
London • New York

Radcliffe Publishing Ltd
33–41 Dallington Street
London
EC1V 0BB
United Kingdom

www.radcliffepublishing.com

Electronic catalogue and worldwide online ordering facility.

British Library Cataloguing in Publication Data

A catalogue record for this book is available from the British Library.

ISBN-13: 978 184619 342 2

Typeset by Pindar NZ, Auckland, New Zealand
Printed and bound by Cadmus Communications, USA

Contents

Preface

Approximately six years ago Phil Cooper, then an MSc student, was searching for information on mental health–substance use. At that time, there was one journal and few published papers. This led to the launch of the journal *Mental Health and Substance Use: dual diagnosis*, published by Taylor & Francis International. To launch the journal, and debate the concerns and dilemmas of psychological, physical, social, legal and spiritual professionals, Phil organised a conference for Suffolk Mental Health NHS Trust and Taylor & Francis. The response was excellent. An occurring theme was that more information, knowledge and skills were needed – driven by education and training.

Discussion with international professionals indicated a need for this type of educational information and guidance, in this format, and a proposal was submitted for one book. The single book progressed to become a series of six! The concept is that each book will follow on from the other to build a sound basis – as far as is possible – about the important approaches to mental health–substance use. The aim is to provide a 'how to' series that will be interactive with case studies, reflective study and exercises – you, as individuals and professionals, will decide if this has been achieved.

So, why do we need to know about mental health–substance use? International concerns related to interventions, and the treatment of people experiencing mental health–substance use problems, are frequently reported. These include:

➤ 'the most challenging clinical problem that we face'[1]
➤ 'substance misuse is usual rather than exceptional amongst people with severe mental health problems'[2]
➤ 'Mental health and substance use problems affect every local community throughout America'[3]
➤ 'The existence of psychiatric comorbidities in young people who abuse alcohol is common, especially for conditions such as depression, anxiety, bipolar disorder, conduct disorder and attention-deficit/hyperactivity disorder'[4]
➤ 'Mental and neurological disorders such as depression, schizophrenia, epilepsy and substance abuse . . . cause immense suffering for those affected, amplify people's vulnerability and can lead individuals into a life of poverty'.[5]

There is a need to appreciate that mental health–substance use is now a concern for us all. This series of books will bring together what is known (to some), and what is not (to some). If undertaken correctly, and you, the reader will be the judge – and those individuals you come into contact with daily will be the final judges – each book will build on the other and be of interest for the new, and the not so new, professional.

The desire to provide services that facilitate best practice for mental health–substance use is not new. The political impetus for this approach to succeed now exists. We, the professionals, need to seize on this momentum. We need to bring about the much-needed change for the individual who experiences our interventions and treatment, be that political will because of a perceived financial benefit or, as we would hope, the need to provide therapeutic interventions for the individual. Whatever the motive, now is the time to grasp the initiative.

Before we (the professionals) can practise, research, educate, manage, develop or purchase services, we must commence with knowledge. From that, we begin to understand. We commence using our new-found skills. We progress to developing the ability to examine practice, to put concepts together, to make valid judgements. We achieve this level of expertise though education, training and experience. Sometimes, we can use our own life experiences to enhance our skills. But knowledge must come first, though is often relegated to last! Professionals (from health, social, spiritual and legal backgrounds) – be they students, practitioners, researchers, educators, managers, service developers or purchasers – are all 'professionals' (in the eye of the individual we meet professionally), though each has differing depths of knowledge, skills and expertise.

What we need to remember is that the individual (those we offer care to), family and carers bring their own knowledge, skills and life experiences – some developed from dealing with ill health. The individual experiences the illness, lives with it, manages it – daily. Therefore, to bring the two together, individual and professional, to make interventions and treatment outcome effective, to meet whatever the individual feels is acceptable to his or her needs, requires mutual understanding and respect. The professionals' skills and expertise '*are founded on nothing less than their complete and perfect acceptance of one, by another*'.[6]

David B Cooper
January 2011

REFERENCES

1 Appleby L. *The National Service Framework for Mental Health: five years on*. London: Department of Health; 2004. Available at: www.dh.gov.uk/prod_consum_dh/groups/ dh_digitalassets/@dh/@en/documents/digitalasset/dh_4099122.pdf (accessed 29 August 2010).

2 Department of Health. *Mental Health Policy Implementation Guide: dual diagnosis good practice guide*. London: Department of Health; 2002. Available at: www.substancemisuserct. co.uk/staff/documents/dh_4060435.pdf (accessed 29 August 2010).

3 Substance Abuse and Mental Health Service Administration. *Results from the 2008 National Survey on Drug Use and Health*. 2008. Available at: www.oas.samhsa.gov/ nsduh/2k8nsduh/2k8Results.cfm (accessed 2 August 2010).

4 Australian Government. *Australian Guidelines to Reduce Health Risks from Drinking Alcohol*.

2009. Available at: www.nhmrc.gov.au/publications/synopses/ds10syn.htm (accessed 29 August 2010).

5 World Health Organization. *Mental Health Improvements for Nations Development: the WHO MIND Project.* World Health Organization; 2008. Available at: www.who.int/mental_health/policy/en (accessed 29 August 2010).

6 Thompson F. *Lark Rise to Candleford: a trilogy.* London: Penguin Modern Classics; 2009.

About the Mental Health–Substance Use series

The six books in this series are:
1 *Introduction to Mental Health–Substance Use*
2 *Developing Services in Mental Health–Substance Use*
3 *Responding in Mental Health–Substance Use*
4 *Intervention in Mental Health–Substance Use*
5 *Care in Mental Health–Substance Use*
6 *Practice in Mental Health–Substance Use*

The series is not merely for mental health professionals but also the substance use professionals. It is not a question of 'them' (the substance use professional) teaching 'them' (the mental health professional). It is about sharing knowledge, skills and expertise. We are equal. We learn from each fellow professional, for the benefit of those whose lives we touch. The rationale is that to maintain clinical excellence, we need to be aware of the developments and practices within mental health and substance use. Then, we make informed choices; we take best practice, and apply this to our professional role.[1]

Generically, the series Mental Health–Substance Use concentrates on concerns, dilemmas and concepts specifically interrelated, as a collation of problems that directly or indirectly influence the life and well-being of the individual, family and carers. Such concerns relate not only to the individual but also to the future direction of practice, education, research, service development, interventions and treatment. While presenting a balanced view of what is best practice today, the books aim to challenge concepts and stimulate debate, exploring all aspects of the development in treatment, intervention and care responses, and the adoption of research-led best practice. To achieve this, they draw from a variety of perspectives, facilitating consideration of how professionals meet the challenges now and in the future. To accomplish this we have assembled leading, international professionals to provide insight into current thinking and developments, from a variety of perspectives, related to the many varying and diverse needs of the individual, family and carers experiencing mental health–substance use.

REFERENCE

1 Cooper DB. Editorial: decisions. *Mental Health and Substance Use*. 2010; **3**: 1–3.

About the editor

David B Cooper
Sigma Theta Tau International: The Honor Society of Nursing Award
Outstanding Contribution to Nursing Award
Editor-in-Chief: *Mental Health and Substance Use*
Author/Writer/Editor

The editor welcomes approaches and feedback, positive and/or negative.

David has specialised in mental health and substance use for over 30 years. He has worked as a practitioner, manager, researcher, author, lecturer and consultant. He has served as editor, or editor-in-chief, of several journals, and is currently editor-in-chief of *Mental Health and Substance Use*. He has published widely and is *'credited with enhancing the understanding and development of community detoxification for people experiencing alcohol withdrawal'* (Nursing Council on Alcohol; Sigma Theta Tau International citations). Seminal work includes *Alcohol Home Detoxification and Assessment* and *Alcohol Use*, both published by Radcliffe Publishing, Oxford.

List of contributors

CHAPTER 2 AND USEFUL CONTACTS   **Jo Cooper**
Former Macmillan Clinical Nurse Specialist in Palliative Care
Horsham
West Sussex
England

Jo spent 16 years in Specialist Palliative Care, initially working in a hospice inpatient unit, then 12 years as a Macmillan Clinical Nurse Specialist. She gained a Diploma in Oncology at Addenbrooke's Hospital, Cambridge, and a BSc (Hons) in Palliative Nursing at The Royal Marsden, London, and an Award in Specialist Practice. Jo edited *Stepping into Palliative Care* (Radcliffe Medical Press; 2000) and the second edition of *Stepping into Palliative Care*, Books 1 and 2 (Radcliffe Publishing; 2006). Jo has been involved in teaching and education for many years. Her specialist subjects include management of complex pain and symptoms, terminal agitation, communication at the end of life, therapeutic relationships, and breaking bad news.

CHAPTER 3   **Poppy Buchanan-Barker**
Director, Clan Unity International Ltd
Newport-on-Tay
Fife
Scotland

Poppy is Director of Clan Unity International – a public limited company offering mental health recovery-focused seminars and workshops, internationally. As a social worker, she spent more than 25 years leading innovative community developments for people with multiple disabilities and their families. Poppy began training as a counsellor in the 1980s, working with individuals and families, in the areas of suicide, alcohol and crisis resolution. She is widely published and has presented her work at many international conferences. In 2008, Poppy was the joint winner of the Thomas S Szasz Award for Outstanding Contributions to the Cause of Civil Liberties, in New York.

Professor Phil Barker
Honorary Professor
Faculty of Medicine, Dentistry, and Nursing, University of Dundee
Psychotherapist
Newport-on-Tay
Fife
Scotland

Phil is a psychotherapist. He was the UK's first Professor of Psychiatric Nursing Practice at the University of Newcastle (1993–2002); elected a Fellow of the Royal College of Nursing in 1995; awarded the Red Gate Award for Distinguished Professors at the University of Tokyo in 2000; awarded an honorary Doctorate of the University at Oxford Brookes University in 2001; and has been visiting professor at several international universities. In 2008, Phil was the joint winner of the Thomas S Szasz Award for Outstanding Contributions to the Cause of Civil Liberties, in New York.

CHAPTERS 4 AND 5   Professor Larry D Purnell

Professor Emeritus, University of Delaware
Adjunct Professor, Florida International University Consulting Faculty
Excelsior College Funded Professor, Universita di Modena, Italy
Newark, DE
USA

Larry has published over 100 refereed journal articles, 75 book chapters, and 13 books. His model, the Purnell Model for Cultural Competence, has been translated into Arabic, Flemish, French, Korean, Portuguese and Spanish. Larry's textbooks have won the American Journal of Nursing and Brandon Hill Book awards. He has made presentations in 14 countries on four continents. Larry is an American Academy of Nursing and Luther Christman Fellow. In addition, he has been the US Representative to the European Union Commission on Intercultural Communication resulting from the Salamanca, Sorbonne, Bologna and WHO Declarations.

CHAPTER 6   Professor Carlo C DiClemente

Professor of Psychology
Psychology Department
Director of Maryland Resource Center for Quitting Use and Initiation of Tobacco (MDQUIT)
University of Maryland, Baltimore County
Baltimore, MD
USA

Carlo is the co-developer of the Transtheoretical Model of behaviour change, and the author of numerous scientific articles and book chapters on motivation and behaviour change and the application of this model to a variety of problem behaviours. Carlo's book *Addiction and Change: how addictions develop and addicted people recover* was released in paperback in 2006. For over 25 years, Carlo has conducted funded research in health and addictive behaviours. He has received a number of awards, including the Innovators Combating Substance Abuse award by the Robert Wood Johnson Foundation and the McGovern award from the American Society of Addiction Medicine.

Kristina Schumann
Graduate Research Assistant
Psychology Department
University of Maryland, Baltimore County
Baltimore, MD
USA

Kristina is a doctoral student in the Human Services Psychology Program at the University of Maryland, Baltimore County (UMBC). She received a BA in Psychology from the University of Connecticut in 2002 and an MA in Psychology from American University in 2006. Her master's research project was titled 'Motivational subgroups: exploring behavior change variables and drinking outcomes among at risk drinkers admitted to a trauma unit'. She is currently researching chronic illness and behaviour change and is particularly interested in the psychosocial components of diabetes self-management.

Preston A Greene
Graduate Research Assistant
Center Specialist, Maryland Resource Center for Quitting Use and Initiation of Tobacco (MDQUIT)
Psychology Department
University of Maryland, Baltimore County
Baltimore, MD
USA

Preston is a doctoral student in the Human Services Psychology Program at the University of Maryland, Baltimore County (UMBC). He received a BS in Psychology from Virginia Commonwealth University in 2005. His MA was conferred in 2010 from UMBC, and his master's thesis was titled, 'Self-efficacy as a mechanism of change during alcoholism treatment'. His research interests include the psychological mechanisms underlying the successful resolution of problematic drinking.

Michael D Earley
Graduate Research Assistant
Habits Laboratory
Psychology Department
University of Maryland, Baltimore County
Baltimore, MD
USA

Michael is a doctoral student in the Clinical Psychology/Behavioral Medicine program at the University of Maryland, Baltimore County. He completed both his BA in English and MEd at the University of Notre Dame in 2000 and 2002 respectively. Michael's research interests include the role of personality and spirituality in engaging the process of intentional behaviour change. He is currently employed by the Center for Integrative Medicine at the University of Maryland and assists in research exploring the efficacy of mindfulness interventions for trauma survivors.

CHAPTER 7   Dr Jennifer E Hettema

Assistant Professor
University of Virginia
Department of Psychiatry and Neurobehavioral Sciences
UVA Center for Addition Research and Education
Richmond, VA
USA

Jennifer is a licensed clinical psychologist and assistant professor in the Department of Psychiatry and Neurobehavioral Sciences at the University of Virginia. She conducts research on the applications of motivational interviewing to a variety of health-related disorders and is interested in the dissemination and implementation of evidence-based practices. She is also a member of the Motivational Interviewing Network of Trainers.

Joshua T Kirsch

Clinical Social Worker
The Permanente Medical Group, Inc.
Pleasanton, CA
USA

Joshua is a psychiatric social worker at Kaiser Permanente and is a member of the Motivational Interviewing Network of Trainers. He has more than 10 years' experience working with adults who have co-occurring disorders, and several years providing clinical supervision. He has extensive experience training clinicians in the use of motivational interviewing.

CHAPTER 8   Dr Catherine Lock

Lecturer in Public Health Research (Evaluation of Complex Interventions)
Fuse – the UKCRC Centre for Translational Research in Public Health
Institute of Health and Society
Newcastle University
Newcastle upon Tyne
England

Catherine specialises in the development and evaluation of complex interventions, particularly those targeted at different stages of the life course including children, young people, working professionals and older people and is interested in the use of social marketing theory and methods. She also has over 10 years' experience of conducting research into alcohol, including involvement in a series of World Health Organization collaborative studies on screening and brief alcohol intervention in primary healthcare. Experienced in both qualitative and quantitative techniques, including randomised controlled trials and systematic reviews, Catherine has over 30 peer-reviewed publications.

Professor Eileen Kaner
Professor of Public Health Research
Director, Institute of Health and Society
Newcastle University
Newcastle upon Tyne
England

Eileen's research aims to understand the nature and extent of alcohol-related risk and harm across populations, and to promote evidence-based interventions to reduce these problems. To date, she has published 88 peer-reviewed papers and won over £12 million in research income. She currently co-leads three national Screening and Intervention Programme for Sensible Drinking (SIPS) trials that are evaluating screening and brief alcohol intervention approaches in primary care, accident and emergency departments and criminal justice settings. Eileen's research also includes funded projects on substance use in pregnancy and in young people. Eileen recently led a national review of liver disease epidemiology and treatment effectiveness in England and a review of the impact of alcohol consumption on young people. The latter formed the scientific basis of national guidance for parents on alcohol consumption in their children. Eileen is a Trustee of the Alcohol Education and Research Council and an honorary fellow of the Royal College of Physicians. Lastly, she is the Chair of the National Institute for Health and Clinical Excellence (NICE) programme development group whose work is focused on the prevention of alcohol use disorders in adults and adolescents.

Professor Nick Heather
Emeritus Professor of Alcohol and Other Drug Studies
Department of Psychology
Northumbria University
Newcastle upon Tyne
England

After working for 10 years as a clinical psychologist in the UK National Health Service, in 1979 Nick developed and led the Addictive Behaviours Research Group at the University of Dundee. In 1987, he became founding Director of the National Drug and Alcohol Research Centre at the University of New South Wales, Australia. He returned to the UK at the beginning of 1994 to take up a post as Consultant Clinical Psychologist at the Newcastle City Health NHS Trust and as Director of the Centre for Alcohol and Drug Studies in Newcastle. Nick has a long-standing interest in research on addictive disorders, with an emphasis on the treatment of alcohol problems. He has accumulated over 400 publications, was lead investig-ator on a recently completed World Health Organization Collaborative Project concerned with the implementation of screening and brief intervention for alcohol problems in primary healthcare and, with colleagues, was commissioned by the UK Government to produce the *Review of the Effectiveness of Treatment for Alcohol Problems*, published in 2006.

CHAPTER 9   Kathleen Sciacca

Consultant; Executive Director
Sciacca Comprehensive Service Development for Mental Illness, Drug Addiction and Alcoholism
New York, NY
USA
http://users.erols.com/ksciacca

Kathleen is a consultant, trainer, speaker and programme developer. She developed the first treatment interventions for people with co-occurring mental and substance disorders and integrated services in 1984. She is a former director of the Mentally Ill Chemical Abusers and Addicted (MICAA) training site for programme and staff development – NYS Office of Mental Health. She implements programmes and workforce competencies across systems, state, city and agency-wide, throughout the USA and internationally. Kathleen is author of the *MIDAA Service Manual*, articles/chapters/reports and producer of the video *Integrated Treatment*. Kathleen is a trainer of motivational interviewing (member of MINT since 1995), group leading and cognitive behavioural therapy. She is also a guest lecturer at Columbia University, Hunter College and various college courses.

CHAPTER 10   Anne Garland

Nurse Consultant Psychological Therapies
Nottingham Psychotherapy Unit
Nottinghamshire Healthcare NHS Trust
Nottingham
England

Anne has been practising cognitive behaviour therapy (CBT) in the NHS for the last 20 years. Anne has worked as a cognitive therapist in two Medical Research Council-funded trials investigating the efficacy of using cognitive therapy in the treatment of chronic depression and bi-polar disorder. Anne is an active researcher in the area of chronic depression and has published widely in this field. Anne is also recognised nationally and internationally as a cognitive therapy trainer and has presented cognitive therapy skills-based workshops and academic papers at both a national and international level.

CHAPTER 11   Professor Alexander L Chapman

Assistant Professor; Chair, Graduate Program
Department of Psychology

Simon Fraser University
Burnaby, BC
Canada

Alex received his bachelor's degree in psychology from the University of British Columbia and his MS and PhD in clinical psychology from Idaho State University. After his internship at Duke University Medical Center, Alex completed a two-year postdoctoral fellowship with Dr Marsha Linehan at the University of Washington, where he received training and supervision in dialectical behaviour therapy (DBT) and in clinical research. Alex's research focuses on understanding borderline personality disorder, emotion regulation problems, self-harm and suicidal behaviour, and impulsivity, and includes research on DBT. He regularly gives workshops on DBT, consults with clinicians in both Canada and the US, and teaches students how to treat persons with borderline personality disorder. Alex has published numerous articles and book chapters and has given over 70 presentations on borderline personality disorder, self-harm, DBT, and impulsive behaviour, among other topics. In 2007, he received the Young Investigator's Award of the National Education Alliance for Borderline Personality Disorder (NEA-BPD) for his research on BPD. He has co-authored a book on borderline personality disorder (*The Borderline Personality Disorder Survival Guide*; 2007), as well as a book on behaviour therapy (*Behavioral Interventions in Cognitive-Behavior Therapy: practical guidance for putting theory into action*; 2007). In addition, Alex is the president and co-founder of the DBT Centre of Vancouver (www.dbtvancouver.com), a treatment centre for persons who struggle with BPD and related problems.

Katherine L Dixon-Gordon
Graduate Student
Department of Psychology
Simon Fraser University
Burnaby, BC
Canada

Katherine is a doctoral student in the Clinical Psychology programme at Simon Fraser University, where she completed her MA working with Dr Chapman. She received her bachelor's degree in psychology from the University of Washington, where she completed a research assistantship with Dr Marsha Linehan. Her research focuses on borderline personality disorder (BPD), psychophysiological measures of emotion regulation, and how emotion dysregulation impacts social problem-solving and impulsivity.

Brianna J Turner
Graduate Student
Department of Psychology
Simon Fraser University
Burnaby, BC
Canada

Brianna is a graduate student in the Clinical Psychology programme at Simon Fraser University working with Dr Chapman, where she completed her bachelor's degree in psychology. Her research focuses on the identification of risk and relapse factors associated with self-injury and other self-damaging behaviours.

CHAPTER 12   Susan H Brown

Private Practice
Licensed Social Worker; EMDRIA Approved Consultant and Facilitator for the EMDR Institute and EMDR Humanitarian Assistance Program
La Mesa, CA
USA

Susan is a licensed Board Certified Diplomate in Clinical Social Work. She has been in clinical practice in San Diego, California since 1979, specialising in the treatment of trauma and substance abuse with adults. She has published and presented nationally on addictions and eye movement desensitisation and reprocessing (EMDR). She was one of the principal investigators in a pilot research study field-testing an Integrated Trauma Treatment Program (ITTP) using EMDR and Seeking Safety with Co-occurring Trauma and Substance Use Disorder in a Drug Court Program in Olympia, WA. She is an EMDRIA Approved Consultant and Facilitator for EMDR Humanitarian Assistance Program and the EMDR Institute.

Julie E Stowasser

Private Practice – Calm Clear and Connected
Licensed Marriage and Family Therapist; EMDRIA Approved Consultant; EMDR Institute/EMDR-HAP Facilitator; Certified Batterer Intervention Provider
Calm, Clear, and Connected, San Luis Obispo and Atascadero, California
San Luis Obispo, CA
USA

Julie is an EMDR Institute and Eye Movement Desensitisation and Reprocessing Humanitarian Assistance Programs (EMDR-HAP) Facilitator; an EMDRIA Approved Consultant who founded and co-moderates the EMDRIA Approved Consultants Email Discussion List; and EMDRIA Approved Credit Unit Provider and presenter on domestic violence and EMDR. She wrote the domestic violence chapter in the *Handbook of EMDR and Family Therapy Processes* (2007), and is a Certified Batterer Intervention Provider who founded and moderates the American Psychological Association's DV Treatment Provider email discussion list. Julie offers consultation in EMDR, the treatment of domestic violence victims and perpetrators, children, ethics, and general clinical concerns. Julie practises in San Luis Obispo, California.

Dr Francine Shapiro

Senior Research Fellow, Mental Research Institute, Palo Alto, CA, USA
Executive Director, EMDR Institute
President Emeritus, EMDR Humanitarian Assistance Programs

Francine is the founder of the EMDR Humanitarian Assistance Programs (a non-profit organisation coordinating services worldwide), and advisor to a wide variety of trauma treatment and outreach organisations. Francine is a recipient of the International Sigmund Freud Award of the City of Vienna for distinguished contribution to psychotherapy, the American Psychological Association Division 56 Award for Outstanding Contributions to Practice in Trauma Psychology, and the Distinguished Scientific Achievement in Psychology Award, from the California Psychological Association. Francine wrote the primary text on EMDR, entitled *Eye Movement Desensitization and Reprocessing: basic principles and procedures.*

CHAPTER 13 David S Manley

Clinical Director Substance Misuse Services
Nurse Consultant in Dual Diagnosis
Senior Fellow of the Institute of Mental Health
Substance Misuse Services
Nottinghamshire Healthcare NHS Trust
Carlton, Nottingham
England

David is currently studying for a PhD in nursing, examining the treatment experiences of individuals with a dual diagnosis and quality outcomes for this service user group. He is a member of the editorial board for Advances in Dual Diagnosis, and has published widely on issues related to dual diagnosis. David has a particular interest in cognitive behavioural interventions in substance misuse including cue reactivity. In the past, David has chaired the East Midlands Clinical Advice Network on Dual Diagnosis.

CHAPTER 14 Dr Andrew Rosenblum

Director, Principle Investigator
Institute for Treatment and Services Research (ITSR)
National Development and Research Institute, Inc. (NDRI)
New York, NY
USA

Andrew has considerable experience developing, implementing and evaluating behavioural substance abuse interventions for diverse at-risk populations and conducting prevalence surveys of prescription opioid abuse and chronic pain among populations of chemical dependency patients. Current work includes developing and evaluating web-based cognitive behavioural interventions for chronic pain patients and post-traumatic stress disorder (PTSD) symptomatic-substance misusing veterans.

Dr Stephen Magura
Director
Evaluations Center
Western Michigan University

Kalamazoo, MI
USA

Stephen is a former Deputy Executive Director and Director of Science and Research at National Development and Research Institutes, Inc., New York City. He has designed and directed drug-dependency clinical trials, treatment evaluation studies, health services research, social epidemiology studies, HIV prevention research and policy analyses. He has been the Principal Investigator of many studies sponsored by the National Institutes of Health and other agencies.

Dr Alexandre B Laudet
Director; Principal Investigator
Center for the Study of Addictions and Recovery (C-STAR)
National Development and Research Institute, Inc. (NDRI)
New York, NY
USA

Alexandre is a recognised expert in addiction recovery. Her federally funded research focuses on elucidating what helps people quit drinking or getting high and how they stay in recovery. A social psychologist, her goals are to build and help translate the science of recovery into services and policy that create opportunities for long-term recovery and improved quality of life for people with substance problems. She has published numerous scientific articles, presents regularly at conferences, serves on the editorial board of several peer-reviewed publications and community-based organisations, and provides consultancy on promoting opportunities for recovery.

Howard Vogel
Executive Director
Double Trouble in Recovery
Brooklyn
New York, NY
USA

Howard is the founder of Double Trouble in Recovery (DTR), which began in New York State in 1989. Dually diagnosed and in recovery for more than 20 years, he has worked towards disseminating information about the special needs of dually diagnosed persons, giving presentations about DTR at hospitals, community agencies, and conferences nationwide, starting new groups, and seeing to many members' progression in recovery. He was/is a collaborator on several research studies of DTR and is the author of *Double Trouble in Recovery: basic guide* and *How to Start a Double Trouble in Recovery Group*.

CHAPTER 15 Catherine Dixon
Therapist and Empowerment Coach
London
England
www.energyroots.co.uk

Catherine is a well-being coach, therapist and teacher. She has been in professional practice for nine years. She currently works within the NHS, other public bodies and in the private sector. Catherine created an employability foundation course called Empower Your Life! This was first introduced as a goal-setting programme in January 2008 as part of the aftercare strategy for a rehabilitation organisation. Catherine graduated in shiatsu in 2001 and acquired further qualifications to practise acupuncture for common ailments and ear acupuncture. Catherine is a Chi Kung teacher (London College of Chi Kung) and a licensed trainer of energy therapies (the AMT). She runs postgraduate training programmes for therapists and is a clinical supervisor for the Ear Acupuncture Register. Catherine trained in cognitive hypnotherapy at the Quest Institute and is a registered member of the National Council of Hypnotherapy, the General Hypnotherapy Register and the General Hypnotherapy Standards Council. She is a member of the NHS Directory of Complementary and Alternative Practitioners (No. 6378).

Terminology

Whenever possible, the following terminology has been applied. However, in certain instances, when referencing a study and/or specific work(s), when an author has made a specific request, or for the purpose of additional clarity, it has been necessary to deviate from this applied 'norm'.

MENTAL HEALTH–SUBSTANCE USE

Considerable thought has gone in to the use of terminology within these texts. Each country appears to have its own terms for the person experiencing mental health and substance use problems – terms that includes words such as dual diagnosis, coexisting, co-occurring, and so on. We talk about the same thing but use differing professional jargon. The decision was set at the outset to use one term that encompasses mental health *and* substance use problems: *mental health–substance use*. One scholar suggested that such a term implies that both can exist separately, while they can also be linked.[1]

SUBSTANCE USE

Another challenge was how to term 'substance use'. There are a number of ways: abuse, misuse, dependence, addiction. The decision is that within these texts we use the term *substance use* to encompass all (unless specific need for clarity at a given point). It is imperative the professional recognises that while we may see another person's 'substance use' as misuse or abuse, the individual experiencing it may not deem it to be anything other than 'use'. Throughout, we need to be aware that we are working alongside unique individuals. Therefore, we should be able to meet the individual where he/she is.

ALCOHOL, PRESCRIBED DRUGS, ILLICIT DRUGS, TOBACCO OR SUBSTANCES

Throughout this book *substance* includes alcohol, prescribed drugs, illicit drugs and tobacco, unless specific need for clarity at a given point.

PROBLEM(S), CONCERNS AND DILEMMAS OR DISORDERS

The terms *problem(s)*, *concerns and dilemmas* and *disorders* can be used interchangeably, as stated by the author's preference. However, where possible, the term 'problem(s)' or 'concerns and dilemmas' had been adopted as the preferred choice.

INDIVIDUAL, PERSON, PEOPLE

There seems to be a need to label the individual – as a form of recognition! Sometimes the label becomes more than the person! 'Alan is schizophrenic' – thus it is Alan, rather than an illness that Alan lives with. We refer to patients, clients, service users, customers, consumers, and so on. Yet, we feel affronted when we are addressed as anything other than what we are – individuals! We need to be mindful that every person we see during our professional day is an individual – unique. Symptoms are in many ways similar (e.g. delusions, hallucinations), some need interventions and treatments are similar (e.g. specific drugs, psychotherapy techniques), but people are not. Alan may experience an illness labelled schizophrenia, and so may John, Beth and Mary, and you or I. However, each will have his/her own unique experiences – and life. None will be the same. To keep this constantly in the mind of the reader, throughout the book series we shall refer to the *individual*, *person* or *people* – just like us, but different to us by their uniqueness.

PROFESSIONAL

We are all professionals, whether students, nurses, doctors, social workers, researchers, clinicians, educationalists, managers, service developers, religious ministers – and so on. However, the level of expertise may vary from one professional to another. We are also individuals. There is a need to distinguish between the person with a mental health–substance use problem and the person interacting professionally (at whatever level) with that individual. To acknowledge and to differentiate between those who experience – in this context – and those who intervene, we have adopted the term *professional*. It is indicative that we have had, or are receiving, education and training related specifically to help us (the professionals) meet the needs of the individual. We may or may not have experienced mental health–substance use problems but we have some knowledge that may help the individual – an expertise to be shared. We have a specific knowledge that, hopefully, we wish to use to offer effective intervention and treatment to another human being. It is the need to make a clear differential, for the reader, that forces the use of 'professional' over 'individual' to describe our role – our input into another person's life.

REFERENCE

1 Barker P. Personal communication; 2009.

Cautionary note

Wisdom and compassion should become the dominating influence that guide our thoughts, our words, and our actions.[1]

Never presume that what you say is understood. It is essential to check understanding, and what is expected of the individual and/or family, with each person. Each person needs to know what he/she can expect from you, and other professionals involved in his/her care, at each meeting. Jargon is a professional language that excludes the individual and family. Never use it in conversation with the individual, unless requested to do so; it is easily misunderstood.

Remember, we all, as individuals, deal with life differently. It does not matter how many years we have spent studying human behaviour, listening and treating the individual and family. We may have spent many hours exploring with the individual his/her anxieties, fears, doubts, concerns and dilemmas, and the illness experience. Yet, we do not know what that person really feels, how he/she sees life and ill health. We may have lived similar lives, experienced the same illness but the individual will always be unique, each different from us, each independent of our thoughts, feelings, words, deeds and symptoms, each with an individual experience.

REFERENCE

1 Matthieu Ricard. As cited in: Föllmi D, Föllmi O. *Buddhist Offerings 365 Days*. London: Thames and Hudson; 2003.

Acknowledgements

I am grateful to all the contributors for having the faith in me to produce a valued text and I thank them for their support and encouragement. I hope that faith proves correct. Thank you to those who have commented along the way, and whose patience has been outstanding. Thank you to Jo Cooper, who has been actively involved with this project throughout – supporting, encouraging, listening and participating in many practical ways. Jo is my rock who looks after me during my physical health problems, and I am eternally grateful.

Many people have helped me along my career path and life – too many to name individually. Most do not even know what impact they have had on me. Some, however, require specific mention. These include Larry Purnell, a friend and confidant who has taught me never to presume – while we are all individuals with individual needs, we deserve equality in all that we meet in life. Thanks to Martin Plant (who sadly died in March 2010), and Moira Plant, who always encouraged and offered genuine support. Phil and Poppy Barker, who have taught me that it is OK to express how I feel about humanity – about people, and that there is another way through the entrenched systems in health and social care. Keith Yoxhall, without whose guidance back in the 1980s I would never have survived my 'Colchester work experience' and the dark times of institutionalisation, or had the privilege to work alongside the few professionals fighting against the 'big door'. He taught me that there was a need for education and training, and that this should be ongoing – also that the person in hospital or community experiencing our care sees us as 'professional' – we should make sure we act that way. Thank you to Phil Cooper, who brought the concept of this book series to me via a conference to launch the journal Mental Health and Substance Use: dual diagnosis, of which he was editor. It was then I realised that despite all the talk over too many years of my professional life, there was still much to be done for people experiencing mental health–substance use problems. Phil is a good debater, friend and reliable resource for me – thank you.

To Gillian Nineham of Radcliffe Publishing, my sincere thanks. Gillian had faith in this project from the outset and in my ability to deliver. Her patience is immeasurable and, for that, I am grateful. Thank you to Michael Hawkes and Jessica Morofke for putting up with my too numerous questions! Thank you to Jamie Etherington, Editorial Development Manager, and Dan Allen of the book marketing department, both competent people who make my work look good. Thanks also to Mia Yardley, Natalie Mason, Camille Lowe and the production team at Pindar,

New Zealand, for bringing this book to publication, and the many others who are nameless to me as I write but without whom these books would never come to print; each has his/her stamp on any successes of this book.

My sincere thanks to all of you named, and unnamed, my friends and colleagues along my sometimes broken career path: those who have touched my life in a positive way – and a few, a negative way (for we can learn from the negative to ensure we do better for others).

A final heartfelt statement: any errors, omissions, inaccuracies or deficiencies within these pages are my sole responsibility.

Dedication

This book is dedicated to Caroline and John Hall. Caroline is a truly dedicated mother and wife. Her sense of humour and willing smile lights up the heart. Despite her discomfort and pain from a progressive back problem, Caroline always moves forward – never giving up. All these things and more make Caroline the daughter we love, and are so very proud of. John is a dedicated supporter of Caroline in all she strives to achieve in life. It is clear he thinks the world of Caroline, and she of him. Together, they are a perfect match – may their love and light continue to shine.

CHAPTER 1

Setting the scene

David B Cooper

It seems that when problems arise our outlook becomes narrow.[1]

INTRODUCTION

The difficulties encountered by people who experience mental health–substance use problems are not new. The individual using substances presenting to the mental health professional can often encounter annoyance and suspicion. Likewise, the person experiencing mental health problems presenting to the substance use services can encounter hostility and hopelessness. 'We cannot do anything for the substance use problem until the mental health problem is dealt with!' The referral to the mental health team is returned: 'We cannot do anything for this person until the substance use problem is dealt with!' Thus, the individual is in the middle of two professional worlds and neither is willing to move, and yet, both professional worlds are involved in 'caring' for the individual.

For many years, it has been acknowledged that the two parts of the caring system need to work as one. However, this desire has not developed into practice. Over recent years, this impetus has changed. There is now a drive towards meeting the needs of the individual experiencing mental health–substance use problems, pooling expertise from both sides. Moreover, there is an international political will to bring about change, often driven forward by a small group of dedicated professionals at practice level.

Some healthcare environments have merely paid lip service, ensuring the correct terminology is included within the policy and procedure documentation, while at the same time doing nothing, or little, to bring about the changes needed at the practice level to meet the needs of the individual. Others have grasped the drive forward and have spearheaded developments at local and national level within their country to meet such needs. It appears that the latter are now succeeding. There is a concerted international effort to improve the services provided for the individual, and a determination to pool knowledge and expertise. In addition, there is the ability of these professional groups to link into government policy and bring about the political will to support such change. However, this cannot happen overnight. There are major attitudinal changes needed – not least at management and practice level. One consultant commented that to work together with mental health–substance use problems would be too costly. Furthermore, the consultant believed it would create 'too much work'! Consequently, there is a long way to go – but a driving force to succeed exists.

Obtaining in-depth and knowledgeable text is difficult in new areas of change. One needs to be motivated to trawl a broad spectrum of work to develop a sound grounding – the background detail that is needed to build good professional practice. This is a big request of the hard-worked and pressured professional. There are a few excellent mental health–substance use books available. However, this series of six books is groundbreaking, in that each presents a much needed text that will introduce the first, but vital, step to the interventions and treatments available for the individual experiencing mental health–substance use concerns and dilemmas.

These books are educational. However, they will make no one an expert! In mental health–substance use, there is a need to initiate, and maintain, education and training. There are key principles and factors we need to bring out and explore. Some we will use – others we will adapt – while others we will reject. Each book is complete. Conversely, each aims to build on the preceding book. However, books do not hold all the answers. Nothing does. What is hoped is that the professional will participate in, and collaborate with, each book, progressing through each to the other. Along the way, hopefully, the professional will enhance existing knowledge or develop new concepts to benefit the individual.

The books offer a first step, relevant to the needs of professionals – at practice level or senior service development – in a clear, concise and understandable format. Each book has made full use of boxes, graphs, tables, figures, interactive exercises, self-assessment tools and case studies – where appropriate – to examine and demonstrate the effect mental health–substance use can have on the individual, family, carers and society as a whole.

A deliberate attempt has been made to avoid jargon, and where terminology is used, to offer a clear explanation and understanding. The terminology used in this book is fully explained at the beginning of the book, before the reader commences with the chapters. By placing it there the reader will be able to reference it quickly, if needed. Specific gender is used, as the author feels appropriate. However, unless stated, the use of the male/female gender is interchangeable.

BOOK 4: INTERVENTION IN MENTAL HEALTH AND SUBSTANCE USE

Case study

My life was good, a home, family, work. I lived for work because that provided me with the money to keep my family – my responsibility. But things were going wrong; I lost control of my perceived destiny. Ill health took control. Initially, I coped, I had hope, it will get better – no need to adapt. However, the system was slow – stepped care meant that I could not get back my usual good health. I had to try this before I could try that – even though I knew 'that' would help me! Then I entered my 'abyss'. The darkness as I call it took over. This may take days, weeks, months, years, maybe never – at that time I did not know! 'Eventually you will find a way to cope and accept.' At this stage this was just a myth put about by 'them'. Just something your family and friends tell you. Slowly, they stepped back, unable to cope with my behaviour and actions. I was angry, sad, despaired, happy, unreasonable and obnoxious! I built a brick wall around me. Each meeting with the specialist brought initial hope – then hopelessness. I tried to recreate what I had – cocoon myself in my own safe world. My income dropped – disappeared altogether – but the bills did not! But society and state perceive people like me as a scrounger – work dodgers – a burden. In my mind I was begging for money. But my income was not as it was. I needed money to keep things as they were. I created my own empire – borrowed money I could not pay back in the misguided belief that this would bring normality back to my life, and I would then pay my debts. My debtors were after me, my family wanted me to change – but there was no way out or so I believed. I felt ashamed. I hid things – my feelings – my life was a lie, because no one would understand. I sank into a hole, maybe sought thrills; I would buy something that I believed would make me happy. I did not need it, and the happiness passed as soon as I bought the expensive 'treat'! Nobody cared – or that is how I felt – I will die. Indeed, I wanted to die. I acted in ways I did not understand – and again the shame, the despair – no way out, so what, who cares! Some sort of self-harm, self-gratification – all was doomed, I would get the punishment I deserved for being ill – not like normal hard-working people. I wanted to be punished – needed to be punished – punished for being weak and ill – not normal. At some point I accepted that I needed to change – to adapt – to take control of 'it'. It cannot be in charge of me. I accepted my position in life – the illness – its potential route. Slowly, I came out of my abyss. I looked around and saw the damage I had done. I was aware of the destruction, but helpless. I tried to make amends and build bridges with those I had hurt along the way. Some may forgive – others may accept – while others will never forgive or accept. It lives alongside my illness. But I saw a light – my own light of acceptance. I accepted the progression of my illness. Of course, many people have helped me along the way, but that goes unacknowledged. I needed to do this for myself. Now I accept the good days – and the bad. I know the damage to me is progressive – and the damage to others cannot be corrected, but I can only accept my future. Yes, there are down days – black, cold and empty days. But I look for hope. Hang on to the hope – for that is my way forward – my way out. Until the end! Of course, this is my story – my life. We are all different – I suppose we handle things differently. But that is how it was for me – then and now.

The case study above offers a glance inside the life of the individual experiencing mental health–substance use problems. We do not know how it is for him/her but we listen to the individual's story. The professional's role is to see where the individual is in his/her life. To support and steer that individual to a level of stability that is acceptable to him/her. You may not be able to 'fix', but maybe encourage acceptance and bring hope.

The professional listens to the individual and takes action to work alongside the movement towards his/her goals. Sometimes one way does not work and so the professional will try another way. However, the good professional never gives up on the individual – no one 'deserves it'. The door should always be open, accepting of the individual at whatever point she/he enters your care (*see* Book 1, Chapter 7).

To achieve this, the professional needs an understanding of what is available to aid the individual to attain his/her own goals: where he/she wants to be, what is acceptable to him/her – not what is acceptable to the professional! To do this we need the basics, then we develop that knowledge into practice and skill.

As mentioned in the Preface, the ability to learn and gain new knowledge is the way forward. As professionals we must start with knowledge, and from there we can begin to understand. We commence using our new-found skills, progressing to develop the ability to examine practice, to put concepts together and to make valid judgements.[2] This knowledge is gained through education, training and experience, sometimes enhanced by own life experiences.

Those we offer care to, and their family members, bring their own knowledge, skills and life experiences, some developed from dealing with ill health. Therefore, making interventions and treatment outcome effective requires mutual understanding and respect.

We need to appreciate and understand the concerns and dilemmas that face the person before she/he comes to the service, and professional, for intervention and treatment. We have to adapt the service to respond to those individual needs. It is important to remember that each person is unique. Yes, there may be similarities in symptoms, and specific needs addressed for sex and age. However, we must accept and acknowledge that each will have variations and specific needs that have to be considered when developing appropriate services, and when interacting with the individual. Moreover, we must be aware of the needs of the family and carers who have their own specific needs.

To get to this level of skills we need a grounding: a sound knowledge of the theories behind the treatment, how they work, who may benefit, the principles behind the interventions. This must be research-led practice and be fluid in that we take onboard the updates and modifications to the intervention as knowledge and skills progress. These are the philosophies, ethics – the grounding – from which effective interventions are introduced and developed. This book describes the various models that can be used to address the concerns and dilemma faced by the individual and family. To provide effective care there is a need for a 'starting point', of intervention – then an understanding of the types of interventions that may improve the quality of life for the person and family. Thus, Book 4 provides the theoretical basis of current practice. In Chapter 2, Jo Cooper looks at how imperative the therapeutic relationship is between the individual and professional. This is the starting point of all good practice. If we get this right, we are commencing the journey alongside the individual to his/her chosen goals.

Chapter 3, the Tidal Model, builds on this chapter and offers a humanistic model of care. In Chapters 4 and 5, Larry Purnell offers an insight into the Purnell Model for cultural competence and the application of transcultural theory in mental health–substance use. Like the preceding chapters, they highlight the importance of the individual as the centre of our interventions and treatments – each unique. Carlo DiClemente and colleagues (Chapter 6) 'describes how to use the principles and concepts of the Transtheoretical Model to address multiple diagnoses and problems and adaptations or limitations when using it' with the individual experiencing mental health–substance use problems. Chapter 7 builds upon this by examining the role of motivational interviewing (MI) when working with people experiencing mental health–substance use problems. 'Motivational Interviewing is a therapeutic technique with specific and teachable skills'; these are discussed throughout the chapter. 'The chapter focuses on general techniques for working alongside' the individual experiencing mental health–substance use problems rather than 'providing specific details about the application of MI to all possible combinations of problems'.

Chapter 8 (Catherine Lock and colleagues) charts the development of brief interventions 'both empirically and in terms of their theory base'. The chapter looks at the effects of brief interventions on substance use and the evidence of the effect of brief interventions on mental health–substance use concerns.

The book then examines specific interventions that may aid the individual experiencing mental health–substance use concerns and dilemmas. Kathleen Sciacca (Chapter 9) draws on her vast consultancy experience across systems of care, programme models and state-wide initiatives. Her chapter covers theme-centred interaction, stages of change, and person-centred reflective listening to explore the role of integrated group treatment.

Anne Garland (Chapter 10) looks at the role of cognitive behavioural therapy (CBT). The chapter aims to describe the fundamental principles of cognitive behaviour therapy, the theory, and the basic treatment rationale and process for making psychological sense of a person's problems.

Alexander Chapman and colleagues (Chapter 11) describe the role of dialectical behaviour therapy (DBT). This chapter offers practical guidance on the evidence for DBT in the treatment of substance use problems and offer suggestions on how to incorporate DBT into the treatment of people experiencing such problems.

Eye movement desensitisation and reprocessing (EMDR) has had considerable success when working alongside people experiencing post-traumatic stress disorders and Susan Brown and colleagues (Chapter 12) expand on the role of EMDR intervention in mental health–substance use.

Relapse prevention plays a pivotal role when working with the person experiencing mental health–substance use problems. While this is explored further in Book 6, Chapter 16 (and for mental health Chapter 15), here David Manley looks at the role of cues and triggers in craving and subsequent lapse and relapse, which is an integral consideration in the relapse process, and deals with the main principles of cue reactivity.

It is important that we achieve an intervention that is right for the individual – what works for one person may not work for another. Matching the intervention to the person leads to a more effective intervention. The individual working with others experiencing similar problems and experiences in a supportive environment should not be overlooked as an effective intervention. In Chapter 14, Andrew Rosenblum and colleagues put forward the role of the mutual aid group for the individual experiencing mental health–substance use problems. Mutual aid groups are based on the premise that a group of individuals sharing a 'common problem can collectively support each other and mitigate or eliminate that problem and its personal and social consequences. Members learn about their problem and share their experiences, strengths and hopes for recovery.'

To conclude Book 4, Catherine Dixon explores a complementary therapy and personal development coaching foundation programme referred to as 'Empower Your Life'. This interesting concept focuses on what the individual is going to do with his/her life now that he/she is no longer dependent on alcohol or other substances. As the author exhorts, Empower Your Life is not therapy or counselling but an educational programme that delivers a methodology for change and transformation. Clearly, this approach deserves more research, and a broadening of the impact of its therapeutic benefits for the individual experiencing mental health–substance use problems.

CONCLUSION

We must remember that there is a constant theme throughout in relation to the need for properly funded education and training, not just for the professional but also for the individual. Just as important, there is constant reinforcement of why we need to know about mental health–substance use. This book is aimed at the professional, educator, service developer, manager and student, for we all need to be aware of the unique needs of the individual and interventions available if our practice is to be effective.

It is hoped that this book is helpful and informative. One would hope that we feel sufficiently stimulated to further develop our knowledge and skills, having extended . and developed this grounding in mental health–substance use. We can build upon our knowledge using the 'To learn more' sections as a guide to further study and knowledge. As one enters each new area of knowledge, so understanding improves of what is needed – and what is not – and how we can apply this knowledge in practice and service development. With that comes the ability to use an open, non-judgemental and accepting approach to the problems identified by the individual presenting for intervention, treatment, advice or guidance.

Our knowledge and understanding constantly change. The challenge is to remain open and accessible to the knowledge and information that will help each of us provide appropriate therapeutic interventions:
➤ at the appropriate level of expertise
➤ at the appropriate time
➤ at the appropriate level of understanding of the individual, and her/his presenting concerns and dilemmas
➤ at the appropriate cost.

We cannot afford to be solid in the belief that all individuals are the same. If this book encourages us to be wise and flexible in practice and the development and provision of services, it has achieved its aim. If it helps us to appreciate some of the problems encountered by the individual, family and carers, it has achieved its aim. We can bring about much-needed changes for the individual experiencing mental health–substance use problems.

Respect leads to caring – a quality of impeccability in what we do. Respect and faith nourish each other and give birth to many skilful actions. As we foster the quality of respect in our lives, we can also begin to see the world in a different light. The tone of caring that arises from giving respect can transform how we interact with society. We begin to explore the possibility of service, of taking an active role in seeing what needs doing and lending our energy to those endeavours. Compassion motivates us to act, and wisdom ensures the means are effective.[3]

REFERENCES

1 The 14th Dalai Lama. As cited in: Föllmi D, Föllmi O. *Buddhist Offerings 365 Days*. London: Thames and Hudson; 2003.

2 Bloom BS, Hastings T, Madaus G. *Handbook of Formative and Summative Evaluation*. New York, NY: McGraw-Hill Book Company; 1971.

3 Joseph Goldstein. As cited in: Föllmi D, Föllmi O. *Buddhist Offerings 365 Days*. London: Thames and Hudson; 2003.

CHAPTER 2

The therapeutic relationship

Jo Cooper

COMMENT

The author worked as a Macmillan clinical nurse specialist in palliative care. However, the following can be applied in any clinical situation and has no boundaries in terms of specialism. There are many parallels within the field of palliation and mental health–substance use. It is something we all can learn from and apply in our own clinical environment. The case representations are in the first person to emphasise the human interactions between two people and the therapeutic relationship that has evolved.

LEARNING OUTCOMES

- Define the terms therapeutic and relationship.
- Understand the elements of a therapeutic relationship.
- Recognise the importance of being human.
- Apply therapeutic relating in everyday life.

INTRODUCTION

This chapter will focus on:
- the meaning of the therapeutic relationship
- our understanding of this relationship.

The work we do is primarily concerned with the essence and quality of the relationships we make, whether this is with the individual, the family, carers, or with other health professionals. It is not something that we 'do' to people. It is a way of 'being', and should be part of our everyday life with each other: a human-to-human experience.

The essence of the relationship is the engagement, the identification of the professional with the person, the instant recognition of another's distress, identifying with that person's human experience.[1] Such relationships have been described as being rewarding for both parties, and the reciprocal nature of the relationship should reduce rather than increase risk of burnout in the professional.

There are two aspects to consider in the theory and practice of caring. For the individual, we are both health professionals and fellow human beings. In the context of caring, we must use both aesthetic and empirical knowledge to diagnose and manage illness. Alongside, we must try to understand the person as a unique individual.

A fundamental premise of 'caring' is that professionals use themselves as therapeutic instruments.[2] The reason for this strong emphasis on the therapeutic relationship is the fact that when people are ill, they often have problems in communicating and forming relationships.[3]

By definition, the relationship needs both professional and personal closeness in order for a meaningful connection to be made. However, there must be a balance between human closeness and professional distance.[4]

REFLECTIVE PRACTICE EXERCISE 2.1

Time: 15 minutes
- What does the term 'therapeutic relationship' mean to you?
- Think about a person in your care that you have worked with recently where you had a good relationship. Consider:
  —What made it 'good'?
  —Why was it different from other relationships?

What does the term 'therapeutic relationship' mean?

The word 'therapy' comes from the Greek word *therapeia*, meaning to care. The word 'relationship' comes from the Latin *relatus*, which denotes a 'connection'. Therefore, to work effectively with the individual and their family, we need to make a caring connection.[5] There is potential for the professional to act as the 'therapeutic tool'. The therapeutic nature of the relations is not so much *what* we say, but *how* we say it. It is a set of behaviours around a way of 'being', which should be practised in our everyday life. The therapeutic relationship is dependent on the effectiveness of our interpersonal communication, both verbal and non-verbal.

In her seminal work on relationships, Muetzel[6] provides us with a simple framework which clarifies the elements within the relationship:
- reciprocity
- intimacy
- partnership.

These elements make up the therapeutic process. Communication and interpersonal skills link the elements forming dynamic fluidity. In addition, it has been proposed that the following 'conditions' are central to the therapeutic relationship:
- genuineness
- empathy
- unconditional positive regard.[7]

REFLECTIVE PRACTICE EXERCISE 2.2

> **Time: 5 minutes**
> - Is there anything that you would like to add?
> - Consider the possibility of adding compassion.

RECIPROCITY

REFLECTIVE PRACTICE EXERCISE 2.3

> **Time: 10 minutes**
> In reviewing the elements of Muetzel's framework,[6] consider the meaning of *'reciprocity'*.
> - How does this fit with your idea of the 'therapeutic relationship'?

The people for whom we care are constantly negotiating with us. They want to know a little about us as people. Can I relate to this person? Can I trust them? It is about making the connection; investing in the relationship, being 'in touch' and entering their world.[8] Exploring their situation, being available and making a quick response is central to connecting. We could say that reciprocity is about sharing together. It needs us to remain functional and not fall 'into the pit', while acknowledging and understanding the pain and distress of another.

REFLECTIVE PRACTICE EXERCISE 2.4

> **Time: 5 minutes**
> - What might you share with this person?
> - Consider what is and what is not appropriate to share.

Often all we have is ourselves and simply saying, *'Thank you, I can see how hard that was for you'*; it is more important to genuinely care than to get the right words.

In examining the concept of reciprocity, one author suggests its therapeutic properties lie in its mutual exchange, an action or relation given in return. In assuming therapeutic value, reciprocity becomes positive in its effect for both the professional and the individual in terms of sharing.[9]

We can share everyday events, something simple and ordinary. Acknowledgement of feelings and difficulties shows that you are 'present', that you have heard. This enables the individual to feel understood and legitimises their feelings. Being present to, and in contact with, the other person is at the heart of the therapeutic nursing relation.[10] 'Presencing' highlights the need to think of communication as more than just speaking. We all communicate differently: sometimes by just being 'present' and saying nothing. Silence is useful and of great value. It allows the gathering of thoughts, giving both sides the time to reflect and consider. It is a 'mindful' silence.

It is tempting to fill every silence with words. Try to sit quietly and calmly – 'less is more'. Allow the person to have space to hear themselves. There is a right time to talk about trivialities, but try to 'allow' the silence.

REFLECTIVE PRACTICE EXERCISE 2.5

Time: 5 minutes
- Reflect on the word 'present'.
- Think about absence of presence.
- How could you show someone you are present?

Sometimes, being present just involves sitting with someone, saying very little, being silent. This is not an empty silence but, rather, contains acceptance and understanding. It lets the person know that you value them and what they are telling you about their experience. It also tells the person, without words, that you know they must struggle to find their own words.[11] As you listen and give attention they will begin to trust you not to rush in with thoughtless words. People take a risk when they share their feelings with us.

REFLECTIVE PRACTICE EXERCISE 2.6

Time: 15 minutes
- With a colleague, discuss how your silence with an individual you are 'caring' for is different to the silence of people just sat in a waiting area.
- Try to think of the 'quality' of your silence and how this could be helpful.

The reciprocity of sharing

Case study 2.1

Bob was dying. He had metastatic prostate carcinoma. He was referred for management of intractable pain. He had been a keen gardener and every year had grown runner beans in his small garden. On one of my visits to Bob, he was showing his wife Gill how to plant the beans as he was no longer able to do this. I shared with him how much I had always wanted to grow them, but did not know where to start. Bob carefully explained to me exactly what I needed to know, sharing his knowledge generously with me. Later I planted my beans, not really expecting great results. On each visit to Bob, he would ask, with great interest, how they were doing and always wanted to know if they were as good as his! I was able to share my stories about how the beans were coming along, what I should have done to them; how I forgot last night to water them; how my granddaughters had loved to pick them for dinner, etc. Bob and I shared a mutual interest unrelated to his medical diagnosis. It provided an opportunity for our relationship to grow; he learned to trust me and found out a little about what sort of a person I was, without my disclosing any 'personal' information. In a big way, this made it a little easier for Bob to disclose some of his own distress and fears around dying. I was not just the professional; I was also a human being. I had knowledge (about Bob's condition and treatment needed); Bob had knowledge that I did not have (about growing vegetables!). I told Bob that I would never forget him – for many reasons. Mostly because of his inordinate faith and courage and also for sharing his knowledge with me about growing runner beans. In turn, he thanked me for taking an interest and being a good 'student'. Long after his death, the story of the beans remains with Gill, his wife, and will always remain with me.

Reciprocity does not mean that we share everything about ourselves. This would not be helpful to the relationship. Some basic essentials for therapeutic encounters lie within the nature of being human. Human qualities are ordinary in that they are commonplace. The foundations of genuine helping lie in being ordinary, 'nothing special'.[12] The relationship requires us to think about ourselves: who we are, and what we are. It gives us the opportunity of self-reflection, a chance to be honest with what and whom we see. If we have a guest in our house, we remember to act with courtesy and respect for our guest. The same principles can be applied to those we care for.

Ordinariness has been offered as having the potential to describe everyday human qualities and activities. When professionals and individuals were 'just themselves' in clinical settings, they were happier with each other. Ordinariness is therapeutic, through the effects of genuine human relationships.[12] There is reciprocity in 'allowingness': allowing individuals to disclose or not to disclose if they so wish. We have an opportunity of opening up possibilities for connectedness, because the everyday dramas of caring for ill and unhappy people encourage us to 'get over' feeling important and superior. The foundation for this related connection lies in the authenticity of the helping relationship. It starts and ends with being open and honest not only with our own self but with other professionals with whom we work.

PARTNERSHIP

REFLECTIVE PRACTICE EXERCISE 2.7

Time: 20 minutes
- What do you think partnership involves?
- Think about your association within the therapeutic encounter.
- How were you a partner in the care you gave?
- What made this a partnership?
- How might you gain from the partnership?
- Is the partnership an equal one?
- What happens to the balance of power?

- Is there a difference in caring for the individual in their home, as opposed to caring for them on the hospital ward?
- Consider the individual's need for privacy.
- How might we invade this?

Meutzel[6] considers partnership as a working association between two parties, implying a gain for both sides. There is so much gain for us when working with individuals and their families. If we remain open, we can learn so much; people have so much to teach us. In the case of 'Bob', knowledge was gained, not only on a practical level, but insightful knowledge on how a person copes when their world is threatened. In turn, this helps when working with others, and when you can say, 'Yes, your feelings are a normal reaction – other people often feel like this too', this can alleviate emotional isolation, normalising and validating their own perceptions and feelings.

Often the little things count. Benner[13] describes these as the 'hallmark of nursing expertise':

- making someone comfortable – takes time and is a skill in itself
- helping the person to eat or drink – a fundamental, rather than a basic skill
- admiring a family photo – part of making the connection
- accepting the offer of a cup of tea – says I am not rushing off; I am here to listen
- attention to detail
- just sitting quietly with someone; words are not always necessary.

All these little things help to build a relationship of trust, of engaging with another. The provision of comfort may be a part and an expression of caring and within the relationship is a key function.[5]

These functions are therapeutic beyond their physical effect. They provide psychological and emotional comfort and are an expression of 'caring'. Development of these skills is essential if we are to work therapeutically and effectively with those in our care. Research suggests that individuals put a high value on physical comfort and information sharing.[14] Information sharing, with the focus on not only what is shared but how and when, is perceived as being an important enabler in the development of both optimal therapeutic relationships and care outcomes.[15] Being honest and genuine when sharing information was also perceived as important. Through the exchange of information, the sharing of humour, the silences, the exploration of thought and spoken word, mutual trust, respect and the recognition of humanness is affirmed.

We cannot claim to know what is 'best' for people. We are human ourselves, and have many frailties. We can only be alongside and help the individual to choose what they feel is best. We can show respect in acknowledging that each individual has the right to choose what is best for them and their family. Each has their own unique journey and story and each must be given time and encouragement to relate it, if they wish.

When appropriate, encourage the person to work with us in planning their care, identifying and achieving realistic goals. Their road to recovery may encounter many difficult setbacks. Hope is an important enabler in fostering a sense of optimism and achievement. This is very difficult when a person feels at their most hopeless, and it lies with us, as the professional, to maintain a sense of hope, even when things seem hopeless.

INTIMACY

REFLECTIVE PRACTICE EXERCISE 2.8

Time: 5 minutes
- What do you think intimacy involves?
- Is this an area that you have given thought to?

Intimacy implies closeness, a friendship – both professional and compassionate. It is about having the opportunity to have meaningful communication, the central focus to a therapeutic relationship. Acting as an authentic person with competence as a professional and as a person does not mean that the relationship is a friendship.[20] A true friendship is characterised by mutuality. Each party has equal rights and obligations for the needs of the other. In contrast, the needs of the individual are the primary concern. Emotional closeness is based on trust, not exclusiveness. There is no ownership. Sometimes, as health professionals, we behave as if we own the person for whom we are caring. This approach is unhelpful and not therapeutic, even though it is probably based on our innate need to provide loving care for that individual. Working together within the professional team, attending supervision and self-reflection, helps us to maintain emotional equilibrium, so that we share more openly, and address together, the needs of the individual.

Intimacy is about being human, about treating the other with respect and compassion; much how we would like to be treated ourselves. We do not have to have all the answers or have to be something that we are not. It is about getting close to the world of the individual, formed often by the caring and intimate physical care, which often provides opportunities and a level of trust that supports psychological closeness.

REFLECTIVE PRACTICE EXERCISE 2.9

Time: 5 minutes
Reflect on what being 'human' means to you.

Perhaps our human purpose is to provide warmth, companionship and acceptance of our fellow women and men, rather than trying to control, contain or 'fix' them.[17]

Insight into our own vulnerabilities and limitations will teach us that we cannot 'fix' the other person's problems. We cannot make their world, their life, their illness or their death different. We can only be 'alongside'. It is their journey, their story, and they are taking big courageous steps in sharing it with us. It is in this sharing and within our listening that takes place that we can make a difference. Some may feel that they have never been truly heard.

Can we make people 'feel' better, rather than 'get' better?

We can be 'ourselves', giving something of ourselves, working alongside that person, listening with compassion, and understanding from within. In order to practise an act of compassion, we need to be compassionate to ourselves. It is easy to forget our own needs when we are dealing with the grief and distress of others, but it is by looking after ourselves that we maintain emotional stamina needed to care for others. Acknowledge and accept our own weaknesses and vulnerabilities, learning from our fears and our own personal distress.

REFLECTIVE PRACTICE EXERCISE 2.10

Time: 10 minutes
- Think about 'compassion'.
- What does this mean to you?
- How can we practise it – for ourselves and for others?

It is not simply warmth of heart, or a sharp clarity of recognition of the individual's needs and pain, it is also a sustained and practical determination to do whatever is necessary and possible to help alleviate suffering.[18] Suffering has been described as a state of severe distress caused by events that threaten the integrity of a person.[19] Suffering is an inevitable and inescapable part of life, for the individual, for their family and for ourselves. Although pain is often associated with physical hurt, the perception of the discomfort is always modified by the person's cognitive and emotional reaction.[20] Therefore, what we think must be a major cause of suffering for the individual may not be so. It is important not to assume. It can be helpful to ask, '*What causes you the most suffering at the moment?*' Suffering, distress, grief – all human experiences – sometimes offer an opportunity for learning and change.

When an individual is deeply distressed, their ability to see or to think clearly is often impaired. With a 'muddled' and often tormented mind, they are often unable to express verbally their troubled thoughts. Sometimes, it can be helpful to ask, '*What do you feel in your heart?*' We know what is in our heart, even if our mind is chaotic and confused.

Case study 2.2

Harry lived in a mobile home. He had few possessions, and his home was his pride and joy. He was elderly, frail, ill and was becoming intermittently confused. He had no family and had been a loner throughout his life. It was clear that he could not remain in his home and needed full-time care. It was such a tremendously difficult decision for Harry to make. He had no one to guide or help him make the decision and it was difficult for him to see a future outside of his home.

> He was bewildered and at a loss of how to express his obvious grief and sadness. His mind was in turmoil. One day as we sat together, I asked, 'What do you feel in your heart Harry?' He sat for several moments as if he had not really heard me, then looked directly at me and, with a degree of resignation, acknowledged that he needed to be cared for.

This does not work every time. It was helpful for Harry. It is about 'knowing' something about the person you are working with, and taking a risk, in order to help reduce emotional distress. It is also about truthfulness. As professionals, we were honest with Harry about his social and medical situation; we did not want to destroy his hope or make him feel that he had 'no choice'. Truth is one of the most powerful therapeutic agents available to us, but we need to develop a proper understanding of its clinical pharmacology, and to recognise optimum timing and dosage in its use.[21]

In mental health and substance use, often on a daily basis, we work alongside despairing and distressed individuals. In order to work closely with them, we need to repair and maintain our own mental and physical well-being. We try to avoid thoughts of having serious illness for ourselves, of body or mind. Illnesses, such as those affecting mental or physical health, disrupt life, taking away our 'assumed' world. In our own mind, we each hold a picture of our assumed future, as we would like it to be. We have hopes and dreams for our future, which become the foundation for a 'certain' way of living. However, nothing in life is certain – only the finality of it. We live only with the illusion of certainty. It is important that we focus on the *person* and not the illness.

Being able to think about our own feelings and being able to imagine the feeling of others is the cognitive basis for empathy and understanding.[11]

REFLECTIVE PRACTICE EXERCISE 2.11

Time: 15 minutes
- Think about a time in your life that was painful. Try to recall the event.
- Think about how other people responded.
- What was helpful? What was not helpful?
- Consider both the practical and emotional elements.
- Notice what feelings arise in you.
- Think about how using your own experience could help you to work alongside others, using the components of compassion and empathy.

FINDING MEANING

REFLECTIVE PRACTICE EXERCISE 2.12

Time: 5 minutes
Consider how you find meaning and purpose in your own life.

Illness often provides strength and opportunities for change. People work hard to make sense of their situation. As professionals, we try to help this process by exploring difficulties and dilemmas. In providing a space for the individual to talk, they will often find their own answers. Speaking openly about a problem is often liberating. Exploration helps in the development of coping strategies and saying something like *'Tell me what is the worst thing for you at the moment . . .?'* stops us from assuming that we know and understand their dilemma before we have thoroughly explored it. Sometimes, people and families have differing goals, or make different choices, causing family tensions and conflict to arise. Respectful and compassionate negotiation between the parties will allow each person to say how they feel; expressing their thoughts, hopes and expectations, enabling family unity and thereby reducing tensions. This is not as simple as it may sound. It takes a great deal of time, patience, effort, tolerance and understanding.[22]

Where both parties are able to remain open to the feelings generated by the meanings of a particular situation, valuable information for coping with the inevitable stresses of help seeking is gained and the humanity of both is affirmed.[22]

Where the relationship is therapeutic, the authentic exchange transforms care into shared experiences that can produce positive growth. Where shared meanings and experiences are positive ones, genuine caring will have occurred, generating therapeutic outcomes for those concerned. Acknowledging the difficulties of another show that you have heard and understood. The most important point is that the individual feels heard, understood and accepted in the place where they are at that moment in time.

Valuing the individual, and ourselves, is the overriding concept in any relationship. Treating people with respect because they are human maintains a supportive relationship. Each person is *worthwhile*.

How can we show respect for those within our care?

REFLECTIVE PRACTICE EXERCISE 2.13

Time: 5 minutes
How can we show simple respect for those within our care?

This comes down to the small, perhaps seemingly insignificant things that are nevertheless important. They include the following.
➤ Introduce ourselves by name.
➤ Ask each individual how she/he would like to be addressed.
➤ Remember the individual's name.
➤ Give full attention – people know if we check our watch.
➤ Do not interrupt or talk over the individual.
➤ Do not assume you know what the individual will say – do not finish the individual's sentence.
➤ Do not assume you know best – help the individual to make his/her own choices and decisions.

The ethical foundation of the therapeutic relationship is grounded in a sincere respect for the dignity of human life.[23]

LISTENING

As part of the communication process, listening is at the heart of therapeutic caring. The focus must be on what the person is telling us, both by their verbal and non-verbal language. It is only by truly listening, clearing our mind of our own concerns and thoughts, that we will hear clearly what is being said. If we feel anxious about what we are going to say or do next, or we are not mindfully relaxed, we will fail to hear and to see how we can help. Sometimes, the best option is to do nothing. We will often not have a solution. This does not mean that we do not make a response to what we have heard. Having no solution is not the same as having no response; responses may be more profound than answers.[24] Even when we have no answer to questions posed, always something can be done, such as 'being there'. Questions can be talked about and explored, even if not answered with finality – using the words:

➤ **HOW** – how do you feel you are coping at the moment? How have you coped in the past?
➤ **WHY** – why did you cry just then?
➤ **WHAT** – what does this mean for you?

People value us for our *presence*, just as much as for our knowledge and our skills:

Case study 2.3

Frank was very ill. He no longer wanted or needed to talk. Management of his physical and psychological symptoms had been a priority. He had done all his talking in the last few months. Was there a need to visit? What could reasonably be achieved at this stage? He was settled and stable. I asked the family how they felt about further visits. Were they needed? Would further visits be too intrusive? Their response was: 'You may not be needed, but you are wanted and we would value it, so yes please.'

How and where we sit in a room makes a difference to how we interact with the individuals present. Can we see each other properly? Can we give appropriate eye contact? Sitting close to someone reduces physical barriers and enables the use of appropriate touch. Holding a hand while we listen says, 'We are here and we understand.'

Listening is a skill, which takes 'time'. It is time well spent and is the basis for a relationship of mutual trust and support. When we are busy it is easy to concentrate on 'doing' rather than' being', and often easier to do a task, rather than *sit* with pain and distress. Closely linked to the tenet of holistic care, listening is characterised by a climate of trust and a sense of being with the person, rather than merely the performance of caring tasks.[25] If we do not ask, we will not know. We should not underestimate the value of listening.

Case study 2.4

John had worked as a mercenary, working almost alone. It had been a solitary life and one where he had ended many lives. His own life was now coming to the end. John carried an enormous amount of unexpressed guilt. I asked him what was the most helpful thing for him. His response was: '*Being listened to!*' . . . 'You are like a little bird. You fly in, sit calmly on my bed, listen to all my worries and problems. Then, you go. And I feel better!'

REFLECTIVE PRACTICE EXERCISE 2.14

Time: 5 minutes
- Reflect on the possible distractions to listening.
- Consider both external and internal.
- Think about your own feelings, attitudes and behaviours.

The art of compassionate caring requires us to be still and to listen. Sometimes people will time the asking of questions when they sense you have no time to answer or to explore. You have your hand on the door ready to go; you have children to meet from school or you are on a busy ward and another is in need of attention. Rather than answering in haste, say that you will explore that at a later date or time. It may be better to take time for reflection and come back to the person when you can give full attention to the matter.[26]

When we are really ourselves, as authentic beings, and when we truly listen, something happens. Listening is *not* a passive exercise; we have to act on what we have heard. The use of silence gives us time to reflect and think about what is needed.

REFLECTIVE PRACTICE EXERCISE 2.15

Time: 5 minutes
- Think about what it means to be authentic and to have an authentic relationship.
- How could this enhance your practice?

One of the consequences of a therapeutic relationship is the trust gained for each party; both in their own ability to relate effectively in the help-seeking situation, and in each other as fellow human beings.[9]

SUPPORT FOR OURSELVES

Working in intensive situations with both individuals and families in the mental health and substance–use setting creates demands on us. We have to find ways to support and maintain our own integrity. We must have belief in our own worth.

Formal and informal supervision from peers will enable difficult issues to be worked through.

Supervision should be actively pursued, demonstrating commitment to improving practice and providing the very best service to the people we work with. It provides the opportunity for us to reflect deeply on ourselves and our practice and explore what is happening in our relationships with others. This openness is the prerequisite for true learning and for the relationship with people to be in any sense therapeutic. The ability to 'simply' sit with painful or distressing feelings is the mark of a competent professional. Understanding the need for, and the value of, silences means they are no longer threatening and we can provide a reassuring presence for people who are struggling.

CONCLUSION

Learn to have the courage to accompany others as they experience unknown and often scary territory. Engaging fully in the supervision process, either on a one to one basis, or within the group setting, is one way of doing this. This leads to greater understanding of ourselves and gives meaning to the way in which we act. In understanding our own frailties and vulnerabilities, we learn how to move forward, creating a helping relationship with others.

Caring for individuals in distress needs knowledge, skills, attention to detail, respect for our fellow human beings and the attitude to work both professionally (empirical knowledge) and from the heart (aesthetic knowledge) creating a deep sense of compassion. It is working from the heart that enables therapeutic relating to take place.

REFERENCES

1 Morse JM, Bottorf J, Anderson G, *et al.* Beyond empathy: expanding expressions of caring. *Journal of Advanced Nursing.* 1992; **17**: 809–21.

2 Hem MH, Heggen K. Being professional and being human: one nurse's relationship with a psychiatric patient. *Journal of Advanced Nursing.* 2003; **43**: 101–8.

3 Peplau H. Interpersonal relations: a theoretical framework for application in nursing practice. *Nursing Science Quarterly.* 1992; **5**: 13–18.

4 Strand L. *Fra kaos mot samling, mestring og helhet. Psykiatrisk sykepleie til psykotiske pasienter.* [From Chaos to Wholeness and Empowerment. Professional care of psychotic patients.] Oslo: Gyldendal; 1990.

5 McMahon R, Pearson A. *Nursing as a Therapy.* 2nd ed. Gloucester: Stanley Thornes; 1998.

6 Muetzel PA. Therapeutic nursing. In: Pearson A, editor. *Primary Nursing: nursing in the Burford and Oxford Nursing Development Unit.* London: Croom Helm; 1988.

7 Rogers C. *Dialogues.* London: Constable; 1990.

8 Davies B, Oberle K. Dimensions of the supportive role of the nurse in palliative care. *Oncology Nursing Forum.* 1990; **17**: 87–94.

9 Marck P. Therapeutic reciprocity: a caring phenomenon. *Advances in Nursing Science.* 1990; **13**: 49–59.

10 Kirby C. The therapeutic relationship. In: Basford L, Slevin O, editors. *Theory and Practice of Nursing: an integrated approach to caring practice.* 2nd ed. Gloucester: Nelson Thornes; 2003.

11 Lendrum S, Syme G. *Gift of Tears: a practical approach to loss and bereavement in counselling and psychotherapy*. 2nd ed. Hove: Brunner-Routledge; 2004.

12 Taylor BJ. Ordinariness in nursing. In: McMahon R, Pearson A, editors. *Nursing as a Therapy*. Gloucester: Stanley Thornes; 1998.

13 Benner P. *From Novice to Expert: excellence and power in clinical practice*. Menlo Park, CA: Addison-Wesley; 1984.

14 Skilbeck J, Payne S. Emotional support and the role of clinical nurse specialist in palliative care. *Journal of Advanced Nursing*. 2003; **43**: 521–30.

15 Seymour J, Ingleton C, Payne S, *et al*. Specialist palliative care: patients' experiences. *Journal of Advanced Nursing*. 2003; **44**: 24–33.

16 Martocchio BC. Authenticity, belonging, emotional closeness, and self representation. *Oncology Nursing Forum*. 1997; **14**: 23–7.

17 Barker P, Buchanan-Barker P. Mental health in an age of celebrity: the courage to care. *Medical Humanities*. 2008; **34**: 110–14.

18 Rinpoche S. *The Tibetan Book of Living and Dying*. Gaffney P, Harvey A, editors. London: Rider; 1992.

19 Cassell EJ. *The Nature of Suffering and the Goals of Medicine*. Oxford: Oxford University Press; 1991.

20 Twycross R. *Introducing Palliative Care*. Oxford: Radcliffe Medical Press; 2003.

21 Simpson M, as cited in: Twycross R. Death without suffering? *European Journal of Palliative Care*. 2005; **12**: 14–17.

22 Benner P, Wrubel J. *The Primacy of Caring: stress and coping in health and illness*. Menlo Park, CA: Addison-Wesley; 1988.

23 Kirby C. The therapeutic relationship. In: Cooper J, editor. *Stepping into Palliative Care: relationships and responses*. 2nd ed. Oxford: Radcliffe Publishing; 2006.

24 Lunn L. Having no answer. In: Saunders C, editor. *Hospice and Palliative Care, an Interdisciplinary Approach*. London: Edward Arnold; 1990.

25 Canning D, Rosenberg JP, Yates P. Therapeutic relationships in specialist palliative care nursing practice. *International Journal of Palliative Nursing*. 2007; **13**: 222–9.

26 Houtepen R, Hendrikx D. Nurses and the virtues of dealing with existential questions in terminal palliative care. *Nursing Ethics*. 2003; **10**: 377–87.

TO LEARN MORE

- Cooper J. *Stepping into Palliative Care: relationships and responses*. 2nd ed. Oxford: Radcliffe Publishing; 2006.
- Jeffrey D. *Patient-centred Ethics and Communications at the End of Life*. Oxford: Radcliffe Publishing; 2006.
- Lendrum S, Syme G. *Gift of Tears*. 2nd ed. Hove: Brunner-Routledge; 2004.
- McMahon R, Pearson A. *Nursing as Therapy*. 2nd ed. Cheltenham: Stanley Thornes; 1998.
- Rinpoche S. *The Tibetan Book of Living and Dying*. Gaffney P, Harvey A, editors. London: Rider; 1992.

CHAPTER 3

The Tidal Model

Poppy Buchanan-Barker and Phil Barker

FOCUS AND ASSUMPTIONS

First developed in England in the late 1990s, the Tidal Model[1] is recognised, internationally, as a key mid-range nursing theory[2] but is practised widely by a range of disciplines. The Tidal Model focuses on helping people, who have experienced some metaphorical 'breakdown', recover their lives as fully as possible, by reclaiming the story of their distress and difficulty.

The Tidal Model can be distinguished from other 'recovery' models, popular in most Western countries. It is:

➤ the *first* recovery-focused model developed *by* mental health nurses *for* mental health nursing practice
➤ the *first* mental health recovery model developed *conjointly* by mental health professionals *and* people in their care
➤ the *first* mental health recovery model developed for use in the most challenging situations, i.e. where people are 'at their lowest ebb'
➤ the *first* mental health recovery model to be *evaluated* rigorously in public sector practice
➤ the *first* model to be used as the basis of recovery-focused care across the *hospital-community spectrum* – from child and adolescent services to older persons.[3,4]

The proper focus of caring

The Tidal Model assumes that all health and social problems are best viewed as 'problems in living'.[5] Practitioners should seek to provide the person with 'the necessary conditions for the promotion of growth and development'.[6] To begin this process, practitioners help people to describe and name their experience of such problems in their *own language*, rather than in the language of medicine or psychology. This leads to exploring how people might begin to deal better with, if not completely resolve, such problems in living.

The tidal metaphor

Traditionally, people with problems in living have been encouraged to think of themselves as being in some fixed state, e.g. 'I am an alcoholic' or 'I have schizophrenia'. The Tidal Model recognises that all human experience is ephemeral – ebbing and flowing like the tide. Sometimes a person is like 'this' and at other times is like 'that'. The experience of 'breakdown' and 'recovery' often seems to 'come and go'; 'two steps forward, one step back'. Most languages have nautical metaphors to describe such uncertain or dramatic states, e.g. drifting, washed up, wrecked or drowning. Tidal practitioners try to discover and employ the person's own preferred metaphors, which best represent an experience, thus respecting the language the person uses to tell her or his own unique story.

REFLECTIVE PRACTICE EXERCISE 3.1

Time: 15 minutes
- Recall *three* 'problems in living' that you have experienced recently.
- Reflect on how they *interfered* with the everyday living of your life.

The tidal theory of the person

The Tidal Model views the person as living in three *domains*:

➤ **Self domain**: where people maintain all their 'private' experiences, e.g. thoughts, feelings and other aspects of consciousness
➤ **World domain**: where people *bring out* some of these 'private' experiences into the world, sharing them, selectively, with others
➤ **Others domain**: where people *act out* their life story with others; influencing, and being influenced by them, through an infinite range of social encounters.

All any person ever can *be* is a story. We only 'know' who people are by the stories *they* tell us about themselves. People grow and develop through storytelling. The Tidal Model uses storytelling as the key means of helping people to 'know themselves' and to 'know better' what is troubling them. This represents a vital step towards working out what might *need to be done* to begin to resolve these problems.

THEORY INTO PRACTICE

Tidal Model practice is focused upon *individual* and *group* processes of care, each related to one of the three *domains*.

➤ **Self**: If the person is perceived to be in any way a risk or threat to her or himself or others, a person-centred **Personal Security Plan** is developed. This identifies the *personal* and *interpersonal* resources the person might use to address current 'risks or threats'.
➤ **World**: When people first enter the service the focus is upon helping them 'tell the story' of how they came to be in need of care. The **Holistic Assessment** is an in-depth conversation, aimed at helping the person explore and describe how problems or difficulties have developed. This leads to a discussion about what might 'need to be done', to begin to address these problems.

    Further conversations, within **One-to-One Sessions**, focus on helping the person identify and discuss *current* issues, problems or difficulties; identifying what the person might do and what help might be received from others, to begin to address them.

➤ **Others**: Three forms of group work aim to help people reclaim their personal power and identify personal and interpersonal resources. The **Discovery Group** helps people become more aware of aspects of life experience, which have shaped who and what they are, as persons. The **Information Sharing Group** helps people learn more about services, issues or other topics, which the person has *chosen* to explore. Finally, the **Solution Group** helps people become more aware of how they can draw support and encouragement from their peers – who are 'in the same boat' as themselves. These groups help to build a sense of community, which hopefully will act as a bridge to supportive communities in the natural social world.

REFLECTIVE PRACTICE EXERCISE 3.2

Time: 15 minutes
- Recall a time, recently, when you felt in any way 'threatened' on a personal level.
- Identify *two* things, which you did *on your own*, that appeared to reduce your sense of 'threat'.
- Identify *two* things, which you *received from other people*, that appeared to minimise your sense of 'threat.

Live storytelling and live recording

Traditionally, stories about the person's care and treatment are written up by practitioners, in the form of histories and clinical notes, in private offices. When a person is discharged, the service will have amassed a large file of such 'notes', but the person often goes home with little more than an appointment card. Tidal assumes that if the person is to make the most of the experience of care they must hold their own record of their interactions with practitioners, which they can use to develop their own 'self-management'. All Tidal processes involve *active conversations*, recorded *live*, confirming the *collaborative* nature of the professional–person relationship. These 'stories' are written in the person's own voice, rather than translated into clinical or bureaucratic language. The person receives a copy at the end of each interaction. This confirms the person's position at the heart of the caring encounter, and the owner of the life story.

REFLECTIVE PRACTICE EXERCISE 3.3

Time: 15 minutes
- Is it important for you to feel that you 'own' the story of your life?
- If so, reflect on why is this important to you.
- If not, reflect on why this is not important.

The beginnings of self-management

User/consumer consultants describe the Tidal Model as the 'beginnings of *self-management*'.[7] Unlike many 'recovery models', the Tidal Model emphasises that 'self-management' should begin at the point of *entry* into the service – *not* at discharge. This helps the person *rehearse* the kind of decisions and actions that might be needed as part of everyday living, on return to ordinary life in the community.

The Tidal Model in practice

Practitioners need to collaborate closely with the people in their care. Six guiding principles underpin the Tidal practitioner's relationship with the person in care.

1 **Curiosity**: The person's life story is a mystery, which requires careful exploration if needs are to be identified and met. The practitioner seeks to understand what the person thinks, feels and knows about her or his self, and the problems which have brought them into the healthcare setting.
2 **Resourcefulness**: People in care settings are often defined in terms of their problems, deficits, diagnosis or illness. While recognising the existence of such 'problems', the Tidal Model is concerned mainly with how the person manages to live with these problems *now*. How might these personal and interpersonal resources be brought to bear to influence the person's recovery?
3 **Respect**: Care and treatment programmes are often based on what the care team believes is 'best' for the person. However, given that the person is the centre of the whole story of care and treatment, it is obvious that she/he should be the final judge as to what is, or is not, helpful.
4 **Crisis as an opportunity**: Traditionally, a crisis is something that needs to be 'managed' or 'contained'. The Tidal Model believes that crises are signs that something needs to change: natural indications that something 'needs to be done'. The crisis is an 'opportunity for change'.
5 **Think small**: Care and treatment programmes often emphasise the end point of the care process, e.g. cure, resolution or discharge. The Tidal Model emphasises the small steps a person needs to take to move away from the circumstances which brought them into care in the first place. What simple, specific actions might help the person begin to move forward, or move away from the problem in living?
6 **Think simple**: Care and treatment programmes are often framed by professional jargon, and may involve multiple layers of action by different agencies. The Tidal Model stresses the need to identify the simplest action which might 'make a difference' for the person. Such a simple action can be understood and 'owned' by the person, thus representing the beginnings of 'self-help'.

The Tidal Model philosophy

The Tidal philosophy involves asking four basic questions.

➤ **Why this, why now?** Why is the person experiencing this particular problem in living *now*? The focus is on what the person is experiencing *at this moment* and what *needs to be done now* to begin to address the situation.
➤ **What works?** Rather than offer advice or counsel, the Tidal practitioner seeks

to establish what the person believes has worked in the past or what might work in the immediate future.

➤ **What is the personal theory?** What does the person think is happening now; what is it all about; and what it might mean? What 'sense' does the person make of their problems? Rather than offering a 'professional' explanation of their difficulties – in the form of psychological theory or diagnosis – the practitioner tries to understand the experience from the person's perspective. 'What is the person's theory of what is going on?'

➤ **How to limit restrictions?** To avoid fostering dependency, practitioners should aim to do as little as is necessary to help people begin to address their problems in living. The main focus is on identifying what the *person* needs to do, which is supplemented by a negotiated form of support from the team.

Case study 3.1: a personal story

Jay lost touch with his family years ago. He used to take various street drugs but now he can afford to drink only cheap wine and cider. He is a 'sociable drunk' but suspicious of people when sober. He is in his early thirties and has a long-standing diagnosis of schizophrenia. He has been receiving depot injections of antipsychotic drugs for over 10 years. Recently, he was sectioned under the Mental Health Act (UK), following a violent outburst in a supermarket café, where he was refused service.

Escorted to hospital by police, Jay refuses to talk with the admitting doctor and nurse. Two days later Mike, a young staff nurse, tries to engage him, but receives the same mix of hostility and silence. Mike comes back six times over the next three days, to try to open a dialogue. Finally, Jay asks him angrily: 'What do you want from me?' Mike is uncertain. 'I'm not sure I want anything *from* you, but I feel that I should be doing something to help you. I don't know how I'm going to do that if I don't know you . . . don't know what's bothering you . . . don't know what *you want from me*'.

Over the next few days, Mike visits Jay and slowly opens up a conversation. From casual talk about weather, TV news and life on the ward, the conversation turns to Jay and the circumstances of his admission. With some difficulty, he begins to talk about the 'stuff going on in my head'.

Mike thinks of himself as a novice. However, honesty is important to Jay, who has never met a nurse or doctor who 'wasn't a smart-arse'. Mike talks about the team's approach and brings two copies of the Holistic Assessment to their next meeting, one for each of them. Mike explains: 'This is just a bunch of questions that might help me learn a bit about what's been happening for you, so we can talk about what *you* might find useful right now.'

When Mike offers him a pen to 'write down some of your answers as we talk', Jay becomes uncomfortable. Mike explains: 'I want to understand what is happening for you, and the best way to do that is to get the story "right from the horse's mouth", in your own words. When we are finished, I'll give you a copy, so you'll know what we've been talking about. It's your life after all. This is your stuff, not mine.'

Jay insists that Mike do the writing: 'It's your job anyway.' Slowly, he gets into his stride, and begins to talk.

Over the next few days Mike and his colleague Jenny spend dedicated time with Jay in one-to-one sessions. They discuss what is on Jay's mind and explore practical ways that he might deal with these issues or problems. A record of these conversations is also made, in Jay's own words, and he keeps a copy as a reminder of what he needs to do to deal with his problems.

Jenny also helps Jay develop a Personal Security Plan. This addresses his feelings of fear and insecurity, which are associated with his violent outbursts. Jay is helped to identify how he managed these feeling in the past, or imagine what might help in the future. Again, he takes away a record of this conversation, in his own words, to use as an aide-memoire.

With some encouragement, Jay agrees to go with Jenny to the Discovery Group she is facilitating. He enjoys listening to the other people talk about the things that are important in their life, their hopes and dreams, and the obstacles they have overcome. Although he doesn't speak, he feels quite emotional afterwards. The mix of laughter and poignant stories was a new experience for him: nothing like his past experience of 'therapy groups'.

When discharged Jay says two things made a difference for him.

➤ First, he would never have started to talk about his voices, and the way people scared him, if 'Mike had not kept coming back, over and over again'. Jay couldn't understand why he wanted to know 'what was happening for me. . . . Usually, they only want to talk about my illness and stuff'.

➤ Second, Jay knew that doctors and nurses wrote things about him, but he had never seen what they had written. He was unnerved at first by Mike's willingness to share what he was writing with him, and to make copies for him to take away for reference. This took a lot of getting used to. Gradually, he came to realise that Mike was right: 'This is my life. This is all about me!'

CONCLUSION

The Tidal Model assumes that reclaiming the story of our lives is the first step in recovery – irrespective of the nature of the problem. To negotiate this simple process of reclamation practitioners must help people in their care feel secure within the relationship. Gaining trust is the biggest challenge facing any practitioner.

By laying open the process of storytelling and by continually negotiating the relationship – as Mike illustrated in his relationship with Jay – practitioners can cast aside the trappings of power and authority which hinder the active collaboration needed to help the person 'grow and develop'. The *process* could not be simpler – but its *practice* is often highly complex.

POST-READING EXERCISE 3.1

Time: 15 minutes
- How would you go about finding out who is the person who is Jay; what troubles him; and how might you help him to deal with this?
- How does the offer of a diagnosis, clinical formulation or other 'label' *explain* what people like Jay are·experiencing?

REFERENCES

1 Barker P, Buchanan-Barker P. *The Tidal Model: a guide for mental health professionals.* London: Brunner-Routledge; 2005.
2 Brookes N, Barker P. The Tidal Model of recovery and reclamation. In: Tomey AM, Alligood MR, editors. *Nursing Theorists and Their Work.* 6th ed. St Louis: Mosby; 2005. pp. 696–725.
3 Buchanan-Barker P, Barker P. The Tidal commitments: extending the value base of recovery. *Journal of Psychiatric and Mental Health Nursing.* 2008; **15**: 93–100.
4 Barker P, Buchanan-Barker P. Reclaiming nursing: making it personal. *Mental Health Practice.* 2008; **11**: 12–16.
5 Barker P, Buchanan-Barker P. Mental health in an age of celebrity: the courage to care. *Medical Humanities.* 2008; **34**: 110–14.
6 Barker P. *The Philosophy and Practice of Psychiatric Nursing.* Edinburgh: Churchill Livingstone; 1999. p. 121.
7 Whitehill I. Foreword. In: Barker P, Buchanan-Barker P. *The Tidal Model: a guide for mental health professionals.* London: Brunner-Routledge; 2005.

TO LEARN MORE

- Barker P. The Tidal Model: the lived experience in person-centred mental health care. *Nursing Philosophy.* 2000; **2**: 213–23.
- Barker P. The Tidal Model: developing an empowering, person-centred approach to recovery within psychiatric and mental health nursing. *Journal of Psychiatric and Mental Health Nursing.* 2001; **8**: 233–40.
- Barker P. The Tidal Model: the healing potential of metaphor within the patient's narrative. *Journal of Psychosocial Nursing and Mental Health Services.* 2002; **40**: 42–50.
- Barker P, Buchanan-Barker P. Beyond empowerment: revering the storyteller. *Mental Health Practice.* 2003; **7**: 18–20.
- Barker P, Buchanan-Barker P. Bridging: talking meaningfully about the care of people at risk. *Mental Health Practice.* 2004; **8**: 12–16.
- Buchanan-Barker P, Barker P. The Ten Commitments: a value base for mental health recovery. *Journal of Psychosocial Nursing and Mental Health Services.* 2006; **44**: 29–33.
- Visit: www.tidal-model.com; for a free copy of the Tidal Model training manual, email: tidalmodel@btinternet.com

CHAPTER 4

The Purnell Model for Cultural Competence

Larry D Purnell

PRE-READING EXERCISE 4.1 (ANSWERS ON P. 50)

Time: 15 minutes
- Delivering culturally competent care is exceedingly complex and has at least five levels. Given this simple vignette, how many levels can you envision?
- Pablo Cardenas, a traditional Mexican, is being seen for depression and alcohol use at a large teaching hospital in the UK. The team includes a physician from Pakistan and a nurse from Germany.

REFLECTIVE PRACTICE EXERCISE 4.1

Time: 5 minutes
- What does the term 'cultural competence' mean to you?
- What does the professional need in order to be culturally competent?

THE NEED FOR CULTURALLY COMPETENT HEALTHCARE

The need for cultural competence is one of the most important recent developments because of increased globalisation and travel. In addition, diversity has increased in many countries due to wars, discrimination, political strife, and socioeconomic conditions resulting in increased immigration. The literature on health and healthcare disparities across ethnic, social and economic groups provides compelling evidence for healthcare providers and healthcare organisations to be attentive to diversity and cultural competency.

This chapter, on the Purnell Model for Cultural Competence, provides a guide for assessing cultural beliefs and practices. Professionals who understand the individual's cultural values, beliefs and practices are in a better position to interact with the individual and to provide culturally acceptable care. This improves the opportunities for:

➤ health promotion and wellness
➤ illness, disease and injury prevention
➤ health maintenance and restoration.

To this end, the professional needs both general and specific cultural knowledge. With specific knowledge of a cultural group, the professional will be in a better position to assess the individual and to provide culturally competent care. However, any generalisation made about the behaviours of an individual, or group of people, is almost certain to be an oversimplification. Within all cultures are subcultures and ethnic groups who do not hold all the values of the dominant culture. Subcultures, ethnic groups and ethnocultural populations are groups of people who have experiences different from those of the dominant culture with which they identify. Subcultures differ from the dominant group and share beliefs according to the primary and secondary variants of culture, as described later in this chapter.

Many definitions of culture exist. The important thing is for the professional to have an understanding of culture and choose a definition with which she/he is comfortable.

KEY POINT 4.1

Culture can be defined as the totality of socially transmitted behavioural patterns, beliefs, values, customs, lifeways, arts and all other products of human work and thought characteristics of a population of people that guide their world view and decision-making. These patterns may be explicit or implicit, are primarily learned and transmitted within the family, are shared by most members of the culture, and are emergent phenomena that change in response to global events.[1]

Culture is learned first in the family and then in churches, educational settings and other social organisations. Culture is largely unconscious and has powerful influences on physical and mental health. Each professional adds a unique dimension to the complexity of providing culturally competent care. The professional must recognise, respect and integrate the individual's cultural beliefs and practices into health prescriptions to eliminate or mitigate health disparities and increase satisfaction.

CULTURAL SELF-AWARENESS

Many theorists and diversity trainers attest that self-examination or awareness of personal prejudices and biases is an important step in the deliberate and conscious cognitive process of developing cultural competence.[1,2] However, discussions of emotional feelings elicited by this cognitive awareness are somewhat limited given the potential impact of emotions and conscious feelings on behavioural outcomes.[3] The ability to understand oneself sets the stage for integrating new knowledge related to cultural differences into the professional's knowledge base, perceptions of health, interventions, and the impact these factors have on the various roles of professionals when interacting with multicultural individuals.

The process of professional development and diversity competence begins with self-awareness, sometimes referred to as self-exploration,[3] or critical reflection.[4,5] Before addressing the multicultural backgrounds and unique perspectives of individuals, families and communities, professionals must first address their own personal and professional:

➤ knowledge
➤ values
➤ beliefs
➤ ethics
➤ attitudes
➤ life experiences.

This optimises interactions and cultural assessment of the individual. Culturally competent providers develop an 'awareness of their own existence, sensations, thoughts, and environment without letting them have an undue influence on those from backgrounds different from their own'.[2] This lifelong process includes a commitment to combat prejudice, discrimination, racism, bias and sexism.

Culture and race are not synonymous. However, the controversial term 'race' must be addressed when learning about culture. Race is genetic and includes physical characteristics that are similar among members of the same group, such as:

➤ skin colour
➤ blood type
➤ hair and eye colour.

Although there is less than 1% difference among the races, this difference may be significant when conducting health assessments and prescribing medications and treatments. People from a given racial group may, but not necessarily, share a common culture. Perhaps the most significant aspect of race is social in origin. Race can either decrease or increase opportunities, depending on the environmental context. The author acknowledges that many people do not like the racial and ethnic classifications used by governmental organisations. This chapter does not address these varied classifications for a specific country or among countries, and it is beyond the scope of this chapter.

PRIMARY AND SECONDARY VARIANTS OF CULTURE

Major influences that shape people's world view and the extent to which people identify with their cultural group of origin are called the primary and secondary variants of culture. These cultural variants should not be seen as categorically imperative. What may be a primary variant for one individual may be a secondary variant for another. The primary variants are:

➤ nationality
➤ race
➤ colour
➤ gender
➤ age
➤ religious affiliation.

Primary variants are attributes that either cannot be changed or if they are changed, a significant stigma may occur for the individual or family.

KEY POINT 4.2

People cannot change their nationality, age, race or colour. They can change their gender and religious affiliation. However, if a person changes his or her gender or changes religious preference, e.g. from Judaism to Pentecostal or vice versa, a significant stigma may occur.

The secondary variants include:
➤ educational status
➤ socioeconomic status
➤ occupation
➤ military experience
➤ political beliefs
➤ urban versus rural residence
➤ enclave identity
➤ marital status
➤ parental status
➤ physical characteristics
➤ sexual orientation
➤ gender issues
➤ reason for migration (sojourner, immigrant, or undocumented status)
➤ length of time away from the country of origin.

Immigration status influences a person's world view. For example, people who voluntarily migrate generally, but not always, acculturate and assimilate more easily. Sojourners who immigrate with the intention of remaining in their new homeland for only a short time, or refugees who think they may return to their home country, may not have the need or desire to acculturate or assimilate. Additionally, undocumented individuals (illegal immigrants) may have a different world view from those who have arrived legally.

The literature reports many definitions for the terms cultural awareness, cultural sensitivity and cultural competence. Sometimes these definitions are used interchangeably. However, **cultural awareness** has more to do with an appreciation of the external or material signs of diversity, such as the arts, music, dress or physical characteristics. Cultural sensitivity has more to do with personal attitudes and not saying things that might be offensive to someone from a cultural or ethnic background different from that of the professional.

Increasing one's consciousness of cultural diversity provides cultural leverage and improves the possibilities for professionals to provide culturally competent care.

Cultural competence, as used in this chapter, means:
➤ developing an awareness of one's own existence, sensations, thoughts and environment without letting them have an undue influence on those from other backgrounds
➤ demonstrating knowledge and understanding of the individual's culture, health-related needs and culturally specific meanings of health and illness
➤ continuing to learn cultures of the individual to whom one provides care
➤ recognising that the primary and secondary variants of culture determine the degree to which the individual adheres to the beliefs, values and practices of the dominant culture
➤ accepting and respecting cultural differences in a manner that facilitates the individual's and family's abilities to make decisions to meet their needs and beliefs
➤ not assuming that the professional's beliefs and values are the same as the individual's
➤ resisting judgemental attitudes such as 'different is not as good'
➤ being open to cultural encounters
➤ being comfortable with cultural encounters
➤ adapting care to be congruent with the individual's culture
➤ engaging in cultural competence is a conscious process and not necessarily a linear one
➤ accepting responsibility for one's own education in cultural competence by attending conferences, reading professional literature and observing cultural practices.

The author recognises that some countries and professionals prefer other terms instead of cultural competence. In this case, they should select and adapt terms with which they are most comfortable. Terms and concepts that are essential for understanding culture in an international context include:
➤ cultural humility
➤ cultural safety
➤ transcultural
➤ cross-cultural
➤ cultural awareness
➤ cultural sensitivity
➤ cultural relativism
➤ cultural imposition
➤ cultural imperialism
➤ cultural leverage
➤ ethnocentrism
➤ stereotyping
➤ generalisation.

Cultural humility[6] focuses on the process of intercultural exchange, paying explicit attention to clarifying the professional's values and beliefs through self-reflection, and incorporating the cultural characteristics of the professional and the individual into a mutually beneficial and balanced relationship. This term appears to be most popular with physicians and some professionals from social sciences.

Cultural safety[7] is popular in Australia and New Zealand, although the term is used elsewhere. Cultural safety expresses the diversity that exists within cultural groups, such social determinants of health, religion and gender, and is an addition to ethnicity.

The terms **transcultural**, as opposed to **cross-cultural**, have been hotly debated among experts in several countries, but especially in the United States. Specific definitions of these terms vary. Some attest that they are the same, while others say they are different.

KEY POINT 4.4

Transcultural compares values, beliefs and practices of a culture from the insider and outsider perspectives.

Nursing seems to favour the word transcultural. The term has been credited to a nurse anthropologist, Madeleine Leininger,[8] in the 1950s, and continues to be popular in the United States, United Kingdom and many other European countries. The term **cross-culture** was initially introduced by anthropologist George Murdock in the 1930s,[9] and it is still a popular term used in the social sciences, although the health sciences have used it too. The term implies comparative interactivity between cultures.

Cultural relativism is the belief that the behaviours and practices of people should be judged only from the context of their cultural system. Cultural relativism, relating one's own cultural experiences to those from another setting, requires knowledge about other cultures complemented by cultural values, biases and subjectivity. Proponents of cultural relativism argue that issues such as abortion, euthanasia, female circumcision and physical punishment in child rearing should be accepted as cultural values without judgement from the outside world. Opponents argue that cultural relativism may undermine condemnation of human rights violations, and family violence cannot be justified or excused on a cultural basis.[2,10-12]

Cultural imposition is the intrusive application of the majority group's cultural view upon individuals and families[10] (Universal Declaration of Human Rights, 2001). The practice of prescribing special diets without regard to individuals' cultural food choices borders on cultural imposition.[2,10-12] Professionals must continually recognise that their beliefs and values may not be the same as the individual's.

Cultural imperialism is the practice of extending policies and procedure of one organisation (usually the dominant one) to disenfranchised and minority groups. Proponents appeal to universal human rights values and standards. Opponents posit that universal standards are a disguise for the dominant culture to destroy or eradicate traditional cultures through worldwide public policy.[11,12]

Cultural leverage is a process whereby the principles of cultural competence are deliberatively invoked to develop interventions. It is a focused strategy for improving the health of racial and ethnic communities by using their cultural practices, products, philosophies or environments to facilitate behavioural changes of the individual and professional.[8]

Ethnocentrism is a universal tendency to believe that one's own world view is superior to another's. It is often experienced in the healthcare arena, in particular when the professional's own culture or ethnic group is considered superior to another.[8]

Stereotyping is having a simplified and standardised conception, opinion or belief about a person or group. The professional who fails to recognise individuality within a group is jumping to conclusions about the individual or family. If one concentrates on the primary and secondary variants of culture when assessing the individual, the tendency can be ameliorated. A generalisation begins with assumptions about the individual or family within an ethnocultural group but leads to further information seeking about the individual or family.[26]

THE PURNELL MODEL FOR CULTURAL COMPETENCE
Model assumptions

The Purnell Model for Cultural Competence has been classified as holographic and complexity grand theory. The model and framework can be used as a guide for assessment of all individuals. The major explicit assumptions on which the Purnell Model is based include the following.

➤ All professions need similar information about cultural diversity.
➤ All professions share the metaparadigm concepts of global society, family, person and health.
➤ One culture is not better than another culture; they are just different.
➤ There are core similarities shared by all cultures.
➤ There are differences within, between and among cultures.
➤ Cultures change slowly over time.
➤ The primary and secondary variants of culture determine the degree to which one varies from the dominant culture.
➤ If the individual is a co-participant in the care and has a choice in health-related goals, plans and interventions, compliance and health outcomes will be improved.
➤ Culture has a powerful influence on one's interpretation of and responses to health care.
➤ Individuals and families belong to several subcultures.
➤ Each individual has the right to be respected for his or her uniqueness and cultural heritage.
➤ Professionals need both cultural-general and cultural-specific information in order to provide culturally sensitive and culturally competent care.
➤ Professionals who can assess, plan, intervene and evaluate in a culturally competent manner will improve the care of the individual.

➤ Learning culture is an ongoing process that develops in a variety of ways, but primarily through cultural encounters.
➤ Prejudices and biases can be minimised with cultural understanding.
➤ To be effective, healthcare must reflect the unique understanding of the values, beliefs, attitudes, lifeways and world view of diverse populations and individual acculturation patterns.
➤ Differences in race and culture often require adaptations to standard interventions.
➤ Cultural awareness improves the professional's self-awareness.
➤ Professions, organisations and associations have their own culture, which can be analysed using a grand theory of culture.
➤ Every individual encounter is a cultural encounter.

Overview of the Purnell Model

The Purnell Model for Cultural Competence and its organising framework can be used in all practice settings and by all professionals. The model is a circle, with an outlying rim representing global society, a second rim representing community, a third rim representing family, and an inner rim representing the person (*see* Figure 4.1). The interior of the circle is divided into 12 pie-shaped wedges depicting cultural domains (constructs) and their associated concepts. The dark centre of the circle represents unknown phenomena. Along the bottom of the model is a jagged line representing the non-linear concept of cultural consciousness. The 12 cultural domains and their concepts provide the organising framework. Each domain includes concepts that need to be addressed when assessing the individual in various settings. Moreover, professionals can use these same concepts to better understand their own cultural beliefs, attitudes, values, practices and behaviours. An important concept to understand is that no single domain stands alone; they are all interconnected. The 12 domains are:

1 overview/heritage
2 communications
3 family roles and organisation
4 workforce issues
5 biocultural ecology
6 high-risk health behaviours
7 nutrition
8 pregnancy and the childbearing family
9 death rituals
10 spirituality
11 healthcare practices
12 healthcare practitioners.

CONCEPTS AND DOMAINS
Metaparadigm concepts

The metaparadigm concepts of the model are:
➤ global society
➤ community

➤ person
➤ family
➤ health.

Phenomena related to a global society include:
➤ world communication and politics
➤ conflicts and warfare
➤ natural disasters and famines
➤ international exchanges in education, business, commerce and information technology
➤ advances in health science
➤ space exploration
➤ the expanded opportunities for people to travel around the world and interact with diverse societies.

Global events that are widely disseminated by television, radio, satellite transmission, newsprint and information technology affect all societies, either directly or indirectly. Such events may create chaos while consciously and unconsciously forcing people to change their lifeways.

In the broadest definition, community is a group of people having a common interest or identity and goes beyond the physical environment. Community includes the physical, social and symbolic characteristics that cause people to connect. Bodies of water, mountains, rural versus urban living, and even railroad tracks help people define their physical concept of community. However, today, technology and the Internet allow people to expand their community beyond physical boundaries. Economics, religion, politics, age, generation and marital status delineate the social concepts of community. Sharing a specific language or dialect, lifestyle, history, dress, art or musical interest are symbolic characteristics of a community. People actively and passively interact with the community, necessitating adaptation and assimilation for equilibrium and homeostasis in their world view. Individuals may willingly change their physical, social and symbolic community when it no longer meets their needs.

A family is two or more people who are emotionally connected. They may, but do not necessarily, live in close proximity to each other. Family may include physically and emotionally close and distant consanguineous relatives, as well as physically and emotionally connected and distant non-blood-related significant others. Family structure and roles change according to age, generation, marital status, relocation or immigration and socioeconomic status, requiring each person to rethink individual beliefs and lifeways.

A person is a biopsychosociocultural being who is constantly adapting to his or her community. Human beings adapt biologically and physiologically with the ageing process:
➤ psychologically in the context of social relationships, stress and relaxation
➤ socially as they interact with the changing community
➤ ethnoculturally within the broader global society.

In Western cultures, a person is a separate physical and unique psychological being and a singular member of society. The self is separate from others (*see* Figure 4.1).

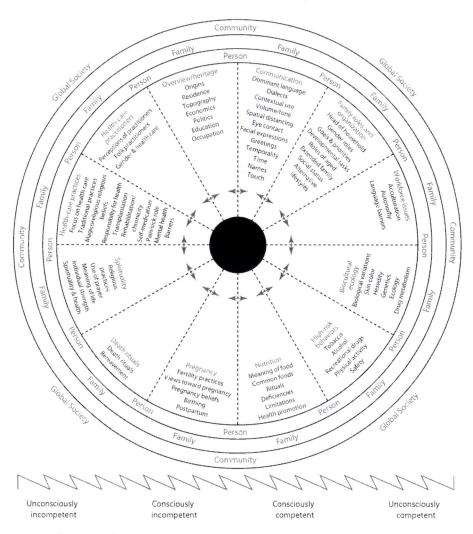

Primary characteristics of culture: age, generation, nationality, race, color, gender, religion

Secondary characteristics of culture: educational status, socioeconomic status, occupation, military status, political beliefs, urban versus rural residence, enclave identity, marital status, parental status, physical characteristics, sexual orientation, gender issues, and reason for migration (sojourner, immigrant, undocumented status)

Unconsciously incompetent: not being aware that one is lacking knowledge about another culture
Consciously incompetent: being aware that one is lacking knowledge about another culture
Consciously competent: learning about the client's culture, verifying generalizations about the client's culture, and providing culturally specific interventions
Unconsciously competent: automatically providing culturally congruent care to clients of diverse cultures

FIGURE 4.1 The Purnell Model for Cultural Competence (© Purnell LD. Reproduced with the kind permission of Professor Larry Purnell)

ASSESSMENT GUIDE

For each of the domains presented below, there is a box that includes suggested questions to ask and observations to make when assessing the individual from a cultural perspective. It is recognised that professionals are not able to complete a thorough cultural assessment for every individual. The list of questions is extensive; thus, the professional must determine what questions to ask according to the individual's presenting symptoms and teaching needs, and the potential impact of culture.

Overview and heritage

Overview and heritage include concepts related to the country of origin and current residence; the effects of the topography of the country of origin and the current residence on health, economics, politics, reasons for migration, educational status and occupations. (*See* Box 4.1.)

BOX 4.1 Overview, inhabited localities, and topography

- Where do you currently live?
- What is your ancestry?
- Where were you born?
- How many years have you lived in the United States (or other country, as appropriate)?
- In what country were your parents born?
- What brought you (your parents/ancestors) to this country (or other country, as appropriate)?
- Describe the land or countryside where you live. Is it mountainous, swampy, etc.?
- Have you lived in other places in the world?
- What was the land or countryside like when you lived there?
- What is your income level?
- Does your income allow you to afford the essentials of life?
- Do you have health insurance? (Depends on country-specific healthcare delivery system.)
- Are you able to afford health insurance on your salary? (As appropriate by specific country.)
- What is your educational level (formal/informal/self-taught)?
- What is your current occupation? If retired, ask about previous occupations.
- Have you worked in other occupations? What were they?
- Are there (were there) any particular health hazards associated with your job(s)?

Questions and observations related to the primary and secondary characteristics of culture not previously covered include the following:
- Have you been in the military? If so, in what foreign countries were you stationed?
- Are you married?
- How many children do you have?

Communications

Communications includes concepts related to the:

➤ dominant language
➤ dialects
➤ contextual use of the language.

Paralanguage variations:

➤ voice volume
➤ tone
➤ intonations
➤ inflections
➤ willingness to share thoughts and feelings.

Non-verbal communications:

➤ eye contact
➤ gesturing and facial expressions
➤ use of touch
➤ body language
➤ spatial distancing practices
➤ acceptable greetings.

Temporality in terms of:

➤ past
➤ present
➤ future orientation of world view
➤ clock versus social time
➤ the amount of formality in use of names.
   (*See* Box 4.2.)

BOX 4.2 Communications

- What is your full name?
- What is your legal name?
- By what name do you wish to be called?
- What is your primary language?
- Do you speak a specific dialect?
- What other languages do you speak?
- Do you find it difficult to share your thoughts, feelings and ideas with family? Friends? Health professionals?
- Do you mind being touched by friends? Strangers? Health professionals?
- How do wish to be greeted? Handshake? Nod of the head, etc.?
- Are you usually on time for appointments?
- Are you usually on time for social engagements?
- Observe the individual's speech pattern. Is the speech pattern high- or low-context? Remember, individuals from highly contexted cultures place greater value on silence.

- Observe the individual when physical contact is made. Does he/she withdraw from the touch or become tense?
- How close does the individual stand when talking with family members? With health professionals?
- Does the individual maintain eye contact when talking with the nurse/physician/etc.?

Family roles and organisation

These include concepts related to:

➤ the head of the household
➤ gender roles (a product of biology and culture)
➤ family goals and priorities
➤ developmental tasks of children and adolescents
➤ roles of the aged and extended family
➤ individual and family social status in the community
➤ acceptance of alternative lifestyles, such as single parenting, non-traditional sexual orientations, childless marriages and divorce.
(*See* Box 4.3.)

BOX 4.3 Family roles and organisation

- Who makes most of the decisions in your family?
- What types of decisions do(es) the female(s) in your family make?
- What types of decisions do(es) the male(s) in your family make?
- What are the duties of the women in the family?
- What are the duties of the men in the family?
- What should children **do** to make a good impression for themselves and for the family?
- What should children **not do** to make a good impression for themselves and for the family?
- What are children forbidden to **do**?
- What should adolescents **do** to make a good impression for themselves and for the family?
- What should adolescents **not do** to make a good impression for themselves and for the family?
- What are adolescents forbidden to do?
- What are the priorities for your family?
- What are the roles of the older person in your family? Are they sought for their advice?
- Are there extended family members in your household? Who else lives in your household?
- What are the roles of extended family members in this household? What gives you and your family status?
- Is it acceptable to you for people to have children out of wedlock?
- Is it acceptable to you for people to live together and not be married?

- Is it acceptable to you for people to admit being gay or lesbian?
- What is your sexual preference/orientation? (If appropriate, and then later in the assessment after a modicum of trust has been established.)

Workforce issues

This includes concepts related to:

➤ autonomy
➤ acculturation
➤ assimilation
➤ gender roles
➤ ethnic communication styles
➤ healthcare practices of the country of origin.

Because this handbook is intended for use in the clinical setting with the individual, this domain is not discussed. (*See* Box 4.4.)

BOX 4.4 Workforce issues

- Do you usually report to work on time?
- Do you usually report to meetings on time?
- What concerns do you have about working with someone of the opposite gender?
- Do you consider yourself a 'loyal' employee?
- How long do you expect to remain in your position?
- What do you do when you do not know how to do something related to your job?
- Do you consider yourself to be assertive in your job?
- What difficulty does English (or another languge) give you in the workforce?
- What difficulties do you have working with people older (younger) than you?
- What difficulty do you have in taking directions from someone younger/older than you?
- What difficulty do you have working with people whose religions are different from yours?
- What difficulty do you have working with people whose sexual orientation is different from yours?
- What difficulty do you have working with someone whose race or ethnicity is different from yours?
- Do you consider yourself to be an independent decision maker?

Biocultural ecology

Biocultural ecology includes physical, biological and physiological variations among ethnic and racial groups:

➤ skin colour (the most evident) and physical differences in body habitus
➤ genetic, hereditary, endemic and topographical diseases

➤ psychological make-up of individuals
➤ the physiological differences that affect the way drugs are metabolised by the body.

In general, most diseases and illnesses fall into three categories:
1 **Lifestyle** – causes include cultural practices and behaviours that can generally be controlled (e.g. smoking, diet and stress).
2 **Environment** – causes refer to the external environment (e.g. air and water pollution) and situations over which the individual has little or no control over (e.g. presence of malarial mosquitoes, exposure to chemicals and pesticides, access to care, and associated diseases).
3 **Genetics**: conditions are caused by genes.
  (*See* Box 4.5.)

BOX 4.5 Bioccultural ecology

- Are you allergic to any medications?
- What problems did you have when you took over-the-counter medications?
- What problems did you have when you took prescription medications?
- What are the major illnesses and diseases in your family?
- Are you aware of any genetic diseases in your family?
- What are the major health problems in the country from which you come (if appropriate)?
- With what race do you identify?
- Observe skin colouration and physical characteristics.
- Observe for physical difficulties and disabilities.

High-risk health behaviours

High-risk health behaviours include:
➤ substance, alcohol and tobacco use
➤ lack of physical activity
➤ increased calorie consumption
➤ no use of safety measures, such as seat belts, helmets, and safe driving practices
➤ not taking safety measures to prevent contracting HIV and sexually transmitted diseases.
  (*See* Box 4.6.)

BOX 4.6 High-risk health behaviours

- How many cigarettes a day do you smoke?
- Do you smoke a pipe (or cigars)?
- Do you chew tobacco?
- For how many years have you smoked/chewed tobacco?
- How much do you drink each day? Ask about wine, beer and spirits.

- What recreational drugs do you use?
- How often do you use recreational drugs?
- What type of exercise do you do each day?
- Do you use seat belts?
- What precautions do you take to prevent getting a sexually transmitted disease or HIV/AIDS?

Nutrition

Nutrition is more than satisfying hunger. It includes:
➤ the meaning of food, common foods and rituals
➤ nutritional deficiencies and food limitations
➤ the use of food for health promotion and restoration, and illness and disease prevention.

BOX 4.7 Nutrition

- Are you satisfied with your weight?
- Which foods do you eat to maintain your health?
- Do you avoid certain foods to maintain your health?
- Why do you avoid these foods?
- Which foods do you eat when you are ill?
- Which foods do you avoid when you are ill?
- Why do you avoid these foods (if appropriate)?
- For what illnesses do you eat certain foods?
- Which foods do you eat to balance your diet?
- Which foods do you eat every day?
- Which foods do you eat every week?
- Which foods do you eat that are part of your cultural heritage?
- Which foods are high-status foods in your family/culture?
- Which foods are eaten only by men? Women? Children? Teenagers? Older people?
- How many meals do you eat each day?
- What time do you eat each meal?
- Do you snack between meals?
- What foods do you eat when you snack?
- What holidays do you celebrate?
- Which foods do you eat on particular holidays?
- Who is present at each meal? Is the entire family present?
- Do you primarily eat the same foods as the rest of your family?
- Where do you usually buy your food?
- Who usually buys the food in your household?
- Who does the cooking in your household?
- How frequently do you eat at a restaurant?
- When you eat at a restaurant, in what type of restaurant do you eat?
- Do you eat foods left from previous meals?

- Where do you keep your food?
- Do you have a refrigerator?
- How do you cook your food?
- How do you prepare meat?
- How do you prepare vegetables?
- What type of spices do you use?
- What do you drink with your meals?
- Do you drink special teas?
- Do you have any food allergies?
- Are there certain foods that cause you problems when you eat them?
- How does your diet change with each season?
- Are your food habits different on days you work versus when you are not working?

Pregnancy and childbearing practices

These include:

➤ culturally sanctioned and unsanctioned fertility practices
➤ views on pregnancy
➤ prescriptive, restrictive and taboo practices related to pregnancy, birthing and the postpartum period.
   (*See* Box 4.8.)

BOX 4.8 Pregnancy and childbearing practices

- How many children do you have?
- What do you use for birth control?
- What does it mean to you and your family when you are pregnant?
- What special foods do you eat when you are pregnant?
- What foods do you avoid when you are pregnant?
- What activities do you avoid when you are pregnant?
- Do you do anything special when you are pregnant?
- Do you eat non-food substances when you are pregnant?
- Who do you want with you when you deliver your baby?
- In what position do you want to be when you deliver your baby?
- What special foods do you eat after delivery?
- What foods do you avoid after delivery?
- What activities do you avoid after you deliver?
- Do you do anything special after delivery?
- Who will help you with the baby after delivery?
- What bathing restrictions do you have after you deliver?
- Do you want to keep the placenta?
- What do you do to care for the baby's umbilical cord?

Death rituals

Death rituals include:

➤ how the individual and the society view death and euthanasia
➤ rituals to prepare for death
➤ burial practices
➤ bereavement behaviours.

Death rituals are slow to change. (*See* Box 4.9.)

BOX 4.9 Death rituals

- What special activities need to be performed to prepare for death?
- Would you want to know about your impending death?
- What is your preferred burial practice? Interment, cremation?
- How soon after death does burial occur?
- How do men grieve?
- How do women grieve?
- What does death mean to you?
- Do you believe in an afterlife?
- Are children included in death rituals?

Spirituality

Spirituality includes:

➤ formal religious beliefs related to faith and affiliation and the use of prayer
➤ behaviour practices that give meaning to life
➤ individual sources of strength.
  (*See* Box 4.10.)

BOX 4.10 Spirituality

- What is your religion?
- Do you consider yourself deeply religious?
- How many times a day do you pray?
- What do you need in order to say your prayers?
- Do you meditate? How often?
- What gives strength and meaning to your life?
- In what spiritual practices do you engage for your physical and emotional health?

Healthcare practices

Healthcare practices include:

➤ the focus of healthcare (acute versus preventive)
➤ traditional, magicoreligious, and bio-medical beliefs and practices
➤ individual responsibility for health

➤ self-medicating practices
➤ views on mental illness, chronicity, rehabilitation, acceptance of blood and blood products, and organ donation and transplantation. (*See* Box 4.11.)

BOX 4.11 Healthcare practices

- In what prevention activities do you engage to maintain your health?
- Who in your family takes responsibility for your health?
- What over-the-counter medicines do you use?
- What herbal teas and folk medicines do you use?
- For what conditions do you use herbal medicines?
- What do you usually do when you are in pain?
- How do you express your pain?
- How are people in your culture viewed or treated when they have a mental illness?
- How are people with physical disabilities treated in your culture?
- What do you do when you are sick? Stay in bed, continue your normal activities, etc?
- What are your beliefs about rehabilitation?
- How are people with chronic illnesses viewed or treated in your culture?
- Are you averse to blood transfusions?
- Is organ donation acceptable to you?
- Are you an organ donor?
- Would you consider having an organ transplant if needed?
- Are healthcare services readily available to you?
- Do you have transportation problems accessing needed health services?
- Can you afford healthcare?
- Do you feel welcome when you see a health professional?
- What traditional healthcare practices do you use? Acupuncture, acupressure, cai gao, moxibustion, aromatherapy, coining, etc.?
- What home difficulties do you have that might prevent you from receiving healthcare?

Healthcare professionals

This domain includes the:
➤ status
➤ use
➤ perceptions of traditional, magicoreligious, bio-medical healthcare providers
➤ gender of the health professional.

BOX 4.12 Healthcare practitioners

- What health professionals do you see when you are ill? Physicians, nurses?
- Do you prefer a same-sex health professional for routine health problems? For intimate care?
- What healers do you use beside physicians and nurses?
- For what conditions do you use healers?

CONCLUSION AND RECOMMENDATIONS

As world immigration increases, professionals need to be attentive to the individual's culture if intervention/treatment plans are to be effective, thereby increasing satisfaction and decreasing costs. The professional is ethically bound to provide culturally competent care by adapting interventions/treatments to meet cultural and ethnic needs. Culturally competent care is complex and includes:

➤ the culture of the individual
➤ the culture of the professional(s)
➤ the culture of the profession(s) and specialties
➤ the culture of the health organisation
➤ the culture of the society/county, in which the care is delivered.

KEY POINT 4.5 SOME RECOMMENDATIONS

- Use a comprehensive cultural theory, model or framework to guide practice.
- Learn your own culture and reflect how the primary and secondary variants of culture affect your world view.
- Learn as much as you can about a cultural group so you know specific questions for assessment.
- Remember: every encounter is a cultural encounter.
- Resist ethnocentrism, stereotyping and attitudes such as 'different is not as good'.
- Be open to cultural encounters and learn what respect means in each culture to which you provide care.
- An individualised intervention(s)/treatment plan(s) is a cultural care plan.
- Take responsibility for your own education by attending conferences, reading literature and observing cultural practices. Search the academic literature for evidence-based practice information and guidelines related to culture.

POST-READING EXERCISE 4.1 (ANSWERS ON P. 50)

Time: 5 minutes
- Every individual has a dominant culture heritage with values, beliefs and practices that are first learned at home and then in church, school and social organisations. Within the dominant culture, an individual's beliefs

vary according to the primary and secondary variants of culture. In addition, personality makes a difference.

- How many primary and secondary variants of culture can you cite?

REFERENCES

1 Andrews M, Boyle J. *Transcultural Concepts in Nursing Care*. Philadelphia: Lippincott, Williams and Wilkins; 2008.

2 Purnell L. The Purnell Model for Cultural Competence. In Purnell L, Paulanka B, editors. *Transcultural Health Care: a culturally competent approach*. 3rd ed. Philadelphia: FA Davis; 2008. pp. 19–56.

3 Markus HR, Kitayama S. Culture and self: implications for cognition, emotion, and motivation. *Psychological Review*. 1991; **98**: 224–53.

4 Gardner F. Culture and change management. *The International Journal of Knowledge*. 2008; **6**: 73–80.

5 Teekman B. Exploring reflective thinking in nursing practice. *Journal of Advanced Nursing*. 2000; **31**: 1125–35.

6 Community Partnerships for Older Adults: Robert Wood Johnson Foundation. Available at: www.partnershipsforolderadults.org/index.aspx (accessed 28 July 2010).

7 Nursing Council of New Zealand. *Guidelines for cultural safety, the Treaty of Waitangi and Maori Health in Nursing and Education Practice*. Wellington: Nursing Council of New Zealand; 2009. Available at: http://nur3425s2.handel.2day.com/NC_Cultural%20Safety.pdf (accessed 29 December 2010).

8 Leininger M, McFarland M. *Culture Care Diversity and Universality: a worldwide theory*. 2nd ed. Sudbury, MA: Jones and Bartlett; 2006.

9 New World Encyclopaedia. Murdock, George Peter. Available at: www.newworldencyclopedia.org/entry/George_Peter_Murdock (accessed 28 July 2010).

10 Universal Declaration of Human Rights. 2001. Available at: www.un.org/Overview/rights.html (accessed 28 July 2010).

11 Giger J, Davidhizar R, Purnell L, *et al*. American Academy of Nursing Expert Panel Report: developing cultural competence to eliminate health disparities in ethnic minorities and other vulnerable populations. *Journal of Transcultural Nursing*. 2007; **18**: 95–102.

12 Purnell L. Cultural competence in a changing healthcare environment. In Chaska N, editor. *The Nursing Profession: tomorrow's vision*. Thousand Oaks, CA: Sage; 2001. pp. 451–61.

13 Fisher TL, Burnet DL, Huang ES, *et al*. Cultural leverage: interventions using culture to narrow racial disparities in health care. *Medical Care Research and Review*. 2007; **64** (Suppl. 5): S43–82.

TO LEARN MORE

- Chun KM, Organista PB, Marín G. *Acculturation: advances in theory, measurement, and applied research*. Washington, DC: American Psychological Association; 2003.
- *Culture, Medicine & Psychiatry*. This is an international and interdisciplinary forum for the publication of work in the fields of medical and psychiatric anthropology, cross-cultural psychiatry, and associated cross-societal and clinical epidemiological studies. Available at: www.springer.com/social+sciences/anthropology+&+archaeology/journal/11013
- Douglas M, Uhl Pierce J, Rosenkoetter M, *et al*. Standards of practice for culturally competent care: a request for comments. *Journal of Transcultural Nursing*. 2009; **20**: 257–69.

- Giger JN, Davidhizar, RE. *Transcultural Nursing: assessment and intervention.* 5th ed. St Louis, MO: Mosby; 2008.
- US Department of Health and Human Services. *Healthy People 2010.* 2nd ed. Washington, DC: US Government Printing Office; 2010. Available at: http://nnlm.gov/outreach/consumer/hlthlit.html
- Helman C. *Culture, Health, and Illness.* 5th ed. Oxford: Butterworth Heinemann; 2007.
- Jeffreys MR. *Teaching Cultural Competence in Nursing and Health Care.* New York: Springer Publications; 2006.
- Papadopoulos I. *Transcultural Health and Social Care.* Edinburgh: Churchill Livingston; 2006.
- Purnell L. *Guide to Culturally Competent Health Care.* 2nd ed. Philadelphia: FA Davis; 2009. Additional resources for this book are available at: http://davisplus.fadavis.com/landing_page.cfm?publication_id=2490
- Purnell L, Paulanka, B. *Transcultural Health Care: a culturally competent approach.* 3rd ed. Philadelphia: FA Davis; 2008. Accompanying this textbook is an extensive guide for web resources and includes documents on health disparities/inequalities and cultural information from several countries in Europe, Australia, Canada, New Zealand, the United States, and the World Health Organization. Additional chapters, case studies, a test bank and instructor resources are also included. Available at: http://davisplus.fadavis.com/landing_page.cfm?publication_id=2417
- Purnell L, Davidhizar R, Giger J, *et al.* A guide to developing a culturally competent organization. *Journal of Transcultural Nursing.* Forthcoming (2011; **22**).

ANSWERS TO PRE-READING EXERCISE 4.1

1 The first level is the culture of the individual, who is from Mexico.
2 A second level is the culture of the professional: Pakistani and German.
3 A third level is the culture of the professions, and specialty: psychiatric medicine and psychiatric nursing.
4 A fourth is the culture of the host country: UK.
5 A fifth level is the culture of the organisation: a large teaching hospital.

ANSWERS TO POST-READING EXERCISE 4.1

- Remember, a primary variant of culture for one person can be a secondary variant of culture for another person so, **do not** be concerned about categorisation.
- Primary variants of culture are nationality, age, race, colour, gender and religious affiliation.
- Secondary variants of culture are educational status, socioeconomic status, occupation, military experience, political beliefs, urban versus rural residence, enclave identity, marital status, parental status, physical characteristics, sexual orientation, gender issues, reason for migration (sojourner, immigrant or undocumented status) and length of time away from the country of origin.

CHAPTER 5

Application of transcultural theory to mental health–substance use in an international context

Larry D Purnell

PRE-READING EXERCISE 5.1 (ANSWERS ON P. 67)

Time: 15 minutes

Maria Elena Cabrera Martinez Casilla (Señora Casilla), originally from Panama, was referred to a large physhiatric hospital by her UK employer. Over the last month she reported to work three times but was unable to function. She admits to having a drinking problem and uses marijuana because she is depressed and missing her family in Panama. Her employer has agreed to keep her employed if she seeks help for her problems. Señora Casilla, who speaks minimal English, has agreed to in-hospital treatment. Her psychiatrist comes from Iran, her nurse comes from the United States and her occupational therapist comes from Germany.

1 What concerns do you see without a common culture among Señora Casilla and the health professionals?

2 The primary languages of Señora Casilla and each of the professionals are the languages of their home countries. What concerns do you have?

3 How is mental illness viewed in the cultures of Señora Casilla and each of the health professionals?

INTRODUCTION

This chapter provides a brief review of the international literature on the value of cultural competence in mental health nursing (but is integral to all health professions). Selected domains from the Purnell Model for Cultural Competence and the research literature on individualistic and collectivistic cultures are used as guides for assessing and planning interventions/treatment specific to the culture of the individual. Although all domains (constructs) of the Purnell Model are applicable, space does not permit an extensive review of them here. The reader is encouraged to read Chapter 4 for a more complete description of the Purnell Model and its organising framework before continuing with this chapter. Material culture, such as music, dance, dress, poetry, literature and art, are important and should be incorporated. However, they are not addressed in this chapter, where the focus in on subjective cultural values, beliefs and practices.

CULTURAL COMPETENCE IN MENTAL HEALTH NURSING

Most countries throughout the world are homes to an array of cultural and ethnic groups, each with its unique ways of:

➤ communicating, handling stress, giving meaning to life, and methods for health promotion and wellness

➤ illness, disease and injury prevention

➤ health maintenance and restoration.[1]

Emotional distress and mental illness are embedded within and cannot be separated from language and cultural, social and political contexts.[2]

KEY POINT 5.1

Mental health is fundamental to overall health and productivity and is the basis for successful contributions to family, community and society.

The evidence-based literature reports that cultural stereotypes, perceived racism and discrimination can deter certain cultural groups from seeking help for mental health concerns and dilemmas and substance use.[1–6] In addition, many immigrants and refugees are at particularly high risk for mental health problems when accompanied by one of the following seven conditions:

1 a drop in socioeconomic status following migration
2 inability to speak the language of the host country
3 separation from family
4 lack of friendly reception from the host country
5 lack of a friendly reception by the host population to provide support
6 a traumatic experience prior to migration
7 migrating during adolescence or after age 65 years.[7]

In addition, mental health concerns frequently occur during periods of rapid social change, when people are displaced from their community of origin, or have been devastated by extensive or sudden influx of outside influence, resulting in a loss of ethnic or cultural identity requiring culturally congruent mental health services.

Acculturation, the degree to which an individual identifies with his or her native culture, is thought to be related to substance use. Higher rates of substance use have been found in people who closely identify with non-Native American values and the lowest rates are found in bicultural individuals who are comfortable with both sets of cultural values.[8]

Cultural mandates

A literature review and query to several professional list serves for legislative mandates for cultural competence in Australia, Great Britain, Portugal, Spain and New Zealand revealed many recommendations from professional bodies. However, only two legislative mandates were forthcoming:

1 The US Department of Health and Human Services
2 Some US state-mandated legislation (California, New Jersey and Washington).

The US Department of Health and Human Services has mandated Cultural and Linguistic Standards (CLAS) for health facilities that receive government funds. They must provide interpreter services and the facility cannot charge the individual for such services. Interpreter services include sign language.[9] The other US mandated legislations come from the states of Washington, California and New Jersey, which have mandated that healthcare facilities must certify their physicians as being culturally competent in order to receive insurance reimbursement. Four other states are currently working towards this same mandate.[10] The 'To learn more' section at the end of this chapter lists online documents from diverse countries and professional organisations that have made recommendations for cultural competence in healthcare facilities.

CULTURAL-GENERAL VERSUS CULTURAL-SPECIFIC INTERVENTIONS

A goal of cultural competence is to balance specific cultural facts and information with acquiring sound skills and general knowledge of effective health professional interaction in all encounters.[11] To provide culturally competent care, professionals should integrate, or coordinate, traditional care approaches with conventional evidence-based medical and nursing approaches.[11] However, the concept of normality across cultures does not exist. Health professionals should understand how their attitudes towards culture can affect the provision of satisfactory behavioural health services.[12]

KEY POINT 5.2

Norms from one culture do not necessarily fit the norms for another culture.

Although the information in this chapter is in the form of cultural group averages, a standard scientific practice for illustrating group differences, it should be well-noted that each racial or ethnic group contains the full range of variation on almost every social, psychological and biological dimension presented.[3] Given the primary and secondary variants of diversity (*see* Chapter 4), no one way exists for treating any racial and ethnic group. Thus, a cultural-general framework of interventions is needed that can be individualised and applied in an individual- and family-centred approach.[13]

As an adjunct to having a general approach for cultural assessment, the professional needs to know general and specific characteristics of the individual's dominant culture. This specific knowledge places the professional in a culturally relevant position. The more one knows about a specific culture, the better the questions the professional can ask, resulting in **cultural tailoring** and **cultural leverage**.[1,13] For example, if the professional is not aware that many Hispanic populations use folk healers, such as:

➤ curanderos – traditional folk healer or shaman
➤ sobadores – similar to a chiropractor
➤ masajistas terapéuticos – massage therapists
➤ yerberos – herbalists
➤ espiritistas – spiritualists,

then they do not know to ask this specific question. Cultural tailoring refers to individualised programming that takes into account individuals' personal preferences.[14] Cultural leverage is a focused strategy using the individuals' cultural practices, products, philosophies or environments as vehicles to facilitate behaviour change of person and professional.[13]

Surface characteristics, such as traditional dress, music, colours, etc., are fairly easily incorporated into health materials and programming. However, deeper dimensions, such as shared underlying values and assumptions, may be harder to incorporate but possibly more effective.[15-17] Each ethnic subgroup, by definition, has a common heritage, values, rituals and traditions. However, there is no such thing as a completely homogeneous racial or ethnic group due to the primary and secondary variants of culture.

Whereas value exists in learning cultural variants of the individual's dominant culture, the professional must not stereotype or overgeneralise, and assume that the beliefs, values and health practices for a certain cultural group are true for every individual who self-identifies with that group. They must pay particular attention to the primary and secondary variants of culture, which determine the degree of adherence to their dominant or blended culture.

What is considered substance use is often culturally determined, especially when religion is taken into consideration. Thus, sociocultural beliefs should shape the approach to mental health counselling.[5,6] Those who experience *anomie*, loss of a healthy cultural identity, may occur among populations whose cultures have been affected by a sudden influx of outside influence that sometimes occurs on migration.[18] Moreover, it is important to note what involvement a person has had with her or his host culture, and to what degree the family is involved with their culture.[1] One aspect of recovery that is often overlooked is that of 'cultural recovery'. Cultural recovery involves regaining a viable ethnic identity and acquiring a functional social network committed to the individual's recovery, by:

➤ making a religious, spiritual, or moral recommitment
➤ re-engaging in recreational or vocational activities
➤ gaining a social role in the recovering community, society at large, or both.

Those individuals who fail to make a satisfactory cultural recovery are at increased risk for relapse.[18]

INDIVIDUALISM VERSUS COLLECTIVISM

All cultures vary along the individualism and collectivism scale and are subsets of broad world views. A continuum of values for individualistic and collectivistic cultures includes:

➤ orientation to self or group
➤ decision-making
➤ knowledge transmission
➤ individual choice and personal responsibility
➤ concepts of progress
➤ competitiveness
➤ shame and guilt
➤ help-seeking
➤ expression of identity
➤ interaction/communication style.[19-21]

Elements of individualism and collectivism exist in every culture. People from an individualist culture will more strongly identify with the values at the individualistic end of the scale. People from a collectivist culture will adhere more closely to the values at the collectivist end of the scale. Moreover, individualism and collectivism fall along a continuum, and some people from an individualistic culture will, to some degree, align themselves towards the collectivistic end of the scale. Some people from a collectivist culture will, to some degree, hold values along the individualistic end of the scale. Acculturation is a key component of adapting individualistic and collectivistic values. Those who live in ethnic enclaves usually, *but not always*, adhere more strongly to their dominant cultural values. Acculturation and the primary and secondary variants of culture (*see* Chapter 4) determine the degree of adherence to traditional individualistic and collectivist cultural values, beliefs and practices.

KEY POINT 5.3

Individualism									*Collectivism*
1	*2*	*3*	*4*	*5*	*6*	*7*	*8*	*9*	*10*

The above individualism and collectivism scale can be reversed if the reader prefers.

Counselling with a person from an individualistic culture, where the most important person in society is the individual, may require different techniques than for a person in a collectivist culture where the group is seen as more important than the individual.[1] The professional must not confuse individualism with individuality, the degree that varies by culture and is usually more prevalent in individualistic countries. Individuality is the sense that each person has a separate and equal place in the community and where individuals who are considered 'eccentrics or local characters' are tolerated.[22]

Some examples of highly individualistic cultures are:

➤ *Traditional* American (USA)
➤ British
➤ Canadian
➤ German
➤ Norwegian
➤ Swedish.

Examples of collectivist cultures are:
➤ *Traditional* Arab
➤ Chinese
➤ Filipino
➤ Korea
➤ Japanese
➤ Latin American
➤ Mexican
➤ Native American Indians (and most other indigenous Indian groups)
➤ Taiwanese
➤ Thai
➤ Vietnamese.

Far more world cultures are collectivistic than are individualistic.[23]

THE PURNELL MODEL FOR CULTURAL COMPETENCE

Selected domains from the Purnell Model for Cultural Competence (*see* Chapter 4), and concepts from individualism and collectivism, are used as guides for developing interventions in mental health and behavioural disorders.

Communications

Communications includes:
➤ concepts related to the dominant language, dialects and the contextual use of the language
➤ paralanguage variations such as voice volume, tone, intonations, inflections and willingness to share thoughts and feelings
➤ non-verbal communications, such as eye contact, gesturing and facial expressions, use of touch, body language, spatial distancing practices, and acceptable greetings; temporality in terms of past, present and future orientation of world view
➤ clock versus social time
➤ the amount of formality in use of names.

The diagnosis and treatment of mental disorders greatly depend on verbal communication and trust between individual and professional.[3]

Often, individuals can feel alienated from the host culture if they do not speak the native language fluently, or at all. Thus, the need for a certified interpreter is a necessity. When working with interpreters, establishing trust is a must, and it is attained through verbal and non-verbal communication. Part of establishing trust among the interpreter, the individual and the professional is to obtain the best interpreter available. The ideal interpreter is:

➤ one who is certified
➤ is dialect specific
➤ is unknown to the individual
➤ understands the culture of the individual in addition to the language
➤ is the same gender of the individual if sensitive issues are being discussed
➤ has the same social status of the individual.[1,11]

The professional should, when possible, allow time for the individual and interpreter to have some initial time together before the interview starts.

KEY POINT 5.4

- Maintain eye contact with both the individual and interpreter.
- Direct questions to the individual, not the interpreter.
- Do not use family members as interpreters (*except to obtain non-sensitive demographic information*).
- Do not use children (*this causes role reversal; can create a concern in some families, especially in collectivistic cultures*).

Cultures differ in the extent to which health and information is explicit or implicit. In low-context cultures, great emphasis is placed on the verbal mode and many words used to express a thought. Low-context cultures are individualistic. In high-context cultures much of the information is implicit where fewer words are used to express a thought, resulting in more of the message being in the non-verbal mode. Great emphasis is placed on personal relationships. High-context cultures are collectivistic.[23]

Consistent with individualism, individualistic cultures encourage self-expression, both verbally and non-verbally. Adherents to individualism freely express personal opinions, share many personal issues and ask personal questions of others to a degree that may be seen as offensive to others who come from a collectivistic culture. Direct, straightforward questioning is usually appreciated with individualism. However, the professional should take cues from the individual before this intrusive approach is initiated.[19-21] An initial approach after a formal introduction is to ask: 'What (*not why, which places blame and puts the individual on the defensive*) made you decide to come here today?'

Small talk before getting down to business is not always appreciated. Individualistic cultures usually tend to be more informal and frequently use first names. Ask the individual by what name he/she prefers to be called. Questions that require a 'yes' or 'no' answer are usually answered truthfully from the individual's perspective.

Spatial distancing practices can be problematic if the professional is not aware of cultural expectations. Among most individualistic cultures, conversants usually maintain a distance of 18 to 24 inches (approx. 45–60 cm), unless they are family or good friends, then the distance is closer. However, with people in hierarchal positions, the spatial distancing is usually greater than 24 inches (60 cm). Among Middle Easterners and Arab cultures, conversants, even if they do not know each other, usually stand within 12 to 18 inches (approx. 30–45 cm), of each other.[1,15] The professional should not take offence when spatial distancing practices are different from his or her own.

In Western individualistic cultures, one is expected to maintain eye contact with the conversant regardless of status differences. Not maintaining eye contact (some mental health conditions are excluded) may be interpreted as:

➤ not telling the truth
➤ not listening
➤ not caring
➤ being devious.

Among traditional collectivist cultures, especially among lower socioeconomic and less educated members, eye contact is not maintained with someone in a higher status position, or with older people, as a sign of respect.

Collectivism is characterised by not drawing attention to oneself and people are not encouraged to ask questions.[19-21] When one fails, shame may be extended to the family and external explanations, spiritual, superiors or fate, may be given. To avoid offending someone, people are expected to practise smooth interpersonal communication by not openly disagreeing and being evasive with negative issues.

KEY POINT 5.5

Personal thoughts, opinions, information and feelings are not shared until a modicum of trust is established.

Respect for tradition, protection of one's reputation, and stability are important. In collectivism, the past is venerated and older people are regarded with wisdom and respect. People's relationships, roles and mental health concerns are interdependent with other members of the group. Most collectivistic cultures are more formal and people, regardless of age differences, should be addressed as Mr, Mrs, Ms, or other title such as engineer, doctor, lawyer, etc., until told to do otherwise.

KEY POINT 5.6

Introducing yourself by first name only, or addressing individual by their first name only, is considered rude or offensive. Introduce yourself by your full name and title to show respect.

Among most collectivist cultures, to disagree or to answer the professional with a 'no' response is considered rude. In fact, in some languages a word for 'no' does not exist. Do not ask the individual if he/she knows about what you are asking, understands you, or knows how to do something, because the only option that a person would have is to answer 'yes'. Yes, could mean:

➤ 'I hear you', but I do not understand you.
➤ 'I understand you', but I not agree with what has been said.
➤ 'I agree with you', but I will not necessarily follow recommendations.

Repeating what has been prescribed does not ensure understanding; instead ask for a demonstration or some other response that is more likely to determine understanding.

Family roles and organisation

Family roles and organisation includes concepts related to:

➤ the head of the household
➤ gender roles – *a product of biology and culture*
➤ family goals
➤ priorities
➤ developmental tasks of children and adolescents
➤ roles of the aged and extended family
➤ individual and family social status in the community
➤ acceptance of alternative lifestyles, such as single parenting, non-traditional sexual orientations, childless marriages and divorce.

It is important to note what involvement a person has had with his or her host culture, and to what degree the family is involved with their culture. In non-Western settings, identity is tied to a person's roles, such as mother/husband, daughter/son, wife/husband, grandmother/grandfather, and through work as a nurse/doctor/teacher/etc. This identity provides the individual with a place of respect and honour in society.

Family involvement is an important focus in working with collectivistic cultures. Both the individual's immediate and extended families are significant and should be involved in the intervention process because mental health problems can erode important family and social ties. Restorative efforts to repair an individual's familial and social network can buffer the effects of mental health concerns and dilemmas.[24] Some immigrants leave the protective environment of their family behind and are faced with a new set of cultural norms and values, resulting in increase in high-risk health behaviours.

Individualistic cultures socialise their members to view themselves as *independent*, separate, distinct individuals, where the most important person in society is self. A person feels free to change alliances and not feel bounded by any particular group (shared identity). Although they are part of a group, they are still free to act independently within the group and less likely to engage in 'group think'. In individualism, competition, whether individual or group, permeates every aspect of life. Separateness, independence and the capacity to express one's own views and opinions are both explicitly valued and implicitly assumed.[19–21,24]

In individualistic cultures, a person's identity is based mainly on one's personal accomplishments, career and challenges. A high standard of living supports self-efficiency, self-direction, self-advocacy and independent living. Decisions made by elders and people in hierarchal positions may be questioned, or not followed, because the ideal is that all people expect, and are expected, to make their own decisions about their lives. Moreover, people are personally responsible and held accountable for their decisions. Improving self, doing 'better' than others (frequently focused on material gains) and making progress on a community or national level are expected. If one fails, the blame and shame are on 'self'.[19-21,24]

In collectivistic cultures, people are socialised to view themselves as members of a larger group, family, school, church, educational setting, work, etc. They are bound through the expectations of loyalty and personal and familial lifetime protective ties.[1,19-21] Children are socialised where priority is given to connections and interrelationship with others as the basis of psychological well-being. Older people and those in hierarchal positions are respected, and people are less likely to openly disagree with them. Parents and elders may have the final say in their children's careers and life partners. The focus is not on the individual but on the group.

KEY POINT 5.7

- In some cultures, there is no word for '*individual*' as someone who stands alone.
- In other cultures there is a word for '*individual*'; in this context, it is not seen as negative.

Healthcare practices

The domain of healthcare practices includes:
➤ the focus of healthcare (acute versus preventive)
➤ traditional, magicoreligious and bio-medical beliefs and practices
➤ individual responsibility for health
➤ self-medicating practices
➤ views on mental illness, chronicity, rehabilitation
➤ acceptance of blood and blood products
➤ organ donation and transplantation.

Throughout the lifespan, mental health is the wellspring of thinking and communication skills, learning, resilience and self-esteem.

Although common biological factors underlie some forms of mental illness across all societies, explanatory models for mental illness and emotional distress are embedded within the assumptions and belief systems of the individual's prevailing culture. An 'illness' in one culture may carry a significant stigma, while in another culture that illness might not have a stigma to the same degree. People with mental illness feel shame and fear of discrimination about a condition that is as real and disabling as any other serious physical health condition.[3] The greater the perceived stigma, the more the individual is likely to delay, or to not seek treatment, even if the treatment is available, affordable and accessible.[1] In addition, mistrust of health professionals and fear of treatment, racism, discrimination (real or perceived) and difference in language and communication deter some individuals and families from seeking physical and mental healthcare until the condition is in crisis, at which time the treatment is more complex and accompanied with an increase in cost to the individual, family and society.

The Western, bio-medical approach to mental 'illness' promotes an approach to 'treatment' that is heavily based on pharmacology. While psychotropic medications are beneficial for psychoses and bipolar disorders, the increasing use of pharmacological treatments can undermine approaches to treatment and care that may be more rooted in local culture. Western psychiatry, traditional healing and systems of self-caring have both benefits and limitations. The recent synthesis of differing views by the World Health Organization concludes that there is no consensus regarding the appropriateness of Western-type interventions in non-Western settings. The globalisation of Western approaches sometimes ignores or pathologises the religious and spiritual dimensions of human experience.[26] Interventions that afford only a passive role delivered by outside (or inside) 'experts', who depend on Western knowledge, may aggravate feelings of helplessness and vulnerability, thereby devaluing traditional understandings of distress and undermining local, time-honoured practices that offer protection at a time of crisis.

Instead of 'person with physical or mental concerns and dilemmas', the term 'person with sensory, motor or cognitive impairment' (SMCI), is used in this chapter, and is more consistent with international usage. A person with SMCI may be treated differently in diverse cultures from full incorporation of the person and his or her abilities into general society, to keeping the person hidden from public view because of a potential stigma for the individual, the family or the community. Thus, the first steps for the professional working with people with SMCIs are to determine:

➤ what is seen as impairment
➤ what is seen as the cause, such as naturalistic from an injury, something the mother did during pregnancy, attributed to a parent's sinful behaviour, violation of a cultural taboo, or it is God's Will
➤ what it means to the person with the impairment, the family and their culture
➤ is the impairment due to a war injury, which is more acceptable than if the same injury is due to driving under the influence of alcohol, which is less acceptable.

In individualistic cultures with value placed on autonomy and productivity, one is expected to be a productive member of society and follow the same life cycle as everyone else in their dominant cultural group. An important concept to recognise is that 'disability' is a subculture unto its own. Among collectivistic cultures, people with a SMCI are *more likely* to be hidden from society to 'save face', and because the cultural norms and the values of family means that care is provided by the family at home.[1] However, with worldwide coverage of the United Nation's Year of the Disabled in 1981, the Special Olympics, disability rights movements and deaf pride, attitudes throughout the world are changing to closely resemble the views of individualistic cultures.[25] People with SMCI have in the past – and continue to a lesser degree – undergone discrimination, prejudice, shunning and embarrassment because of the associated stigma. In addition, the primary and secondary variants of culture may have a significant impact on how people with SMCI are seen within their dominant culture.

Even though some societies at a national level have encouraged acceptance of people with a SMCI, some families may still have negative feelings about them, feel ashamed, have pervasive negative attitudes and remain marginalised, which is more likely to occur among collectivist cultures such as India, China and Ethiopia.[25] For present-oriented cultures, where much is seen as 'God's Will', impairment may be seen as evidence of God's displeasure. In highly contexted collectivistic cultures, where focus is not on the individual but on the group, personhood depends more on social identity and the fulfilment of family obligations. Individual accomplishments are not as important as in individualistic cultures. In collectivist cultures, it is absolutely imperative to include the family, and sometimes the community, for effective counselling; otherwise, the treatment plan will not be followed. Among many Middle Eastern and other collectivistic cultures, people with a SMCI are hidden from the public because *'their pollution'* may mean that other children in the family will not be able to obtain a spouse if the condition is known.[1] For other impairments, such as one resulting from HIV, the condition may be kept hidden, not because of confidentiality rights, but for fear that it may spread to other family members and the community. Even though they are all primarily collectivistic cultures, Asian cultures and Native indigenous cultures are more likely to stigmatise a person with a SMCI than their African American or Latin American counterparts. The greater the cultural stigma for a person with a SMCI, the more likely the delay in seeking counselling, resulting in the condition being more severe at the time of treatment.

HEALTHCARE PRACTITIONERS

The domain of healthcare practitioners – 'Professionals' – (*see* Chapter 4) includes the status, use and perceptions of traditional, magicoreligious and bio-medical professionals, providers and the gender of the professional. A greater appreciation of the strengths of indigenous or traditional healing practices, and their underlying cultural assumptions, could help lead to a more appropriate integration of, and synergy between, different systems and models of care. The concept of treatment from the traditional healer's (TH) point of view often transcends the physical, emotional and psychological to include the social and spiritual parameters. It involves man's relationship with the past, the present and the future and with spirits, especially of ancestors. During treatment, some individuals continue consulting THs, while others consult them after discharge to perform certain rituals or ceremonies. A common belief among the majority of some cultures is that witchcraft, sorcery, the evil eye, the breaking of taboo, or the neglecting of rituals for ancestral spirits cause mental distress. THs occupy a key position in the community. They see and treat many people with mental concerns by reciting incantations and wearing of prescribed amulets.[1]

CONCLUSION AND RECOMMENDATIONS

KEY POINT 5.8

- Mental health is fundamental to health.
- The mind and body are inseparable.

A number of theories and models exist to assess the individuals' cultures, and they range from very simplistic to complex and incorporate research from nursing, medicine, sociology, anthropology and communication, to name a few. A few are culturally specific with non-prescriptive recommended interventions. The literature reports few intervention research studies, although there are more over the last decade. The following 'Do's and 'Do not's may be helpful to the reader.

Do

✔ Reframe health assessment using a cultural model/theory or approach.

✔ Make a concerted effort to learn more about your culture.

✔ Make a concerted effort to learn about the cultures of the individuals and other professionals with whom you work.

✔ Greet the individual formally until told to do otherwise.

✔ Provide counselling in the individual's preferred language, whenever possible.

✔ Provide a dialect-specific interpreter, whenever possible.

✔ Provide a same gender interpreter and/or professional if the individual prefers. This is especially important for many collectivist cultures.

✔ Check voice volume. A loud voice volume may be interpreted as anger by some, especially among collectivist cultures.

✔ Engage in small talk and get to know the individual before getting down to business. This may be especially important with high-context collectivist cultures.

✔ Remember that many people from collectivist cultures may not maintain eye contact with older people or people in hierarchal positions, such as the professional.

✔ Determine the degree of stigma around mental health concerns and dilemmas in the individual's culture and dispel myths that surround mental illness.

✔ Incorporate material culture in translations and the physical environment whenever possible. If the organisation has a large Bangladeshi population, incorporate their art and other material culture to make the individual feel welcome.

✔ Use caution on asking questions that require a 'yes' or 'no' answer. In collectivistic high-context cultures, giving a 'no' answer may be considered rude.

✔ With permission from the individual work with, and incorporate, traditional healers and religious leaders.

✔ Determine importance of nuclear, extended and older family members.

With permission, incorporate them into care and counselling. In many collectivist high-context cultures, no action will be taken until the family in included.

✔ Include support networks, such as churches, school groups and social and community-based activities of like cultures. This is especially important for collectivist high-context cultures.

Do not

✗ Let your cultural values and beliefs have an undue effect on the care you provide.

✗ Assume cultural groups are homogeneous and stereotype. Each individual varies according to the primary and secondary variant culture.

✗ Take offence if the individual sits closer or further away than to which you are accustomed.

✗ Openly disagree with the individual. Use smooth interpersonal communication to allow the individual to 'save face'.

✗ Be judgemental on family decision-making patterns. When someone is ill it is not the time to teach egalitarianism and assertiveness.

✗ For some individuals, especially refugees, asking many questions, taking notes, and completing forms in front of the individual increases apprehension. Take notes during assessment and complete forms out of view.

POST-READING EXERCISE 5.1 (ANSWERS ON P. 68)

Mr Li, a 72-year-old from Beijing, moved to England five years ago to live with his daughter, Bing Bing. He speaks and reads some English and most of the time seems to understand what physicians and nurses tell him. Today, he has walked the eight blocks to the clinic for his monthly check-up for a bipolar disorder for which he was prescribed new medications. The professional is giving him instructions on his new medication.

Professional: You can read the instructions on this bottle, can't you?
Mr Li nods his head and quietly says yes.
Professional: You know how to take these medicines and at what time, don't you?
Mr Li nods his head and quietly says yes.
Professional: If you have any problems understanding the written instructions, your daughter can help you, can't she?
Mr Li nods his head and quietly says yes.
Professional: I'll show you how to take the medicine to make sure you know how. You do not mind, do you?
Mr Li: You give me the medicine now, my daughter give me the medicine tomorrow.
Professional: I'll show you now. Open the bottle by pressing down hard and turn it to the right while holding down while you turn the lid. Take two blue pills from this bottle every morning when you get up. You can remember to do that, can't you, Mr Li?
Mr Li: Yes.

With a confused look on his face, Mr Li leaves the clinic reading the instructions on the bottle.

What should the professional have done to assure that Mr Li knows how to take his medicine?

REFERENCES

1 Purnell L, Paulanka B. *Transcultural Health Care: a culturally competent approach.* 3rd ed. Philadelphia: FA Davis; 2008.

2 Prince M, Patel V, Saxena S, *et al.* No health without mental health. *The Lancet.* 2007; **370**: 859–77.

3 *Mental Health: race, ethnicity and culture. A supplement to mental health: a report of the Surgeon General.* US Public Health Service; 1999. Available at: www.surgeongeneral.gov/library/mentalhealth/cre (accessed 29 July 2010).

4 Wood P, Landry C, Bloomfield J. *Cultural Diversity in Great Britain.* York: Joseph Roundtree Foundation; 2006.

5 Purnell L, Foster J. Cultural aspects of alcohol use: Part I. *The Drug and Alcohol Professional.* 2003; **3**: 17–23.

6 Purnell L, Foster J. Cultural aspects of alcohol use: Part II. *The Drug and Alcohol Professional.* 2003; **3**: 3–8.

7 Canadian Taskforce on Mental Health Issues Affecting Immigrants and Refugees. *After the Door has been Opened: mental health issues affecting immigrants and refugees in Canada.* Ottawa: Ministry Supply and Services Canada; 1988.

8 European Commission Culture. *Sharing diversity: national approaches to intercultural dialogue in europe.* Available at: http://ec.europa.eu/culture/key-documents/doc1351_en.htm (accessed 29 December 2010).

9 US Department of Health and Human Services, Office of Minority Health. *National Standards of Cultural and Linguistic Services in Health Care*; 2001. Available at: www.omhrc.gov/templates/browse.aspx?lvl=2&lvlID=15 (accessed 29 July 2010).

10 Quality Interactions. State licensing requirements for cultural competency. Available at: www.qualityinteractions.org/cultural_competence/cc_statelicreqs.html (accessed 29 July 2010).

11 US Department of Health and Human Services Office of Minority Health. Think cultural health: bridging the health care gap through cultural competency continuing education programs. Available at: www.thinkculturalhealth.hhs.gov (accessed 29 July 2010).

12 Pacific Institute for Research and Evaluation. Available at: www.pire.org (accessed 29 July 2010).

13 Fisher TL, Burnet DL, Huang ES, *et al.* Cultural leverage: interventions using culture to narrow racial disparities in health care. *Medical Care Research and Review.* 2007; **64**(Suppl. 5): S243–82.

14 Kreuter MW, Strecher, VJ. Do tailored behavior change messages enhance the effectiveness of health risk appraisal? Results from a randomised clinical trial. Health Education Research. 1996; **11**: 97–105. Available at: http://her.oxfordjournals.org/content/11/1/97.full.pdf.html (accessed 29 July 2010).

15 Kreuter MW, Lukwago SN, Bucholtz DC, *et al.* Achieving cultural appropriateness in health promotion programs: targeted and tailored approaches. *Health Education and Behavior.* 2003; **30**: 133–46.

16 Hall ET. *Beyond Culture.* New York: Anchor Books; 1989.

17 Resnicow K, Baranowski T, Ahluwalia JS, Braithwaite TL. Cultural sensitivity in public health: defined and demystified. *Ethnicity and Disease.* 1999; **9**: 10–21.

18 Bui YN, Turnbull A. East meets west: analysis of person-centered planning in the context of Asian American values. *Education and Training in Developmental Disabilities.* 2003; **38**: 18–31.

19 Kenrick DT, Neuberg SL, Watson JC. *Social Psychology: goals in interaction.* 4th ed. Boston: Allyn and Bacon; 2007.

20 Fu H, Hawkins D, Hui EKP. Personality correlates of the disposition towards interpersonal forgiveness. *International Journal of Psychology.* 2004; **39**: 305–16.

21 Sigelis TM. The measurement of independent and interdependent self-construals. *Personality and Social Psychology Bulletin.* 1994; **20**: 580–91.

22 Condon J, Yousef F. *Introduction to Intercultural Communication.* Upper Saddle River, NJ: Prentice Hall; 1985.

23 Gudykunst WB, Ting-Toomey S, Nishida T. *Communication in Personal Relationships across Cultures.* Thousand Oaks, CA: Sage; 1996.

24 Abbott P, Chase DM. Culture and substance abuse impact of culture affects approach to treatment. *Psychiatric Times.* 2008; **25**. Available at: www.psychiatrictimes.com/substance-abuse/article/10168/1147546 (accessed 29 July 2010).

25 Black-Lattanzi J, Purnell L. *Developing Cultural Competence in Physical Therapy Practice.* Philadelphia: FA Davis; 2006.

26 World Health Organization. *Mental Health Atlas 2005.* Geneva: WHO; 2005. Available at: www.who.int/mental_health/evidence/mhatlas05/en/index.html (accessed 29 July 2010).

TO LEARN MORE

- California Endowment. The California Endowment's work is a multicultural approach to health, which is defined not only by race and ethnicity but financial status, cultural beliefs, gender, age, sexual orientation, geographic location, immigration status and physical or mental abilities. This approach seeks to mobilise the talents, cultures and assets of California's diverse populations to improve the quality of the health systems and to promote health at the level of communities. Available at: www.calendow.org

- CultureMed at the Peter J Cayan Library at SUNYIT is a website and a resource centre of print materials promoting culturally competent healthcare for refugees and immigrants. This project provides support to the healthcare community and newcomers by providing practical information regarding culture and healthcare from both viewpoints. Available at: http://culturedmed.sunyit.edu

- *Diversity in Health and Social Care.* This journal is concerned with all aspects of diversity in health and social care. Diversity is seen as a very broad concept, embracing, e.g. culture, beliefs, disability, race, gender and ethnicity as well as underserved and marginalised populations.

- Douglas M, Uhl Pierce J, Rosenkoetter M, *et al.* Standards of practice for culturally competent care: a request for comments. *Journal of Transcultural Nursing.* 2009; **20**: 257–69.

- Gardner F. Culture and change management. *The International Journal of Knowledge.* 2008; **6**: 73–80.

- *Journal of Transcultural Nursing.* Offers nurses, educators, researchers and practitioners theoretical approaches and current research findings that have direct implications for the delivery of culturally congruent healthcare and for the preparation of healthcare professionals who will provide that care: http://tcn.sagepub.com/

- Markus HR, Kitayama S. Culture and self: implications for cognition, emotion, and motivation. *Psychological Review.* 1991; **98**: 224–53.

- George Peter Murdoch. *New World Encyclopedia*. 2008. Available at: www.newworldencyclo pedia.org/entry/George_Peter_Murdock
- National Pharmaceutical Council Clearinghouse for pharmacological research on specific populations. The aim is to help inform the national debate on how to make reliable evidence the cornerstone of healthcare decisions in order to ensure the best patient outcomes and best value. Available at: www.npcnow.org/
- National Quality Forum. This standards-approving organisation has endorsed 45 cultural competency standards for providing culturally appropriate services, largely in the area of communication, community engagement, and training. 2009. Available at www.qualityforum.org
- Nursing Council of New Zealand. *Guidelines for Cultural Safety, the Treaty of Waitangi and Maori Health in Nursing Education and Practice*. Wellington: Nursing Council of New Zealand; 2009. Available at: www.nursingcouncil.org.nz/download/97/cultural-safety09.pdf
- Papadopoulos I. *Transcultural Health and Social Care*. Edinburgh: Churchill Livingstone; 2006.
- Project Salaam: the Islamic Center of San Diego. San Diego State University, Center for Behavioral and Community Health Studies; 2006. Available at: www.sdsubach.org/
- Purnell L, Davidhizar R, Giger J, Fishman D, Strickland O, Allison D. A guide to developing a culturally competent organization. *Journal of Transcultural Nursing*. Forthcoming (2011; **22**).
- Robert Wood Johnson Foundation. Community partnerships for older adults. Available at: www.partnershipsforolderadults.org
- Sam DL, Berry JW. *The Cambridge Handbook of Acculturation Psychology*. Cambridge: Cambridge University Press; 2006.
- Teekman B. Exploring reflective thinking in nursing practice. *Journal of Advanced Nursing*. 2000; **31**: 1125–35.

ANSWERS TO PRE-READING EXERCISE 5.1

1   What concerns do you see without a common culture among Señora Casilla and her health professional? Each professional comes to the individual encounter with his or her own culture. The first step in this scenario is for the team to determine how depression and substance misuse is viewed in the Panamanian culture, specifically by Señora Casilla, and create a treatment plan that is acceptable and congruent with her views.

2   The primary languages of Señora Casilla, and each professional, are the languages of their home countries, what concerns do you have? If each professional speaks with an accent different from that to which Señora Casilla is accustomed, she may have extreme difficulty in understanding her treatment plan. In addition, mental illnesses are culture-bound without direct translation and meaning in different cultures, especially with the affective domain.

3   How is mental illness viewed in the cultures of Señora Casilla, and each of the professionals? In the Panamanian culture, mental illnesses are tacitly accepted without significant stigma. Substance use concerns and dilemma are not accepted, especially among women, and is not openly talked about. In traditional Iranian culture, mental health issues are strongly denied, fearing genetic transmission of the illness, and may affect future generations for obtaining marriage partners. For the traditional German culture, a minor stigma occurs but the person is expected to seek treatment and make every attempt to be a fully functioning member of society.

ANSWERS TO POST-READING EXERCISE 5.1

Mr Li does not adequately understand the English instructions. The professional should have provided an interpreter to assure understanding. If an interpreter is not available, the daughter should be contacted and taught how Mr Li should take his medications. Written instructions should be provided in the person's preferred language. The professional should ask for Mr Li to demonstrate taking his medication. Asking questions that can be answered with a 'yes' or 'no' response does not assure understanding. In this scenario, the only response Mr Li can give is 'yes'. In addition, having the individual take medication by the colour of the pill can be dangerous because:

- in some languages the colour for blue and green are the same
- with generic medications the colour of a pill may change.

Instructions should be given in a step-by-step approach without using contractions. A suggestion follows.

1 Take the bottle in your left hand.
2 Press down on the lid.
3 Turn the lid while pressing down.
4 Take two pills from the bottle.
5 Put the pills in your mouth.
6 Drink a glass of water with the pills.
7 Take the medicine each morning.

A Transtheoretical Model perspective on change: process-focused intervention in mental health–substance use

Carlo C DiClemente, Kristina Schumann,
Preston A Greene and Michael D Earley

INTRODUCTION

The Transtheoretical Model of intentional behaviour change (TTM) offers a framework for understanding important dimensions of intentional behaviour change rather than a well-defined or manually driven therapy.[1–3] Its utility lies in the fact that the dimensions described in the model (i.e. the stages, processes, context and markers of change) offer concepts and a structure for understanding critical elements of the process of behaviour change that seem relevant for both self-guided/natural change[1,4] and treatment-supported behaviour change.[5,6] The TTM involves a learning perspective of intention and self-regulation and assumes that the individual has to choose which change to make and learn how to manage the change and to sustain change by incorporating the change into one's life. The model is integrative since it incorporates elements and constructs from various theories of therapy, learning and behaviour change, hence the name 'Transtheoretical'. However, the model is not a comprehensive theory and simply tries to identify and describe important elements of the process of intentional behaviour change.

Change of any behaviour, even something simple, is difficult for most people to engineer and accomplish. However, for individuals experiencing mental health–substance use problems, change becomes more complicated and challenging as these problems interact, undermining overall self-regulation and important components of the change process. The presence of each type of problem, the combination of the two disorders, and the interactions among these problems, present the professional with a complicated diagnostic and clinical scenario which poses multiple barriers to change. Barriers such as:

➤ problematic motivation
➤ impaired decision-making

➤ underdeveloped behaviour change skills
➤ lack of planning
➤ the presence of multiple problems

all exist within the context of the lives of individuals experiencing mental health–substance use problems to distress, distract, disable and discourage change. This chapter describes how to use the principles and concepts of the TTM to address multiple diagnoses and problems and adaptations or limitations when using it with these individuals.

Changing substance use and other health behaviours involves voluntary control and choice which are fundamentally the responsibility of the individual. However, it is also true that most change is assisted. Consequences, social and family influences, external pressures, support, and a variety of helping hands promote and support self-change even without the presence of formal treatment or interventions. The role of treatment or interventions for substance use, mental health and mental health–substance use problems is to help the individual use more effective, empirically supported strategies to stimulate, facilitate, assist and support the individual change process. The constructs of the TTM offer a framework to consider how to help.

CRITICAL DIMENSIONS OF CHANGE

Change is complicated and multidimensional. It takes a number of elements to create successful sustained change whether one talks about being 'ready, willing, and able' or having 'motivation, commitment, skills, and support'. The TTM offers a way to identify, organise and sequence these various dimensions of the change process.

Stages and tasks of change

The change process involves critical tasks that need to be accomplished in order to initiate and consolidate behaviour change into a stable pattern. Stages represent a set of tasks that build the foundation for successful change (*see* Table 6.1). The end product is a new sustained pattern of behaviour supported by the adequate accomplishment of each preceding task. Stages bring together the cognitive and motivational, as well as behavioural learning elements of change, to create a larger, more complex and more credible picture of the process of change.[7] Stages also shift the conversation about change from an exclusive discussion of action outcomes to one that increases the focus on motivation, decision-making, commitment and planning.[8,9] Interventions should help individuals to understand the process, to see where they may be having trouble and getting stuck, and to realise the function of relapse and recycling through the stages of change.[6,7,10] In order to successfully traverse stages and accomplish tasks, the individual must engage in a number of cognitive and behavioural activities that promote successful behaviour change. These activities constitute the 'processes of change'.

TABLE 6.1 Stages, tasks, and processes of change

Stages	Tasks	Key processes
Precontemplation	Raising interest, concern, and awareness of the problem	Consciousness-raising, self- and environmental re-evaluation, and emotional arousal
Contemplation	Weighing pros and cons of the target behaviour and of the behaviour change	
Preparation	Planning and committing to a reasonable, accessible, and effective plan	Self-liberation, helping relationships
Action	Implementing the plan and addressing barriers	Stimulus control, counter-conditioning, and reinforcement management.
Maintenance	Making the behaviour change part of daily life, addressing relapse.	

Processes of change and their interaction with the stages

The original insight underlying the TTM was that individuals at different points in the process of change used different processes of change.[3] Processes represent the active ingredients or change engines that enable individuals to accomplish the tasks of the stages, move through the process and achieve successful, sustained behaviour change. The individual experiences, thoughts and actions foster and energise movement through stages and accomplishment of tasks. In order for a substance-dependent individual to become concerned enough about the status quo (precontemplation task) to consider a new way of behaving, and then to engage in a risk–reward analysis (contemplation task), he/she has to increase awareness (consciousness-raising), re-evaluate both the status quo and the new behaviour (self- and environmental re-evaluation), and hopefully get upset about the costs of the current behaviour (emotional arousal). These processes are critical for accomplishing both the precontemplation and contemplation tasks. Additionally, choosing a course of action to change the problem behaviour and committing to that choice (self-liberation) are essential for accomplishing the tasks of the preparation stage. Similarly, learning how to create or deconstruct cues to action (stimulus control), modify conditioned responses to cues (counter-conditioning), and create rewards for new behaviour (reinforcement management) are critical to the action and maintenance stages. As the individual moves through each of the stages, but particularly in the preparation stage, it is helpful if he/she has trusting and open discussions about the problem behaviour with a supportive individual (helping relationships).[1,7,11] Without successful engagement in these processes of change, the individual is unlikely to successfully accomplish the tasks of the stages, modify the target problem behaviour and sustain the new pattern of behaviour. However, the individual does not use processes in a vacuum, uninfluenced by contextual factors.

The context of change: complicating problems and similar solutions

Although many professionals claim to use holistic approaches to healthcare, most treat only diagnosable conditions and treat health and substance use behaviour problems in isolation. However, individuals concerned about or trying to change a single behaviour most often have multiple other concerns. The context of change acknowledges competing problems, complicating issues and environmental and systemic challenges that can interfere with engagement in processes of change, hinder accomplishment of stage tasks and complicate movement through the process of change.[1,2] There also may be resources and protective factors in these contextual areas that can facilitate use of processes and more successful completion of stage tasks. The recent focus on mental health–substance use, and the growing realisation of the importance of dealing with the multiple associated life problems (e.g. employment, family, social), highlights the complexity of the challenges facing many individuals. This enhanced focus also reinforces the need to specify and address the contextual problems surrounding the targeted behaviour change in order to achieve successful change.[12,13] It is important to consider how to address these problems using both empowerment of self-change and engagement in treatment-assisted change. The Context, Stages, and Processes of Change from the TTM provide a framework for understanding how these different types of change interact and overlap.

TREATMENT-ASSISTED CHANGE FROM A TTM PERSPECTIVE

Stages of change create a dynamic view of the change process. Individuals can move forwards, backwards and recycle through the stages. Some people become stuck in certain stages like precontemplation and contemplation for long periods of time. Others consider change, then reject it and return to precontemplation. Still others make a decision and a plan but fail to implement it. The path to successful behaviour change seems to involve accomplishing stage tasks well enough to be effective in creating a new pattern of behaviour, and each person has a personal change history.

Successful behaviour usually includes:
➤ significant concern
➤ solid decision-making
➤ sufficient planning
➤ significant commitment
➤ change-plan implementation intention
➤ behavioural enactment
➤ generalisation of the behaviour.

Relapse (*see* Book 6, Chapters 15 and 16) is an event that signals the individual and the intervener that one or more stage tasks have not been completed adequately. Rather than indicating failure and implying that an individual cannot change, relapse is a marker of inadequate learning and problematic completion of stage tasks. Relapse can be part of the process of change and represents the learning by successive approximations, allowing the individual to get closer to a change goal by learning how to get all the parts of the process right.[1,5]

This dynamic framework makes it imperative that behaviour change specialists be aware of both the critical tasks and stages necessary for change, where individuals are in this process, and what tasks they have accomplished in this process thus far. Professionals can then focus their efforts on helping people with the parts of the process of change where they are having difficulty trying to use one or more of these types of assistance.

Specific types of process assistance include:

➤ influence and advice
➤ inspiration and motivation
➤ ambivalence reduction
➤ decision-making support
➤ commitment enhancement
➤ planning and prioritising
➤ skills building
➤ implementation support
➤ maintenance support.

The goal of treatment is to engage and influence appropriate processes that can help people accomplish tasks. Interventions should be constructed, materials created and techniques taught to assist the individual in accomplishing critical stage tasks needed for success, or to learn from recycling how to be more successful in moving through the stages. Processes of change refocus us on the individual's coping activities and again offer a dynamic view of change. However, individuals differ significantly based on:

➤ education
➤ ethnicity (*see* Chapters 4 and 5)
➤ social connections and networks
➤ economic standing
➤ age
➤ cultural values.

Knowing how to activate appropriate processes for individuals with diverse cultural backgrounds, ethnic traditions and values is essential for creating effective interventions (*see* Chapters 4 and 5).[1]

A benefit of looking at behaviour change within the TTM framework is that the same process model can be used to understand and promote change in many different areas of the individual's life. The problems may be multiple and varied, but the process seems common and isomorphic.[3,6,14] Table 6.2 offers a view of the types of problems that are often seen in people experiencing mental health–substance use problems and the target behaviours that could serve as the focus of change. If there is a target behaviour that needs to be started, modified, or stopped, these contextual problems would also require individuals to accomplish the tasks of the stages and engage the processes of change. For any of the target behaviours in the person's profile, the counsellor can look at the dimensions of the TTM perspective to see how to assist the individual to make a change in that area. These contextual problems are often interconnected, and the challenge is not to lose sight of which one may be a key target behaviour, and not to get distracted by one problem while not addressing another that can undermine a desired change.

TABLE 6.2 Target problems in the context of change

Contextual area	Target behaviours
Symptom/Situation	
• Psychiatric	• Depression medication
• Financial	• Enrolling in SSI
• Homelessness	• Temporary or permanent housing
• High-risk health behaviours	• Diet, exercise, safe sex
Beliefs	
• Medication views	• Medication compliance
• Cultural beliefs	• Acceptable goals
Interpersonal	
• Marital	• Effective communication
• Aggression	• Anger management
• Intimacy	• Sexual dysfunction
Systemic	
• Employment	• Job training
• Family/children	• Parent effectiveness
• Family of origin	• Changing family dynamics
• Legal	• Managing consequences
Interpersonal	
• Self-esteem	• Sense of self
• Sexual identity	• Coping with identity

WHAT WE KNOW AND WHAT WE SHOULD DO
Individual factors and the TTM

There is solid evidence that personal process variables like motivation, intentions, expectancies and commitment are important in treatment outcomes and successful change for individuals with and without multiple diagnoses.[12,15,16] However, the individual experiencing mental health–substance use problems faces special challenges. The following sections highlight key motivational dimensions and special considerations needed when addressing this population.

Motivation to change is a significant predictor of treatment engagement and outcome in substance use problems and psychotherapy outcome studies.[17-19] Individuals closer to the 'action' stages of change (i.e. action and maintenance) seem to do better in treatment than individuals who are in a 'pre-action' stage of change (i.e. precontemplation, contemplation and preparation). Multiple problems, neurocognitive complications and stress make it challenging to evaluate and use motivation and stage-based approaches with individuals experiencing mental health–substance use problems. Although the experience of moderate levels of distress has often been seen as a motivator to get individuals concerned and invested in making changes in their behaviours,[20] higher levels of distress can interfere with the ability of an individual to engage in and sustain a behaviour change. For example, individuals experiencing mental health–substance use problems may have more difficulty sustaining change than those without a mental health diagnosis, particularly during periods of high psychiatric distress.[21] Given that motivation and readiness to change are so important in predicting treatment outcome, how do we evaluate and intervene on motivation to change with individuals experiencing mental health–substance use problems?

Cognitive deficits of individuals with serious mental illness impact their ability to express motivation to change and participate in the tasks of the stages. Professionals must take cognitive deficits into account as they assess motivation and develop appropriate intervention strategies and treatment plans with the individual experiencing mental health–substance use problems. For example, individuals with schizophrenia often have deficits in attention, memory and higher order processes such as abstract reasoning (*see* Book 3, Chapter 8).[22] Although there are studies that have used the University of Rhode Island Change Assessment (URICA) to evaluate stage status and readiness to change among individuals experiencing mental health–substance use problems,[12,23] it may be difficult to use because it requires abstract reasoning to answer the complex questions. Measures that are simpler to understand or administer like readiness rulers or the non-verbal, cartoon readiness-to-change measure developed by Wells and colleagues[24] can be useful for people with serious mental illness.[22] However, a sensitive motivational interview that allows people to express their attitudes, intentions, goals and decisional consideration may be the best way to evaluate where someone is in terms of the tasks of the stages of change and a person's readiness to make a change. Table 6.3 summarises a variety of methods for assessing motivation/readiness to change.[25]

Self-efficacy, described as an individual's confidence to remain abstinent or modify substance use in the face of temptation, seems to be extremely important in predicting treatment success.[17] In Project MATCH, individuals with *higher levels of confidence and lower levels of temptation* at the end of treatment were more likely to remain abstinent at the three-year follow-up.[19] Efficacy is situation specific, as are temptation or craving to use. When experiencing significant psychiatric distress, individuals experiencing mental health–substance use problems are more likely to feel tempted to use a problematic substance, especially in response to negative affect cues like frustration, anxiety, depression and anger. Clinical assessment and interventions, therefore, should focus on the individual's experiences of temptation and on mood management as well as providing the person with a number of tools to deal with negative mood states other than 'self-medicating' with alcohol or drugs, and should focus on determining which behavioural processes and strategies to engage and what skills to focus on in treatment.

As described earlier, use of *processes of change* has been associated with successful outcomes.[15,29] Although some processes may be more or less difficult for individuals with mental health problems to use, most people are capable of using various processes of change even when they have both psychiatric and substance use diagnoses.[21,30] Although the conversation may differ based on factors such as language comprehension, capacity for complex thinking, social norms and cultural considerations, professionals should teach the individual about the processes of change and develop skills needed to engage each of the processes of change.

TABLE 6.3 Ways to assess motivation

Measure	Description
University of Rhode Island Change Assessment (URICA)	Assigns individuals to a particular stage based on endorsed attitudes and behaviours (e.g. 'I've been thinking that I might want to change something about myself' is reflective of the Contemplation stage).
	Different versions exist for different target behaviours (i.e. smoking, alcohol, drug use).[25,26]
Cartoon Stage of Change Measure (C-SOC)	Assigns individuals to a particular stage based on their endorsement of specific cartoon pictures reflective of four of the stages of change (i.e. Precontemplation, Contemplation, Action, Maintenance). This measure is particularly useful for individuals with low literacy or cognitive deficits.[22]
Readiness Ruler	Assesses how far along the individual is in the change process ranging from precontemplation to maintenance. The ruler can also be used to measure how important change is to the individual.[27]
Readiness to Change Questionnaire (RCQ)	Assigns individuals to a particular stage based on their views of which stage best describes them (e.g. 'I am actually changing my drinking habits right now' is reflective of the Action stage).
	This measure is designed specifically for assessing readiness to change drinking behaviour.[28]
Clinical Interview	Open-ended, non-standardised probing questions to elicit information about the individual's motivation to change. This interview can be used throughout treatment to keep a pulse on the individual's dynamic change process.

Decisional balance deliberations, considering the pros and cons of a current or future behaviour, influence the shifts in stage status and are related to process use.[31] Decisional considerations are associated with successful treatment, particularly in the early stages of change.[14,32] For individuals experiencing mental health–substance use problems it is especially important to realise that decisional considerations are uniquely personal.

Case study 6.1: decision-making

One example from a clinician working with homeless individuals experiencing mental health–substance use problems illustrates the uniqueness and idiosyncratic nature of these considerations. While discussing the need for more permanent housing with one homeless individual living under a large bridge in California, the outreach worker heard the following argument against more permanent housing. 'I cannot understand you people wanting me to go to an apartment that costs 500 US dollars a month when I already live under a bridge that costs more than five million US dollars.'

Professionals must be sensitive to these 'unique' reasons and the interaction of the two problems as they attempt to influence the decisional balance of each individual. Interventions should focus on developing personal pros and cons related to substance use, medication compliance, and other target behaviours (employment, housing, anxiety management strategies) in order to influence decision-making.

TREATMENT AND THE TTM: PROBLEM- AND PROCESS-FOCUSED INTERVENTIONS

Controversies exist about whether treatments tailored to each individual stage are always better than control comparisons[33,34] and whether stage-specific treatments have shown differential effects for individuals who begin treatment in different stages.[35] However, there is a significant body of knowledge that supports a motivational, multidimensional, process-oriented and tailored approach to working with individuals experiencing mental health–substance use problems. However, that label encompasses a very heterogeneous population. Individuals experiencing mental health–substance use problems vary significantly in the type and severity of both mental health and substance use problems.[32] Process-focused interventions evaluate and consider individual problems, symptom severity, levels of motivation and readiness when designing a treatment plan for any individual experiencing mental health–substance use problems.

Important dimensions of process-focused interventions
Enhancing motivation
Motivational enhancement is critical for treatment engagement and retention, as well as predicting behavioural outcomes.[36] Many current clinical studies of interventions with individuals experiencing mental health–substance use problems incorporate a motivational approach.[36] A recent review[12] highlighted the need to address motivational dimensions related to the stages of change in treating individuals not only during the initial phase of treatment but also when transitioning between various types of programmes to prevent individuals from falling through the cracks of the system of care.[37] Programmes that include interventions tailored specially to motivational enhancement, rapport building[38] and stage of change[39] have produced better outcomes in substance use problems and also reductions in hospitalisations and psychopathology.[40] Some include an early engagement component in their inpatient or intensive outpatient programmes. Assertive outreach and case management as well as intensive residential treatment (e.g. therapeutic communities) also have begun to focus on and address motivational considerations to become promoters of the process of change.

Mutual support and residential options with gradual integration into the larger community often are used to support individuals with compromised and weakened self-efficacy and self-regulation. Integrated treatment programmes and intensive outreach can offer structure for individuals experiencing mental health–substance use problems. Such structure supports compromised self-regulation while promoting engagement in the processes and tasks needed to achieve sustained behaviour change.[12] These supports need to be kept in place until the necessary skills and capacities can be developed that enable compromised individuals to become more self-sufficient in creating change.

Tailoring treatments

Studies of health behaviour change indicate that interventions tailored to key individual characteristics, circumstances and problems, and that include personalised feedback, are generally best received, most personally relevant and most successful.[41,42] Tailored information encourages decisional conversations that are more personally relevant and compelling compared to generic information about health hazards.

Tailoring treatment, providing feedback and using Motivational Interviewing strategies (*see* Chapter 7) to evoke and elicit important decisional considerations, ambivalence, change talk and commitment language are as relevant for individuals experiencing mental health–substance use problems as for the substance-dependent individuals who were the first beneficiaries of such approaches. There is growing evidence that the dimensions of the stages, processes and markers of change for various types of substance dependence operate in a manner similar for those with mental health problems as it does in those without the complications of mental health–substance use problems.[23,26,43]

Interventions that address the entire context of change

Ideal integrated treatment for mental health–substance use problems does not simply address substance use and mental illness but also the multiple co-occurring contextual problems that can exacerbate and complicate or promote recovery. The work of McClellan and colleagues[44] recent reviews[45] and commentaries[46] indicate that multiple problems are the norm for these individuals, and that more serious contextual problems are associated with more severe mental illness and substance use problems. Homeless and marginally housed individuals demonstrate greater severity of mental health and substance use, and deficits in social support, compared to those with housing.[47] Choi and Ryan[48] note that substance abuse of women with children '*reflects a coalescence of complex interlocking layers of psychological, legal, medical, social, and cultural issues*', reinforcing the need to pay attention to the context of change.

Access to services for drug-free housing, medical care, legal services, parenting support and employment services improves outcomes for individuals with multiple problems. However, motivation for change for each of these dimensions as well for the various types of drugs an individual[36] uses varies greatly.[1,49] Comprehensive programmes that include:

➤ motivational components (*see* Chapter 7)
➤ harm reduction approaches (*see* Chapter 13 and Book 3, Chapter 15)
➤ social learning
➤ skills building
➤ contingency contracts
➤ realistic goal-setting

seem to produce better outcomes for the individuals experiencing mental health–substance use problems.[50] Addressing not only the existence of multiple associated problems in the life context but also the individual's motivation and need for assistance in these areas appears critical for substantive and sustained recovery.

PROCESS-FOCUSED INTERVENTIONS FOR INDIVIDUALS AND GROUPS

How can professionals apply constructs of the Transtheoretical Model with the individual experiencing mental health–substance use problems? Although there is no single manualised approach that captures all of the various dimensions of the model, there are a number of examples of clinical practices that thoughtfully integrate the multiple facets of the TTM.

Individual treatment approaches

Drake,[36] Carey[51] and Bouis[52] and their colleagues offer recommendations for assisting individuals experiencing co-occurring substance use and other mental health concerns consistent with a process of change-focused intervention approach. More programmatic approaches describe *phases* of treatment that demarcate treatment providers' strategies based on important milestones of treatment related to the stages and processes of change. Stages mark the various steps and tasks of the personal process of change; phases indicate key points in the intervention when providers need to shift focus and strategies based on the individual's progress.

Initial phase

Important therapist tasks of the initial phase are:
➤ building a strong, trusting therapeutic relationship
➤ assessing readiness to change in a variety of problem areas
➤ facilitating motivational enhancement and providing feedback and education
➤ facilitating concern, interest and decision-making
➤ use of motivational enhancement approaches, feedback and some education.

This may be the most lengthy and challenging phase since few people enter in a similar stage of readiness for mental illness and substance use problems and many enter treatment to manage contextual problems such as accessing social services, gaining financial support and finding housing. In addition, many individuals may need stabilisation, such as housing, symptom management, etc.[36,51] before they can be engaged. Individuals presenting for one issue or concern are often unconcerned or uninterested in change for problems that the clinician considers more important. The challenge is to adequately assess each domain or problem area, and to respond to each area according to the stage of readiness. Individuals need not be motivated to change all problem areas at once in order to become engaged in treatment or for substantial progress to be made in treatment. In fact, having some success in changing one problem area may be a powerful motivator to consider attempting change in other areas.

Intermediate phase

Important therapist tasks of the intermediate phase are:
➤ solidifying the individual's commitment to changing a target behaviour

➤ identifying realistic goals
➤ aiding in formulation of a change plan
➤ supporting implementation and revision of the change plan.

Individuals often signal when to proceed to this phase when they are stabilised and committed to treatment.[52] Whereas the initial phase is characterised by cognitive processes composed of experiences and realisations leading to recognition of the problem and creating interest, concern and motivation to change, the intermediate phase challenges individuals to engage in behavioural processes and learn and practise behavioural coping skills.

Many empirically supported treatments and components of manualised treatments can be implemented during this phase. However, as individuals implement change, it is important to reassess readiness and stage tasks recognising that people may move backwards in the stages of change or recycle through the stages for one or more problems. Treatment strategies and phases need to track or follow movement in the process of change and not jump ahead or rigidly follow a preordained set of techniques or plans disregarding readiness and success. Managing people experiencing mental health–substance use problems requires greater flexibility than that needed for individuals with single diagnoses or with more resources and protective factors.

Final phase
Important therapist tasks of the intermediate phase are:
➤ strengthening changes by consolidating them into the individual's lifestyle
➤ strengthening the individual's confidence in sustaining changes
➤ helping the individual shift social networks
➤ preparing for relapse (*see* Chapter 13; and Book 6, Chapters 15 and 16).

Group therapy, mutual help groups (*see* Chapter 14), and 'double trouble' 12-step fellowships addressing mental health and substance use problems can be particularly helpful in providing support and role models of successfully maintained change. Final phase does not mean that support or treatment should be ended. Mental health–substance use treatment should be long term. As individuals progress in one area, additional problems may emerge that complicate and threaten a successful change and need to be addressed.

GROUP TREATMENT APPROACHES WITH A PROCESS OF CHANGE FOCUS
Although a process of change perspective is essentially individually focused and tailored, group treatment approaches can incorporate a process perspective in a variety of ways. Specific groups can be designed to address different parts of the process. Many programmes are developing motivational enhancement, pretreatment or engagement types of group experiences. One programme[53] uses a post-traumatic stress disorder (PTSD) motivational enhancement group to help identify and resolve barriers to successful PTSD treatment such as alcohol use, anger and social isolation. Brief motivational enhancement groups might be used to increase the

individual's readiness to change his/her substance use, increase successful engagement in outpatient psychiatric treatment, or to prevent treatment dropout. Squires and Moyers[54] describe adapting motivational enhancement therapy (MET) for individuals experiencing mental health–substance use problems to address substance use in the context of an integrated treatment setting.

Another group treatment based directly on the Transtheoretical Model more explicitly focuses on stages and designed modules that promote use of specific processes. The *Group Treatment for Substance Abuse* manual[11] offers two sets of modules to be used, one with individuals in 'pre-action' (Precontemplation/Contemplation/Preparation) stages and the other for 'action' (Action/Maintenance) individuals. Pre-action group modules attend to recognition of the problem, decision-making, commitment, and planning and experiential process of change. The action group topics concentrate on change plan implementation and revision as well as behavioural coping strategies. A similar approach could be taken in integrated mental health–substance use settings. Closed or open treatment groups could be conducted using modules sequentially from pre-action to action or with separate pre-action and action-focused groups run simultaneously, transferring individuals from one to another as they become more motivated to change. The latter may be better for the individual experiencing mental health–substance use problems since they may require more time in the pre-action before becoming prepared to make a change attempt.

SYSTEMS APPROACHES WITH A PROCESS FOCUS

Integrated dual diagnosis treatment (IDDT) has been identified as a best practice.[36] However, getting organisations and systems to make the changes needed to adopt IDDT can be just as challenging as assisting individuals experiencing mental health–substance use problems to make desired changes. A process perspective using some of the dimensions of the Transtheoretical Model can be useful in considering systemic and organisational changes, particularly when there is a constellation of behaviour changes that are the goal.

More recently, the TTM has been used to describe organisational changes[1,55] and dimensions of the model are being used to facilitate implementation of IDDT into treatment facilities. The Ohio Substance Abuse and Mental Illness Coordinating Center of Excellence (Ohio SAMI CCOE) has developed materials for organisations to help achieve the organisational change necessary to implement the IDDT model that incorporate stages and processes of change focused at an organisational level. The resources available at www.ohiosamiccoe.cwru.edu document how they are attempting to help community treatment agencies to implement IDDT using a stage-based approach.

THE CHALLENGE OF MULTIPLE PROBLEMS AND DIAGNOSES

The Transtheoretical Model often has been used to assist in describing and intervening on changes for a single problem behaviour (smoking, alcohol use, illegal drug use, medication adherence) or constellations of related behaviours (physical activity, eating a low fat diet, cancer screening). Since individuals can vary in motivation, commitment and implementation for specific behaviours, using this process perspective is best when the focus of change is either on a specific behaviour or on a group of behaviours related to a single goal. For example, abstinence from all substance use including drugs and alcohol is an overarching goal that can bring together a number of behaviours and can be an organising principle for an individual's behaviour change process. However, as providers are painfully aware, individuals often have varying levels of motivation depending on specific parts of such an overarching treatment goal. Individuals, who are ready to stop cocaine use, often are ambivalent about quitting drinking. This motivational dilemma is complicated even further when there are multiple interrelated but separate problems as happens with mental health–substance use problems.

The TTM process perspective assumes that there can be varying levels of motivation for different behaviours but also it can accommodate viewing multiple behaviours under a more overarching and integrating goal so that an individual can bring a specific set of behaviours under a more unified motivational perspective. For example, if an individual can envision his/her recovery as encompassing stopping cocaine use, taking the medication for bipolar disorder, and quitting all excessive alcohol use, there is a synergy in motivational considerations and in the commitment and planning needed to make a successful recovery. However, motivation for these different aspects of recovery is variable with some success in one or another of the target behaviours related to recovery with the long-term goal achieved after many attempts with variable success.

Since the motivation, energy, commitment and completion of multiple changes all reside in the single individual experiencing the multiple problems, the burden of change and the effort needed in the change process is much greater for those individuals experiencing mental health–substance use problems, and especially those for whom these separate but related conditions have resulted in consequences that have created multiple ancillary contextual problems. From a process perspective, it is not only very understandable why treatment and change is so difficult and complex, it is really remarkable that so many have been able to successfully address the dual conditions and recover. Multiple problems compromise the entire self-regulation and self-control operations of the individual.[12] Impaired self-regulation makes successful negotiation of the process of change more challenging since many of the tasks of the stages require attention, organisation, cognitive decisional processes and emotion regulation capacities. This seems to support the need for stability and support and the type of scaffolding that occurs in residential programmes for the most troubled and problematic individuals. The compromised self-regulatory system is one of the biggest challenges to treatment of the individual experiencing mental health–substance use problems and to the utilisation of a process perspective with these individuals.

IMPLICATIONS OF A PERSONAL PROCESS-ORIENTED PERSPECTIVE FOR MENTAL HEALTH–SUBSTANCE USE

Most individuals experiencing mental health *and* substance use problems have multiple target behaviours that require modification in order to manage the diagnosable conditions, the precursors to those conditions, and/or the serious consequences resulting from those conditions. The array of new behaviours that are required for recovery from these chronic conditions can be overwhelming to the professional. The Process of Change perspective offered by the Transtheoretical Model proposes a pathway through this bewildering array by focusing on how to promote accomplishment of the varied tasks and engagement in the processes needed for the self-management and self-regulation of change. Though problems may differ and the target behaviours vary greatly, the process appears similar. In order to modify the behaviours, individuals need to acknowledge some need to make this particular change, make a decision, form an intention and plan, garner commitment and initiate the behaviour and revise the plan to successfully establish a new pattern of behaviour and make it normative. This process seems as relevant for getting a person experiencing schizophrenia to undertake and maintain a needed medication regimen as it is for that same person to stop using cocaine, reduce or eliminate alcohol consumption, use anxiety or anger management strategies, change interactions with key family members, or to gain and maintain employment.

Accomplishing stage tasks is not always as sequential, explicit or complete as in the preceding descriptions. Tasks are often undertaken and abandoned at various points in the sequence. However, if the individual is ultimately expected to function autonomously, she/he must have the motivation, commitment, competence and follow-through needed to make the change happen. Treatment professionals and interventions should be designed to promote successful engagement in the process of change. Professionals must be careful not to co-opt or compromise the personal process of change and should use strategies that engage the individual in activities and processes that can promote task completion, taking responsibility, and autonomy. Individuals experiencing mental health–substance use problems must take charge of the change process and create a sustainable change plan. The professional's treatment plan should be developed to empower and enable the individual's change plan.

Integrated treatment for individuals experiencing mental health–substance use problems should not only integrate the needs into a more coherent and holistic perspective and offer a range of coordinated services but should also focus on engaging the individual in the process of change needed across recovery behaviours. Programmes cannot simply prescribe a course of action without the engagement and involvement of the individual and tailoring interventions to the individual's readiness and perspectives. This argues for programmes and professionals that are flexible, personalised and persistent, ready to adjust when change does not happen or interventions fail and to focus on barriers that undermined the change process.

Adding a process of change perspective to the holistic, comprehensive and integrated approaches currently recommended for the treatment of people experiencing mental health–substance use problems adds a motivational, learning-oriented, task-focused, individualised perspective that can enrich each of the phases of treatment. It also shifts treatment focus from pathology to potential for change, from professional prescriptions to collaborative engagement, and from an exclusive focus on global change to one that is incremental and encompasses both the target and contextual problems of those experiencing conditions encompassed by the term mental health–substance use.

REFERENCES

1 DiClemente CC. *Addiction and Change: how addictions develop and addicted people recover.* New York: Guilford Press; 2003.

2 DiClemente CC, Prochaska JO, Miller WR, *et al. Toward a Comprehensive, Transtheoretical Model of Change: stages of change and addictive behaviors. Treating addictive behaviors.* 2nd ed. New York: Plenum Press; 1998. pp. 3–24.

3 Prochaska JO, DiClemente CC. *The Transtheoretical Approach: crossing the traditional boundaries of therapy.* Homewood, IL: Dow Jones-Irwin; 1984.

4 Klingemann H, Sobell LC. *Promoting Self-Change from Addictive Behaviors: practical implications for policy, prevention, and treatment.* New York: Springer Science & Business Media; 2007.

5 Carbonari JP, DiClemente CC, Sewell KB. Stage transitions and the transtheoretical 'stages of change' model of smoking cessation. *Swiss Journal of Psychology/Schweizerische Zeitschrift fur Psychologie/Revue Suisse de Psychologie.* 1999; **58**: 134–44.

6 Connors GJ, Donovan DM, DiClemente CC. *Substance Abuse Treatment and the Stages of Change: selecting and planning interventions.* New York: Guilford Press; 2001.

7 Prochaska JO, DiClemente CC, Norcross JC. In search of how people change: applications to addictive behaviors. *American Psychologist.* 1992; **47**: 1102–14.

8 Center for Substance Abuse Treatment. *Enhancing Motivation for Change in Substance Abuse Treatment.* Washington, DC: DHHS Publication No. SMA 99–3354; 1999. Report No. 35. Available at: www.motivationalinterview.org/library/TIP35/TIP35.htm (accessed 2 August 2010).

9 DiClemente CC, Velasquez MM. Motivational Interviewing and the stages of change. In: Miller WR, Rollnick S, editors. *Motivational Interviewing.* 2nd ed. New York: Guilford Press; 2002. pp. 201–16.

10 DiClemente CC, Prochaska JO, Fairhurst SK, *et al.* The process of smoking cessation: an analysis of precontemplation, contemplation, and preparation stages of change. *Journal of Consulting and Clinical Psychology.* 1991; **59**: 295–304.

11 Velasquez MM, Maurer GG, Crouch C, *et al. Group Treatment for Substance Abuse: a stages-of-change therapy manual.* New York: Guilford Press; 2001.

12 DiClemente CC, Nidecker M, Bellack AS. Motivation and the stages of change among individuals with severe mental illness and substance abuse disorders. *Journal of Substance Abuse Treatment.* 2008; **34**: 25–35.

13 McLellan AT, Lewis DC, O'Brien CP, *et al.* Drug dependence, a chronic medical illness: implications for treatment, insurance, and outcomes evaluation. *Journal of the American Medical Association.* 2000; **284**: 1689–95.

14 Prochaska JO, Velicer WF, Rossi JS, *et al.* Stages of change and decisional balance for 12 problem behaviors. *Health Psychology.* 1994; **13**: 39–46.

15 Carbonari JP, DiClemente CC. Using Transtheoretical Model profiles to differentiate levels of alcohol abstinence success. *Journal of Consulting and Clinical Psychology.* 2000; **68**: 810–17.

16 Moyers TB, Martin T, Christopher P, *et al.* Client language as a mediator of motivational interviewing efficacy: where is the evidence? *Alcoholism: Clinical and Experimental Research.* 2007; **31**: S40–7.

17 Adamson SJ, Sellman JD, Frampton CMA. Patient predictors of alcohol treatment outcome: a systematic review. *Journal of Substance Abuse Treatment.* 2009; **36**: 75–86.

18 McMurran M, Theodosi E, Sellen J. Measuring engagement in therapy and motivation to change in adult prisoners: a brief report. *Criminal Behaviour and Mental Health.* 2006; **16**: 124–9.

19 Project Match Research Group. Matching alcoholism treatments to client heterogeneity: treatment main effects and matching effects on drinking during treatment. *Journal of Studies on Alcohol.* 1998; **59**: 630–9.

20 Velasquez MM, Crouch C, von Sternberg K, *et al.* Motivation for change and psychological distress in homeless substance abusers. *Journal of Substance Abuse Treatment.* 2000; **19**: 395–401.

21 Velasquez MM, Carbonari JP, DiClemente CC. Psychiatric severity and behavior change in alcoholism: the relation of the Transtheoretical Model variables to psychiatric distress in dually diagnosed patients. *Addictive Behaviors.* 1999; **24**: 481–96.

22 Strong Kinnaman JE, Bellack AS, Brown CH, *et al.* Assessment of motivation to change substance use in dually-diagnosed schizophrenia patients. *Addictive Behaviors.* 2007; **32**: 1798–813.

23 Nidecker M, DiClemente CC, Bennett ME, *et al.* Application of the Transtheoretical Model of change: psychometric properties of leading measures in patients with co-occurring drug abuse and severe mental illness. *Addictive Behaviors.* 2008; **33**: 1021–30.

24 Wells EA, Calsyn DA, Clark LL, *et al.* Motivational enhancement to increase treatment readiness among stimulant users: a pilot evaluation [Abstract]. In: Harris LS, editor. *The College on Problems of Drug Dependence 1998: National Institute of Drug Abuse Research Monograph.* Bethesda, MD: National Institute of Drug Abuse; 1998. p. 97.

25 DiClemente CC, Schlundt D, Gemmell L. Readiness and stages of change in addiction treatment. *The American Journal on Addictions.* 2004; **13**: 103–19.

26 McConnaughy EA, Prochaska JO, Velicer WF. Stages of change in psychotherapy: measurement and sample profiles. *Psychotherapy: Theory, Research and Practice.* 1983; **20**: 368–75.

27 LaBrie JW, Quinlan T, Schiffman JE, *et al.* Performance of alcohol and safer sex change rulers compared with readiness to change questionnaires. *Psychology of Addictive Behaviors.* 2005; **19**: 112–15.

28 Rollnick S, Heather N, Gold R, Hall W. Development of a short 'readiness to change' questionnaire for use in brief, opportunistic interventions among excessive drinkers. *British Journal of Addiction.* 1992; **87**: 743–54.

29 Perz CA, DiClemente CC, Carbonari JP. Doing the right thing at the right time? The interaction of stages and processes of change in successful smoking cessation. *Health Psychology.* 1996; **15**: 462–8.

30 Prochaska JJ, Rossi JS, Redding CA, *et al.* Depressed smokers and stage of change: implications for treatment interventions. *Drug and Alcohol Dependence.* 2004; **76**: 143–51.

31 DiClemente CC, Prochaska JO, Gibertini M. Self-efficacy and the stages of self-change of smoking. *Cognitive Therapy and Research.* 1985; **9**: 181–200.

32 Miller WR, Rollnick S. *Motivational Interviewing: preparing people to change addictive behavior.* New York: Guilford Press; 1991.

33 Davidson R. The Transtheoretical Model: a critical overview. In: Miller WR, Heather N, editors. *Treating Addictive Behaviors.* 2nd ed. New York: Plenum Press; 1998. pp. 25–38.

34 West R. Time for a change: putting the Transtheoretical (Stages of Change) Model to rest. *Addiction.* 2005; **100**: 1036–9.

35 Herzog TA. Analyzing the Transtheoretical Model using the framework of Weinstein, Rothman, and Sutton (1998): The example of smoking cessation. *Health Psychology.* 2008; **27**: 548–56.

36 Drake RE, Mueser KT, Brunette MF, *et al.* A review of treatments for people with severe mental illnesses and co-occurring substance use disorders. *Psychiatric Rehabilitation Journal.* 2004; **27**: 360–74.

37 Hellerstein DJ, Rosenthal RN, Miner CR. A prospective study of integrated outpatient treatment for substance-abusing schizophrenic patients. *The American Journal on Addictions.* 1995; **4**: 33–42.

38 Kavanagh DJ, Young R, White A, *et al.* A brief motivational intervention for substance misuse in recent-onset psychosis. *Drug and Alcohol Review.* 2004; **23**: 151–5.

39 James W, Preston NJ, Koh G, *et al.* A group intervention which assists patients with dual diagnosis reduce their drug use: a randomised controlled trial. *Psychological Medicine.* 2004; **34**: 983–90.

40 Ho AP, Tsuang JW, Liberman RP, *et al.* Achieving effective treatment of patients with chronic psychotic illness and comorbid substance dependence. *American Journal of Psychiatry.* 1999; **156**: 1765–70.

41 Miller WR, Tonigan JS. Assessing drinkers' motivations for change: the Stages of Change Readiness and Treatment Eagerness Scale (SOCRATES). *Psychology of Addictive Behaviors.* 1996; **10**: 81–9.

42 Ryan P, Lauver DR. The efficacy of tailored interventions. *Journal of Nursing Scholarship.* 2002; **34**: 331–7.

43 Martino S, Carroll KM, Nich C, *et al.* A randomized controlled pilot study of motivational interviewing for patients with psychotic and drug use disorders. *Addiction.* 2006; **101**: 1479–92.

44 McLellan AT, Hagan TA, Levine M, *et al.* Does clinical case management improve outpatient addiction treatment? *Drug and Alcohol Dependence.* 1999; **55**: 91–103.

45 Drake RE, Essock SM, Shaner A, *et al.* Implementing dual diagnosis services for clients with severe mental illness. *Psychiatric Services.* 2001; **52**: 469–76.

46 McGovern MP, McLellan AT. The status of addiction treatment research with co-occurring substance use and psychiatric disorders. *Journal of Substance Abuse Treatment.* 2008; **34**: 1–2.

47 Eyrich-Garg KM, Cacciola JS, Carise D, *et al.* Individual characteristics of the literally homeless, marginally housed, and impoverished in a US substance abuse treatment-seeking sample. *Social Psychiatry and Psychiatric Epidemiology.* 2008; **43**: 831–42.

48 Choi S, Ryan JP. Co-occurring problems for substance abusing mothers in child welfare: matching services to improve family reunification. *Children and Youth Services Review.* 2007; **29**: 1395–410.

49 Heesch KC, Velasquez MM, von Sternberg K. Readiness for mental health treatment and for changing alcohol use in patients with comorbid psychiatric and alcohol disorders: are they congruent? *Addictive Behaviors.* 2005; **30**: 531–43.

50 Bellack AS, Bennett ME, Gearon JS, *et al.* A randomized clinical trial of a new behavioral treatment for drug abuse in people with severe and persistent mental illness. *Archives of General Psychiatry.* 2006; **63**: 426–32.

51 Carey KB. Substance use reduction in the context of outpatient psychiatric treatment: a collaborative, motivational, harm reduction approach. *Community Mental Health Journal.* 1996; **32**: 291–306.

52 Bouis S, Reif S, Whetten K, *et al.* An integrated, multidimensional treatment model for individuals living with HIV, mental illness, and substance abuse. *Health and Social Work.* 2007; **32**: 268–78.

53 Murphy RT, Rosen C, Thompson K, *et al. A Readiness to Change Approach to Preventing PTSD Treatment Failure. Advances in the treatment of posttraumatic stress disorder: cognitive-behavioral perspectives.* New York: Springer; 2004. pp. 57–91.

54 Squires DD, Moyers TB. Motivational enhancement for dually diagnosed consumers.

University of Mexico Center on Alcoholism, Substance Abuse and Addictions; 2001. Available at: www.bhrm.org/guidelines/squiresmoyers.pdf (accessed 2 August 2010).

55 Prochaska JM, Prochaska JO, Levesque DA. A transtheoretical approach to changing organizations. *Administration and Policy in Mental Health*. 2001; **28**: 247–61.

TO LEARN MORE

- DiClemente CC. *Addiction and Change: how addictions develop and addicted people recover.* New York: Guilford Press; 2003. Paperback edition 2006.
- DiClemente CC. Conceptual models and allied research: the ongoing contribution of the Transtheoretical Model. *Journal of Addiction Nursing*. 2005; **16**: 5–12.
- DiClemente CC, Nidecker M, Bellack AS. Motivation and the Stages of Change among individuals with severe mental illness and substance abuse disorder. *Journal of Substance Abuse Treatment*. 2008; **34**: 25–35.
- Habits Laboratory website. Available at: www.umbc.edu/psych/habits

CHAPTER 7

Motivational interviewing: mental health–substance use

Jennifer E Hettema and Joshua T Kirsch

The views expressed here are those of the authors, and in no way are meant to reflect those of the organisations they work for. The clinical vignettes presented are completely fictional, and in no way represent clients, alive or dead.

PRE-READING EXERCISE 7.1 (ANSWERS ON P. 100)

Consider Simon, a fictional 28-year-old man diagnosed with paranoid schizophrenia and cocaine dependence. Simon is unemployed, lives with his mother, and is currently receiving government support. Simon does not accept his diagnosis of schizophrenia, attends treatment sessions irregularly, and takes his prescribed medication erratically. Simon uses cocaine when he has money and, following these binges, he has been hospitalised for hearing voices and causing public disturbances. We will return to his situation throughout the chapter.

1 What area or areas should be the primary focus of treatment?
2 Should the professional working with Simon focus on encouraging him to accept the labels of schizophrenic and addict?
3 During his treatment sessions at an outpatient treatment programme, Simon has been withdrawn and non-participatory. When asked about his lack of engagement, Simon replies that he knows that if he opens up the information he shares is going to be reported to the police or leaked to the tabloids. What is the most motivational interviewing consistent *first* response to this statement?
   a If you would take your medications regularly, you probably would not feel so paranoid all of the time.
   b I am a good professional and would never do that.
   c Opening up feels pretty scary and unsafe right now.
   d Let me explain my confidentiality policy to you again, which states that I will not share any information about you with individuals outside of this clinic unless I believe that you are a danger to yourself or others.

INTRODUCTION

Motivational interviewing (MI) has strong conceptual and empirical grounding for the treatment of people experiencing mental health–substance use disorders. Motivational interviewing is a therapeutic technique with specific and teachable skills, which will be discussed throughout this chapter. In addition, MI is an interpersonal style, or way of being with the individual, and much of the effectiveness of the approach is likely a by-product of embodying the 'spirit' of the intervention. MI is often referred to as a guiding approach, in which the professional is encouraged to engage in specific strategies that are designed to mobilise the individual's internal resources. MI also facilitates an integrated approach to treatment, and allows individuals the opportunity to address multiple concerns or problem behaviours within a single setting.

Throughout this chapter, we will refer to Simon, the fictional character described in Pre-reading exercise 7.1. While Simon is a person with co-occurring psychosis and substance use disorder, MI can also be used to work with individuals experiencing co-occurring mood disorders, anxiety disorders and other mental health problems. This chapter will focus on general techniques for working with mental health–substance use, instead of providing specific details about the application of MI to all possible combinations of problems. As you read, please keep in mind that this approach is not meant to be applicable to every clinical situation, and professionals need to utilise clinical judgement and consultation as appropriate.

OVERVIEW OF APPROACH

Motivational interviewing is simultaneously person centred and directive.[1] The person-centred component is influenced by the work of Carl Rogers and holds that people have within them the capacity for change, and that the professional can best facilitate this change through genuineness and non-directive empathic listening.[2] MI maintains Rogers' emphasis on genuineness and empathic listening, but allows and even encourages the professional to use behaviours that differentially elicit and reinforce talk about change. Unlike Rogerian therapy, MI explicitly posits the necessity of a directive approach in many clinical situations. For instance, most individuals who are using cocaine and hearing voices would clearly benefit from behaviour change; in MI the professional is encouraged to interact with such individuals in a way that is most likely to facilitate positive change. Motivational interviewing is directive in its strategic and selective focus on problem areas, provision of information, and encouragement of the individual to articulate his/her reasons for making a change. However, the MI professional avoids aspects of other directive therapies, including direct persuasion, unsolicited advice, labelling and confrontation.

OVERVIEW OF PRINCIPLES

Motivational interviewing has four core principles, which include:
➤ expressing empathy
➤ supporting self-efficacy
➤ rolling with resistance
➤ developing a discrepancy.[1]

Table 7.1 provides an overview of the four principles.

TABLE 7.1 Four principles of motivational interviewing

Principle	Description
Express empathy	Communicate an interest in and understanding of the individual's perspective through reflective listening
Support self-efficacy	Affirm the individual's strengths and efforts and help him or her to verbalise past successes
Roll with resistance	View resistance as a sign to respond differently and make efforts to reflect and empathise with resistant statements
Develop a discrepancy	Help the individual to identify and articulate dissonance between their behaviour and their important goals and values.

1 **Expressing empathy** involves communicating with the individual in a way that allows him/her to feel understood, validated and accepted. The MI professional uses reflective listening techniques to demonstrate and ensure an accurate understanding of the individual's specific situation. Research strongly supports the benefits of emphatic listening within clinical interactions.[3–5]

   In the case of Simon, the MI professional could express empathy by using reflective listening skills to signify understanding of Simon's perspective and specific situation. This would allow a trusting relationship to develop. Once Simon feels confident that the professional understands his perspective, and is able to listen and relate without prescribing corrective courses of action, he will likely feel more comfortable addressing the factors involved in his drug usage and inconsistent medication adherence.

2 **Supporting self-efficacy** is another core principle of MI. Self-efficacy refers to the extent to which a person believes that he/she can accomplish a task. In our case example, Simon is a skilled drummer, and thus has high self-efficacy about his abilities in this area. However, he is not sure whether or not he could stop his cocaine use, and thus has lower self-efficacy in this domain. When individuals have high self-efficacy about making a change, they are more likely to attempt the change. On the other hand, when individuals are unsure about their ability to change, they are less likely to initiate a change. In MI, professionals support self-efficacy by affirming the individual's strengths and efforts, and encouraging the individual to talk about past successes, in addition to other strategies.

3 **Rolling with resistance** is another important principle of MI. When individuals express feelings of dissatisfaction with treatment or argue for reasons why they should maintain their maladaptive behaviour, professionals are often tempted to meet this behaviour head on, by directly confronting or debating with the individual. However, such interactions can often serve to increase rather than decrease resistant behaviour and can damage the therapeutic relationship (*see* Chapter 2). In MI, resistance is not seen as a trait or behaviour, but as a by-product of the interaction between the individual and professional, and as a sign that the professional should switch strategies. Motivational interviewing

encourages understanding of the individual's perspective, and posits that the professional should respond to resistance with reflection and empathic listening.

When Simon presented at the mental health clinic following his last hospital discharge, the mental health professional spent 20 minutes trying to get him to accept the diagnosis of schizophrenia. The interaction became heated, and Simon left the session in anger. Within MI, there is little emphasis on the acceptance of labels, as acceptance of diagnoses does not necessarily lead to behaviour change. Rather than focusing on labelling, the MI professional focuses on action.

4 **Developing discrepancy** describes the professional's attempts to help individuals view maladaptive behaviour in the context of their goals and values. For example, Simon highly values independence, freedom and family. For Simon, cocaine use leads to hospitalisation, preventing Simon from achieving a lifestyle that is high in independence and freedom. It may also interfere with his relationship with his family, who he cares about and wants to please. When individuals engage in maladaptive behaviour, there are, arguably, always goals, values or other areas of importance which do not support the current behaviour. In MI, the professional can explicitly elicit the individual's goals and values through empathic conversation or predesigned exercises and offer the individual the opportunity to consider those values in the context of their current behaviour.

OVERVIEW OF GENERAL SKILLS

In addition to the guiding principles of MI, the intervention involves the strategic use of several clinical skills. The core skills of MI, which are commonly remembered using the acronym OARS, are:

➤ Open-ended questions
➤ Affirmations
➤ Reflections
➤ Summaries.[1]

Table 7.2 provides a summary of these skills.

TABLE 7.2 Core skills of motivational interviewing

Skill	Description
Open-ended questions	Questions that cannot be answered with a 'yes', 'no' or other one-word answer
Affirmations	Statement intended to encourage and support the individual
Reflections	Statements that infer meaning in what the individual has said
Summaries	Statements that tie several aspects of what the individual has said together.

Open-ended questions are questions that cannot be answered with a 'yes' or 'no' response or other one-word answer. They are designed to increase dialogue and the impact that individuals can have on the direction of therapy. Examples of open-ended questions include 'What brings you in today'? and 'What are some of the things you like about cocaine?'

Affirmations are designed to increase the self-efficacy of the individual and can be used to highlight individual strengths or efforts. They emphasise the professional's perspective. Examples of affirmations include 'I can tell you are someone who sticks to your word' and 'I appreciate you taking the time to talk about these difficult issues.'

Reflections are, in many ways, the backbone of motivational interviewing, and serve as a means to ensure understanding and communicate an active interest in the individual's perspective. In many ways, reflections are guesses about the underlying meaning of what a person has said. Good MI reflections are typically complex, and may highlight issues such as ambivalence or underlying affect. In form, reflections are made as statements with inflections that go down at the end. Following are several examples of reflective responses that might be made to Simon:

Reflection example 1

> **Simon**: My mom was pretty frustrated with me when I came home this last time. She says I don't make any sense after I've been gone for days. I just don't know what to say to her when she keeps drilling me. I wish she would just leave me be and let me do my thing.
>
> **MI professional's reflection**: You want to get along with your mom, and you'd like to be able to live your life the way you'd like to.

Reflection example 2

> **Simon**: Why do you guys keep asking me all of these questions about my stupid medications?
>
> **MI professional's reflection**: It really annoys you that this topic keeps coming up, when it seems irrelevant to you.

The last core skill of MI is the use of **summaries**. Summaries are special forms of reflections, in which the professional reflects a larger portion of the person's words. Summaries can be used for transition from one topic to another, provide an overview at the end of a session, or tie together different aspects of what a person has said. The following summary is an example where MI might be used with Simon.

Summary example

> **MI professional summary**: You have been hospitalised several times, which really bothers you. You have been told to take your medications and stop using cocaine; at the same time, you aren't sure you agree with this. You are considering avoiding cocaine, because it makes you paranoid. Plus, the people who use it with you are often greedy and they don't share your belief in God. You are not so sure about medications, because you have not liked how they make you feel.

THE IMPORTANCE OF CHANGE TALK

Research on the processes or mechanisms of action of MI has suggested that eliciting the individual's language about change within sessions may be predictive of positive outcome.[6] Language about change is often referred to as 'change talk' and typically involves the individual's statements regarding desire, ability, reasons, need and commitment to make a change.

Because of this research, an increased emphasis has been placed on recognising, eliciting and responding to change talk within MI. Several of the core skills of motivational interviewing can be used specifically for this purpose. For one, MI professionals may wish to differentially reflect and affirm talk about change when it happens. In addition, open-ended questions can be designed in such a way that they elicit the expression of change talk. Examples include 'What are some of the bad things about using cocaine?' and 'Tell me about some of things you accomplished the last time you were taking your medications consistently?' Open-ended questions can also be used to ask for elaboration of change talk when it occurs. For example, if Simon reports that it felt really good the last time he had a job, he could be encouraged to talk more about that experience and what it felt like. Similarly, if he states that he felt really bad after his mom confronted him about his behaviour, the MI professional could ask him to share more about the interaction. The objective of all of these strategies is to give the individual as many opportunities as possible to talk within session about the drawbacks of their current behaviour and the benefits of change. Following is an example of an MI professional eliciting, elaborating on and reflecting change talk.

Change talk

> **MI professional**: What don't you like about cocaine? (*Asking for change talk*)
> **Simon**: I don't like how it makes me feel.
> **MI professional**: In what ways? (*Asking for elaboration*)
> **Simon**: It makes my voices worse and the police don't like it.
> **MI professional**: You are avoiding cocaine because it increases your anxiety and gets you in trouble with the law. (*Reflecting change talk*)

Questions to elicit change talk

The following are examples of questions to elicit change talk.

➤ What are the benefits of staying sober?
➤ If you did make a change, how might you go about doing it?
➤ What are the advantages of avoiding alcohol?
➤ Can you say more about what happened last time you stopped taking medication?
➤ What do you see happening if you did not make a change?
➤ If you did participate in the programme for three months, how might your life be different?
➤ What are you going to do at this point?

INFORMATION PROVISION

The last MI skill that we will discuss involves the use of information provision. Professionals often have received a great deal of training in the treatment of individuals experiencing mental health–substance use problems and have likely witnessed successes and failures among this treatment population. A sincere desire to help people succeed, coupled with the possession of a vast array of relevant information, skills and resources, can make it very tempting to try to solve problems through persuasion. In MI, professionals are encouraged to share information in a way that is tailored to the readiness level of the individual. For example, within the MI model, if Simon has not yet decided that he is willing to make a change in his cocaine use, teaching him stimulus control and drug refusal skills would be a waste of time and could potentially damage the therapeutic relationship (*see* Chapter 2). At this stage, however, Simon may benefit from information that may impact his readiness to quit or reduce cocaine use, such as personalised feedback about his use or information regarding the impact of cocaine use on feelings of paranoia and confusion.

Information provision can be facilitated using the permission-ask-provide-ask (PAPA) technique. When possible, it can often be helpful to get the individual's implicit or explicit consent prior to sharing information. This can be done by asking *permission*, or by stressing autonomy, saying something such as, 'I'd like to give you some input about your medications, which may or may not be helpful to you.' Of course, permission should only be asked in situations in which the professional is willing and able to accept the individual's response. The MI professional then *asks* what the person already knows about the topic. Information is then *provided* in a way that is tailored to the current knowledge of the individual. Finally, the person is *asked* about his response to the information, by querying what he thinks the relevance of the information is to his situation, or what he plans on doing with the information. As will be discussed later, this second *ask* can also be used as an opportunity to have the individual repeat back his/her understanding of the information, to ensure that she/he has accurately heard the information. This is especially relevant for individuals with psychotic symptoms or who are cognitively impaired. There is an example of using this technique later in the chapter.

Frequently, cognitive behavioural therapy (CBT – *see* Chapter 10; Book 5, Chapters 11 and 12) strategies are utilised to address symptoms. The PAPA technique can be used to integrate MI with such skill-building techniques. If there is not time to use the PAPA technique, simply ask permission to use an intervention, and then, if consent is gained, begin the CBT strategy. This is in keeping with the collaborative spirit of MI.

EVIDENCE BASE

The application of MI to mental health–substance use problems has been studied empirically with some promising results. One early pilot study found that MI increased the outpatient treatment attendance of hospitalised individuals experiencing mental health–substance use problems following discharge.[7] Similarly, another study[8] found that one session of MI increased the treatment attendance and substance use outcomes of people experiencing mental health–substance use problems attending a partial hospitalisation programme. Graeber[9] and colleagues found reductions in alcohol use among people experiencing mental health–substance use problems receiving a brief application of MI, while Steinberg[10] and colleagues found similar results for smoking cessation treatment initiation. Moreover, MI has been combined with other treatment approaches in more prolonged interventions and found improved outcomes in the areas of substance use, treatment engagement and other important psychosocial outcomes.[11–13] However, in addition to these positive studies, several studies have failed to demonstrate improvements.[14,15] Further research is needed to identify reasons for differences in treatment effect across studies.

SPECIAL APPLICATION IN MENTAL HEALTH–SUBSTANCE USE

Motivational interviewing is especially relevant to people experiencing mental health–substance use disorders because it does not assert that readiness to change is a prerequisite of treatment, and explicitly acknowledges that individuals may be at different readiness levels for different problem areas or diagnoses. Individuals often present to treatment with low levels of motivation to change substance use or manage psychiatric illness.[16] In many settings, such individuals are turned away from treatment because they are labelled as not being ready to make a change, or are classified as being 'in denial'.[17] This issue is especially common around issues of medication adherence and illicit drug use.

When using MI with these individuals, the professional is encouraged to start with the behaviour that is most important for the individual. If, for example, the individual is presenting with drug use and depression, the professional could leave it up to the individual which issue to start with. Of course, given the interaction between these conditions, it would be important to use information provision to inform the individual that there is often a connection between substance use and depression. Nevertheless, the professional focuses on the area in which the individual is most interested.

Motivational interviewing is unique in that it differentiates between therapeutic strategies that are designed to prepare the individual to make change, and those that are designed to help facilitate or maintain action once a decision to change has been made. Very often, an internal shift in motivation is needed before behavioural change can occur. With individuals experiencing mental health–substance use disorders, this problem is confounded by the presence of two or more diagnoses, and individuals are often denied treatment or bounced back and forth between treatment systems as professionals become frustrated with their inability to effectively address lack of readiness to change. MI provides an avenue for integrated treatment that is tailored to the unique needs of each member of the heterogeneous population experiencing mental health–substance use problems by encouraging professionals to focus on increasing treatment engagement, developing rapport and increasing motivation to change as the first important steps in a staged treatment approach.

Consider again the case of Simon. Within many mental health settings, Simon is likely to be told by the professional that he is not ready to change, and should come back when he has 30 days abstinent. Simon, who has difficulty trusting others, will likely have no intention of following these instructions. What is needed in this situation is an approach that will allow Simon time to trust the professional, and start to reconsider his actions.

Motivational Interviewing provides a means to provide integrated treatment by simultaneously addressing the numerous problems presented. Minkoff[18] pointed out that because mental health and substance treatment are often delivered by separate agencies, access to services is difficult for people experiencing mental health–substance use disorders. Let us consider Simon again. He is referred by a mental health professional to a substance use treatment centre across town. Although he does not want to go, a family member takes him there. Simon is assessed but the substance use professional is concerned about his psychotic symptoms. He is told that because he hears voices, he is not stable enough to enter treatment. He is referred to another mental health centre. Both systems place prerequisites on Simon in order to access treatment. Motivational interviewing provides a framework for the professional to treat the individual in one location, and permits addressing multiple presenting concerns simultaneously.

SPECIAL ADAPTATIONS FOR INDIVIDUALS WITH SEVERE MENTAL ILLNESS

Martino[19] and colleagues suggest several modifications to motivational interviewing that may be appropriate for individuals with severe mental illnesses and the cognitive impairments that often accompany them. First, the MI professional might simplify open-ended questions and reflections to avoid tracking difficulties or processing deficits. In addition, professionals may wish to avoid reflecting disturbing content, provide sufficient time for people to process, and respond to reflections. Encouraged is the increased use of affirmations with the individual, who may face increased social stigma, invalidation and frustration with the treatment process (*see* Book 1, Chapters 4, 5, 7 and 8).[19]

Motivational interviewing is less focused on correcting delusional beliefs than other approaches. The individual receiving MI therapy would be encouraged to make behavioural change, rather than switching to more conventional beliefs. The reason is pragmatic rather than ideological, as such beliefs are often very difficult to influence, and attempts to do so may increase resistance and damage the therapeutic relationship. When reflecting psychotic content, the MI professional is encouraged to focus on emotions and themes, rather than on disturbing content. Consider the following example from Simon:

> **Simon**: Everywhere I go people are talking about me and misquoting me. It makes it hard for me to get a job.
> **MI professional**: It must be frustrating to deal with that.
> **Simon**: Yes, it is horribly frustrating. It's even worse because they read my thoughts.
> **MI professional**: It's almost like you can't get a break.

By focusing on these feelings and themes, the MI professional can easily switch to a focus from the content of delusions to the individual's motivation to make a change. The permission-ask-provide-ask information provision technique may also be particularly helpful for people experiencing severe mental illness. This technique can be used to ensure understanding, correct misconceptions, integrate the information with the individual's knowledge and link information to future behaviour. Consider another example from Simon:

> **MI professional**: There is something I'm thinking of that may be helpful to you. Is it alright if I tell you about it? (*Permission*)
>
> **Simon**: Sure.
>
> **MI professional**: Many individuals have found that certain medications can help them with concerns like the ones you mentioned. What has been your experience with medication? (*Ask*)
>
> **Simon**: When I took those pills I was sleepy all day and gained 60 pounds.
>
> **MI professional**: Your experience was not so good. (*Reflection*) There are newer medications which do not seem to have those side-effects. They can help people to feel less frustrated and more able to work on other areas of their lives, like getting a job. There are doctors here that you could meet with to discuss medication, if you would like. (*Provide*) How do you think this information might be relevant to you? (*Ask*)
>
> **Simon**: Is there a doctor here now? I could talk to one. But I want you to come with me. Some of them get pharmaceutical money and I don't trust them.
>
> **MI professional**: You are willing to talk to a doctor to find out more. (*Reflection*) It makes sense that you are somewhat sceptical of doctors, given your past experience. (*Affirmation*) In answer to your question, I'll see if the psychiatrist is available. We can meet with her together.

CONCLUSION

Motivational interviewing is a psychosocial technique which is useful for engaging individuals in treatment, addressing resistance and promoting behaviour change. The emphasis on addressing ambivalence, and the ease with which it can be used to address multiple problem areas, makes it a good fit for working alongside individuals experiencing mental health–substance use disorders. There are ways it can be tailored to fit the specific needs of the individual. Finally, it can be combined and integrated with the other psychosocial and pharmacological (*see* Book 5, Chapter 13) interventions that are helpful.

POST-READING EXERCISE 7.1 (ANSWERS ON PP. 100–101)

1 Following are several of an individual's statements followed by the professional's responses. Match each response with the motivational interviewing principles it best describes.

Interaction	MI principles (select one for each interaction)			
Individual: You're out to get me just like everybody else. **MI professional**: It's hard for you to trust me.	*Express empathy*	*Support self-efficacy*	*Develop discrepancy*	*Roll with resistance*
Individual: My kids mean everything to me. **MI professional**: In what ways, if any, does your substance use affect your relationship with your kids?	*Express empathy*	*Support self-efficacy*	*Develop discrepancy*	*Roll with resistance*
Individual: I visited my psychiatrist last week. **MI professional**: You are really working hard to make some positive changes in your life.	*Express empathy*	*Support self-efficacy*	*Develop discrepancy*	*Roll with resistance*
Individual: When I start to panic it is hard for me to believe that I'm not really having a heart attack this time. **MI professional**: Your panic attacks are terrifying and it's sometimes very hard to implement the skills we've been working on.	*Express empathy*	*Support self-efficacy*	*Develop discrepancy*	*Roll with resistance*

2 Name and describe the four core skills of motivational interviewing.

REFERENCES

1 Miller WR, Rollnick S. *Motivational Interviewing: preparing people for change.* New York: Guilford Press; 2002.

2 Rogers CR. *Client-centered Therapy: its current practice, implications, and theory.* Oxford: Houghton Mifflin; 1951.

3 Miller WR, Taylor CA, West JC. Focused versus broad spectrum behavior therapy for problem drinkers. *Journal of Consulting and Clinical Psychology.* 1980; **48**: 590–601.

4 Miller WR, Baca LM. Two-year follow-up of bibliotherapy and therapist-directed controlled drinking training for problem drinkers. *Behavior Therapy.* 1983; **14**: 441–8.

5 Miller WR, Benefield RG, Tonigan JS. Enhancing motivation for change in problem drinking: a controlled comparison of two therapist styles. *Journal of Consulting and Clinical Psychology.* 1993; **61**: 455–61.

6 Amrhein PC, Miller WR, Yahne CE, *et al.* Client commitment language during motivational interviewing predicts drug use outcomes. *Journal of Consulting and Clinical Psychology.* 2003; **71**: 862–78.

7 Swanson AJ, Pantalon MV, Cohen KR. Motivational interviewing and treatment adherence among psychiatric and dually diagnosed patients. *Journal of Nervous and Mental Disorders.* 1999; **187**: 630–5.

8 Martino S, Carroll KM, O'Malley SO, *et al.* Motivational interviewing with psychiatrically ill substance abusing patients. *The American Journal on Addictions.* 2000; **9**: 88–91.

9 Graeber DA, Moyers TB, Griffith G, *et al.* A pilot study comparing motivational interviewing and an educational intervention in patients with schizophrenia and alcohol use disorders. *Community Mental Health Journal.* 2003; **39**: 189–202.

10 Steinberg ML, Zeidonis DM, Krejci JA, *et al.* Motivational interviewing with personalised feedback: a brief intervention for motivating smokers with schizophrenia to seek treatment for tobacco dependence. *Journal of Consulting and Clinical Psychology.* 2004; **72**: 723–8.

11 Barrowclough C, Haddock G, Tarrier N, *et al.* Randomized controlled trial of motivational interviewing, cognitive behavior therapy, and family intervention for patients with comorbid schizophrenia and substance use disorders. *American Journal of Psychiatry.* 2001; **158**: 1706–13.

12 Bellack AS, Bennett ME, Gearon JS, *et al.* A randomized clinical trial of a new behavioral treatment of drug abuse in people with severe and persistent mental illness. *Archives of General Psychiatry.* 2006; **63**: 426–32.

13 Kemp R, Kirov G, Everitt B, *et al.* Randomised controlled trial of compliance therapy. 18-month follow-up. *British Journal of Psychiatry.* 1998; **172**: 413–19.

14 Baker A, Lewin T, Reichler H, *et al.* Evaluation of a motivational interview for substance use within psychiatric in-patient services. *Addiction.* 2002; **97**: 1329–37.

15 Martino S, Carroll KM, Nich C, *et al.* A randomized controlled pilot study of motivational interviewing for patients with psychotic and drug use disorders. *Addiction.* 2006; **101**: 1479–92.

16 Drake RE, Essock SM, Shaner A, *et al.* Implementing dual diagnosis services for clients with severe mental illness. *Psychiatric Services.* 2001; **52**: 469–76.

17 Sciacca K. Removing barriers: dual diagnosis and motivational interviewing. *Professional Counselor.* 1997; **12**: 41–6.

18 Minkoff K. Developing standards of care for individuals with co-occurring psychiatric and substance use disorders. *Psychiatric Services.* 2001; **52**: 597–9.

19 Martino S, Carroll K, Kostas D, *et al.* Dual diagnosis motivational interviewing: a modification of motivational interviewing for substance-abusing patients with psychotic disorders. *Journal of Substance Abuse Treatment.* 2002; **23**: 297–308.

TO LEARN MORE

- For more information *see* www.motivationalinterview.org
- Rollnick S, Miller WM, Butler CC. *Motivational Interviewing in Health Care: helping patients change behavior (applications of motivational interviewing).* New York and London: Guilford Press; 2008.

ANSWERS TO PRE-READING EXERCISE 7.1

1 Simon would likely most benefit from receiving integrated treatment for his mental health–substance use disorders. As is described in the chapter, historically, experiencing mental health–substance use disorders have been bounced between substance use and mental health treatment settings, as the former have required managed psychiatric symptoms and the latter have required abstinence as preconditions of treatment entry. Motivational interviewing provides a means to provide integrative treatment that is tailored to the individual needs and readiness levels of the individual.

2 A professional relying on the MI model would not focus energy on encouraging Simon to accept the labels of schizophrenic and addict. Within MI, the professional instead focuses on behavioural outcomes, such as decreased use or increased medication compliance and partners with the individual to make changes that are beneficial to his health and consistent with his goals and values.

3 The correct answer is (c). Within MI, professionals are encouraged to roll with resistance by reflecting the individual's feelings. This increases rapport and, once the individual feels understood, she/he may feel safe enough to open up more. (d), 'Let me explain my confidentiality policy to you again, which states that I will not share any information about you with individuals outside of this clinic unless I believe that you are a danger to yourself or others', may be an appropriate next response, depending on the particular situation.

ANSWERS TO POST-READING EXERCISE 7.1

1 Please see the correct responses in bold below.

Interaction	MI principles (select one for each interaction)			
Individual: You're out to get me just like everybody else. **MI professional**: It's hard for you to trust me.	*Express empathy*	*Support self-efficacy*	*Develop discrepancy*	**Roll with resistance**

Interaction	**MI principles** (select one for each interaction)			
Individual: My kids mean everything to me. **MI professional**: In what ways, if any, does your substance use affect your relationship with your kids?	*Express empathy*	*Support self-efficacy*	**Develop discrepancy**	*Roll with resistance*
Individual: I visited my psychiatrist last week. **MI professional**: You are really working hard to make some positive changes in your life.	*Express empathy*	**Support self-efficacy**	*Develop discrepancy*	*Roll with resistance*
Individual: When I start to panic it is hard for me to believe that I'm not really having a heart attack this time. **MI professional**: Your panic attacks are terrifying and it's sometimes very hard to implement the skills we've been working on.	**Express empathy**	*Support self-efficacy*	*Develop discrepancy*	*Roll with resistance*

2 The four core skills of motivational interviewing can be remembered using the acronym OARS, which stands for:
- **O**pen-ended questions – questions that cannot be answered with a 'yes', 'no' or other one-word answer.
- **A**ffirmations – statements that focus on the strengths or efforts of the individual.
- **R**eflections – statements that can be used to ensure accurate understanding and communicate interest in the individual's perspective.
- **S**ummaries – special forms of reflections that tie together different aspects of an interaction.

CHAPTER 8

Brief interventions: mental health–substance use

Catherine Lock, Eileen Kaner and Nick Heather

INTRODUCTION

This chapter provides a definition of brief interventions and charts their development both empirically and in terms of their theory base. Evidence is set out regarding the effects of brief interventions on substance use, including alcohol, tobacco, cannabis, stimulants, benzodiazepines, opiates and multiple substance use. For each of these substances the evidence of the effect of brief interventions on mental health–substance use concerns is presented.

WHAT ARE BRIEF INTERVENTIONS?

Brief interventions refer to a range of clinical activities focused on the use of a talk-based therapeutic approach aimed at changing certain health-limiting behaviours (usually smoking, heavy drinking or other drug use) and their associated problems. Brief interventions have been applied opportunistically to non-treatment-seeking individuals, with the core aim of secondary prevention, as well as to those undergoing treatment (sometimes referred to as brief treatments). Key components of brief interventions include simple structured advice, written information, behaviour change counselling and motivational interviewing (*see* Chapter 7) and each of these elements can either occur alone or in combination with each other.[1] Brief interventions have also been delivered either in a single appointment or a series of related sessions. Sessions can last between 5 and 60 minutes, and while brief interventions for non-treatment-seeking individuals do not tend to exceed five sessions in total, those in treatment can have many more than five sessions, including cognitive behavioural therapy (*see* Chapter 10; and Book 5, Chapters 11 and 12) and motivational interviewing.[2] Although there is wide variation in brief interventions activities there are a number of essential principles to delivery; brief interventions should obviously be short and should be deliverable by health professionals without specialist training and who are working in busy healthcare settings. Brief interventions are often based on a fundamental set of ingredients summarised by the acronym FRAMES (*see* Box 8.1).[3]

BOX 8.1 FRAMES

Feedback	Provides feedback on the individual's risk for behaviour
Responsibility	The individual is responsible for change
Advice	Advises reduction or gives explicit direction to change
Menu	Provides a variety of options for change
Empathy	Emphasises a warm, reflective and understanding approach
Self-efficacy	Encourages optimism about changing behaviour.

Given the variability in activity, it is important to explain that brief interventions are *not* merely traditional treatments (psychiatric or psychological) carried out in a short timescale;[4,5] they have more specific properties. Brief interventions are techniques that a variety of health professionals (general practitioners [GPs], nurses, pharmacists, health workers, drug workers, social workers, psychiatrists, etc.) can easily incorporate into their practice in a variety of cultural settings, populations and healthcare systems.[6] Brief interventions are supported by a large body of literature on their efficacy and cost-effectiveness with a wealth of trials and meta-analyses indicating that both opportunistic brief interventions delivered by generalists and brief treatment delivered by substance use specialists are efficacious as a secondary prevention and treatment strategy respectively. Brief interventions are also highly cost-efficient due to the minimal cost of the intervention and the breadth of scope for prevention of more serious and costly problems. Brief interventions are particularly effective in the field of substance use.[7]

ORIGINS OF BRIEF INTERVENTIONS

Brief interventions were first developed in the United Kingdom in the smoking cessation field.[8] A study carried out by Russell and colleagues revealed that a small proportion (5.1%) of patients had stopped smoking one year after a simple intervention provided by their GP.[9] This intervention comprised brief advice to quit smoking plus a leaflet with additional information to help the individual to achieve his/her goals.[9] While the results from this study appeared modest from a clinical perspective the authors estimated that such a simple intervention could easily be delivered by GPs to all smokers who consulted; if implemented by all GPs in the UK, this could potentially result in over half a million smokers quitting each year. They claimed that this figure could not be matched even if the number of specialist withdrawal clinics was doubled. This move towards interventions in non-treatment-seeking individuals was perhaps the key principle supporting the development of brief interventions. The potential impact of brief interventions from a public health perspective was huge and coincided with a growing interest in secondary prevention around this time. A model for brief interventions, derived from this pioneering study, continued to be used within the field of smoking cessation. However, it was further applied to other areas of public health. In particular, brief interventions were applied to excessive alcohol consumption in 1983,[10] as coincidental research had highlighted that lower intensity interventions were often as effective as more intensive treatments coupled with moderate alcohol consumption being accepted as a valid treatment goal. Brief interventions for excessive alcohol consumption have subsequently proved successful in a wide range of published studies.[2]

BRIEF INTERVENTIONS THEORY

Brief interventions are firmly grounded in theory from the field of psychology, which is concerned with understanding, predicting and changing human behaviour. Different theories are relevant to the context for brief interventions and its content or delivery mode.

In general terms, the principles of brief interventions are broadly based on social cognitive theory, which is drawn from the concept of social learning, as proposed by Albert Bandura.[11] He posited that behaviour occurred as a result of a dynamic interaction between individual, behavioural and environmental factors, the last-named including both physical (structural) and social aspects. Thus each individual has personal, cognitive (thinking) and affective (feeling) attributes that affect how they respond to the external world, and they differ in how they think about their own behaviour and are reinforced by it and by other people's actions. In addition, individuals have the capacity to observe and learn from the behaviour of people around them. Thus behaviour change interventions based on social cognitive theory focus on both personal and contextual factors. Important components include individuals' beliefs and attitudes about a behaviour, their self-efficacy or the sense of personal confidence about changing it and their view about how their own behaviour sits in relation to other people's actions (normative comparison). All these factors influence an individual's motivation for, and ability to change, a behaviour. Consequently, brief interventions address, in a structured format, an individual's knowledge, attitudes and skills in relation to behaviour so as to encourage behaviour change for subsequent health benefit.

In terms of therapeutic application, brief interventions in pioneering research[10] were based on principles of cognitive behavioural therapy (CBT – see Chapter 10; and Book 5, Chapters 11 and 12), which was itself closely linked to the social learning perspective. CBT is a talk-based treatment designed to make individuals change how they think (cognitive) and what they do (behaviour). Unlike some other therapies it focuses on 'here and now' problems and difficulties instead of focusing on causes or symptoms in the past. This tradition was continued in the Drink-Less pack,[12] a brief intervention developed for the WHO Collaborative Project, *The Identification and Management of Alcohol-Related Problems in Primary Care.*[6] This was based on a six-step plan consisting of:

1 examining reasons for drinking
2 selecting and endorsing good reasons for cutting down
3 identifying personal high-risk situations for excessive drinking
4 choosing and practising coping skills in preparation for the high-risk situations
5 eliciting social support for a change in drinking
6 planning for relapse prevention.

These elements represent a condensed version of the treatment modality known as *behavioural self-control training.*[13]

Recently, in brief interventions research and practice there has been a move away from condensed CBT towards adaptations of motivational interviewing (MI – *see* Chapter 7).[14] Motivational interviewing is a person-centred interviewing style with the goal of resolving conflicts regarding the pros and cons of change, enhancing motivation and encouraging positive changes in behaviour. The interviewer style is characterised by empathy and acceptance, with an avoidance of direct confrontation. Any statements associated with positive behaviour change that the person brings up in the discussion are encouraged so as to support self-efficacy and a commitment to take action. Although within the time constraints for brief interventions, particularly in general health and social care settings, it is not possible to carry out MI, the general ethos and some of the techniques of MI can be adapted for this purpose.[15] Adapted or condensed versions of MI are often referred to as behaviour change counselling (BCC).

The Transtheoretical (Stages of Change) Model has been widely used to inform the context for brief intervention activities (*see* Chapter 6). Initially developed to describe the stages through which people progress in smoking cessation,[16] this model has since proved influential in guiding treatment across a range of addictive behaviours. Individuals are characterised as belonging to one of six internal 'stages' depending on the individual's awareness of a problem and their readiness to change behaviour to address this problem. The stages consist of:

1   **Precontemplation** (not thinking about change for at least six months)
2   **Contemplation** (planning to change in the next six months)
3   **Preparation** (planning to change in the next month)
4   **Action** (changing behaviour within the last six months)
5   **Maintenance** (having changed for more than six months)
6   **Termination** (permanently changed behaviour).

Individuals progress through these stages sequentially and it may take several cycles around the stages of change (i.e. relapses – *see* Chapter 13; and Book 6, Chapters 15 and 16) before a sustained recovery is achieved. The model also proposed that different self-change strategies or 'processes of change' are involved in moving between different stages and that different stages are associated with different beliefs about a problem. It argued that brief interventions to promote change should be designed so that they are appropriate to an individual's current stage. Although the theory has provided a heuristic model, evaluations to date have not supported its use in improving treatment outcomes.[17]

BRIEF INTERVENTIONS AND ALCOHOL

More than a hundred clinical trials have been conducted to evaluate the efficacy and cost-effectiveness of alcohol screening and brief interventions in both non-treatment and treatment-seeking populations.[18] There is now a very strong evidence base supporting the effectiveness of brief alcohol interventions in reducing alcohol-related problems. Many systematic reviews and meta-analyses have reported beneficial outcomes of brief interventions, compared to control conditions, in terms of reductions in hazardous and harmful drinking.[19–28] In 2007, a review focusing on primary care identified 29 controlled trials of brief interventions, which included over 7000 patients. This review found that brief interventions produced an average reduction of seven standard drinks (UK = 8 g ethanol) per week and there was no significant benefit of longer (more intensive) interventions compared to shorter input.[2] Although the evidence for brief interventions in the adult population is strong, this has not been successfully replicated in adolescent populations. A recent review of the impact of brief interventions on mental health–substance use conditions identified two studies[29,30] which related specifically to alcohol misuse. Both studies found a positive impact of brief interventions on alcohol, reporting positive drinking outcomes at six months in terms of abstinence rates and reduced weekly drinking.[31]

BRIEF INTERVENTIONS AND TOBACCO

There have also been over 41 controlled trials of brief interventions for smoking cessation.[32] Pooled data from 17 trials of brief advice versus no advice or usual care has shown that brief interventions result in significant increases in smoking cessation among patients.[33] Brief interventions are shown to be even more effective if combined with nicotine replacement therapy.[34,35] It has been concluded that when health professionals provide brief interventions for smoking it increases the likelihood that the patient will successfully quit and remain a non-smoker 12 months later.[33] National surveys have demonstrated that smoking is two to three times more common in people with mental health problems than in the general population.[36] A recent review of the impact of brief interventions on mental health–substance use conditions identified two studies which related specifically to tobacco use.[37,38] However, only one study found a positive impact of brief interventions on smoking.[38] This study reported a significant reduction in cigarette use at three months in patients with a range of psychiatric disorders, but this effect had disappeared at one year. However, individuals misusing substances with psychiatric conditions were more likely to attempt to quit smoking compared to those with substance disorders alone.[31]

BRIEF INTERVENTIONS AND CANNABIS

In contrast to the alcohol and tobacco literature, much less research has been conducted on the efficacy of brief interventions for illicit drug use. Nevertheless, cannabis use or dependence appears to be responsive to the same types of treatment as other substance dependencies.[39,40] Although research is limited and of lower quality, a systematic review of randomised controlled trials involving self-identified problem cannabis users in the community has shown brief interventions (including cognitive behavioural, motivational enhancement and contingency management therapies) to be efficacious for reducing cannabis use and associated consequences in adult populations.[39] However, among adolescents involved in the juvenile justice system and those with severe, persistent mental illness, longer and more intensive therapies provided by interdisciplinary teams may be required.[40] A year later, another review concluded that, while there was a general lack of research into brief interventions for cannabis use disorders, with few good quality randomised controlled trials mainly carried out in America and Australia, brief cognitive behavioural therapy had the strongest evidence of success for treatment-seeking adults with cannabis dependence.[40]

Brief interventions for cannabis use appear to be generalisable to adolescent populations, with a recent randomised controlled trial of brief interventions consisting of a single session of motivational interviewing for young (non-treatment seeking) cannabis users (aged 14–19 years) in Australia. This resulted in greater reductions in cannabis use for the brief interventions group compared to a delayed treatment control condition at three-month follow-up.[41,42] When considering brief interventions for mental health and cannabis use, research evidence is again extremely limited. An Australian randomised controlled trial compared a cannabis-focused intervention for young people with first-episode psychosis to a clinical control condition which involved psychoeducation. Although no significant differences were found between the groups, both the specific cannabis-focused intervention and the brief psychoeducation were associated with reduced cannabis use in young people with first-episode psychosis. As neither intervention was found to be superior, relatively simple, brief interventions may be worth implementing in the first instance to reduce cannabis use in this population.[43]

BRIEF INTERVENTIONS AND STIMULANTS

Once more, evidence for brief interventions and stimulant use is relatively limited in the number of well-conducted controlled studies. However, a review of the literature on psychosocial interventions for amphetamine use concluded that brief (cognitive behavioural) interventions were feasible and moderately effective among people using amphetamine but that more research was needed.[44] Brief (cognitive behavioural) interventions have shown their effectiveness in two six-month randomised controlled trials in people regularly using amphetamine in Australia.[45,46] With psychiatric inpatients brief interventions showed a lack of effectiveness, the authors concluding that people with moderate to severe levels of depression may best be offered more intensive interventions for amphetamine use from the outset, with further treatment for amphetamine use and/or depression depending on response.[46] A more recent randomised controlled trial of brief interventions for students (14–19 years old) with methamphetamine use disorders in Thailand found short-term (eight-week) benefits of brief interventions in terms of a decrease in the number of days that methamphetamine was used.[47]

Brief motivationally based interventions may also help people achieve abstinence from cocaine. A randomised controlled trial of peer-delivered brief interventions for non-treatment-seeking people using cocaine in the USA found the intervention group was more likely to be abstinent for cocaine than the control group.[48] However, a randomised controlled trial of a brief (motivational) intervention among young (16–22 years old) adults using ecstasy and cocaine users found positive reactive effects on stimulant use for both the brief interventions and control group who received written health risk information materials.[49]

BRIEF INTERVENTIONS AND BENZODIAZEPINES

While only six randomised controlled trials have evaluated brief interventions to reduce benzodiazepine use, all six studies produced positive effects. Brief interventions, consisting of a GP letter, consultation offer, simple advice and/or self-help booklet, significantly reduced benzodiazepine use compared to control groups.[50–55] A systematic review with meta-analysis of brief interventions (e.g. giving simple advice in the form of a letter or meeting to a large group of people) and systematic discontinuation (defined as treatment programmes led by a physician or psychologist) found both to be significantly more effective than treatment as usual.[56] Using different inclusion and exclusion criteria, a more recent systematic review with meta-analysis assessing the effectiveness of treatment approaches to assist benzodiazepine discontinuation concurred with the observation of Oude Voshaar[56] and colleagues that brief interventions were more effective than routine care. Brief interventions in this review consisted of a letter outlining the need to reduce benzodiazepine use, sometimes accompanied by a self-help booklet.[57] Further research is required to determine the most effective and cost-effective type of brief interventions for mental health benzodiazepine use.

BRIEF INTERVENTIONS AND OPIATES

There have been only two studies of brief interventions and opiate use. However, brief (motivational) interventions do show promise for people using opiates. Opiate using individuals attending a methadone programme who received a brief motivational intervention were more committed to abstaining from their drug use, reported fewer drug-related problems, were more compliant with treatment and were slower to relapse.[58] A randomised controlled trial of peer-delivered brief interventions for non-treatment-seeking individuals using heroin in the USA found the intervention group was more likely to be abstinent than the control group for heroin.[48] Again, there is a need for research to determine the efficacy of brief interventions for mental health opiate use, particularly for those with less severe dependence who are not actively seeking help.

BRIEF INTERVENTIONS AND MULTIPLE SUBSTANCES

Most brief interventions focus on a single behaviour. However, health professionals often work alongside individuals who concurrently drink and smoke or use a combination of other substances. Thus, it is important to determine if brief interventions can be successfully used across multiple areas of behaviour. Much of the evidence regarding brief interventions for multiple substance use focuses on adolescents and young people. A systematic review of brief interventions for adolescents in reducing alcohol, tobacco and other drugs concluded that, across a diverse range of settings and therefore probably diverse individuals, brief interventions conferred benefits to adolescents using substances.[59] In addition, a single session of motivational interviewing (for alcohol, tobacco and illicit drug use) resulted in a reduction in use of these drugs at three-month follow-up among 200 young people in a randomised controlled trial in the United Kingdom.[60] However, the beneficial effects were not maintained at 12 months.[61] An overview of systematic reviews looking at interventions to reduce harm associated with adolescent substance use (including alcohol, tobacco, non-medical use of prescribed medications, cannabis, heroin, cocaine, amphetamine-type substances and hallucinogens) concluded that there was review-level evidence of efficacy of screening and brief interventions but still a need to evaluate them in real-world settings to establish effectiveness.[62] At the same time, a Cochrane review based on findings from 25 randomised controlled trials which assessed the effectiveness of psychosocial interventions (including brief interventions) to reduce substance use by people with a severe mental illness found no compelling evidence to support any one psychosocial treatment over treatment as usual and concluded with the need for more research.[63] A more recent systematic review of the impact of brief interventions on mental health–substance use conditions found that the evidence of positive brief intervention effects in patients experiencing mental health–substance use problems was unconvincing. Brief interventions trials, which targeted more than one type of substance use, of which four were identified, generally reported null findings or a change in just one behaviour.[31] Thus further research is needed on interventions to promote positive change across mental health and multiple substance use domains.

CONCLUSION

Research on brief interventions for alcohol and tobacco has accumulated rapidly during the past two decades. There is now substantial literature on the effectiveness of brief interventions, including both opportunistic brief interventions delivered by generalists and brief treatment delivered by substance use specialists. Not only are the procedures generally effective with a variety of population groups, they can be delivered by a variety of health professionals. Less evidence is available regarding brief interventions for people using other drugs, but several studies show positive effects. There is no reason in principle why some of the findings from the alcohol and tobacco field should not be explored. It could possibly be argued that illicit drug use disorders usually show such a high level of dependence, and/or involve such a strong commitment to a deviant lifestyle, that brief interventions are unlikely to be successful. Needless to say, however, these assumptions should be tested and there will almost certainly be exceptional subgroups that may well respond to brief intervention. As indicated above, one example of generalisation to substances other than alcohol and tobacco is work on the effectiveness of forms of brief interventions directed against long-term benzodiazepine use in primary healthcare populations. Research indicates the global efficacy of brief interventions for illicit and licit drugs in the general population and there is a growing but diverse evidence base covering brief interventions for mental health substance use. However, research findings on brief interventions for people experiencing mental health and substance use problems are currently inconclusive. Thus, further research is needed on interventions to promote positive change across mental health and substance use domains.[31]

REFERENCES

1 Babor TF, Higgins-Biddle JC. Alcohol screening and brief intervention: dissemination strategies for medical practice and public health. *Addiction*. 2000; **95**: 677–86.
2 Kaner EFS, Beyer F, Dickinson HO, *et al*. Effectiveness of brief alcohol interventions in primary care populations. *Cochrane Database of Systematic Reviews*. 2007; **2**: CD004148.

3 Miller WR, Sanchez V. *Motivating Young Adults for Treatment and Lifestyle Change*. Notre Dame, IN: University of Notre Dame Press; 1993.

4 Babor TF. Avoiding the horrid and beastly sin of drunkenness: does dissuasion make a difference? *Journal of Consulting and Clinical Psychology*. 1994; **62**: 1127–40.

5 Miller WR, Rollnick S. *Motivational Interviewing: preparing people to change addictive behaviour*. New York: Guilford Press; 1991.

6 Heather N. A long-standing World Health Organization collaborative project on early identification and brief alcohol intervention in primary health care comes to an end. *Addiction*. 2007; **102**: 679–81.

7 Dunn C, Deroo L, Rivara FP. The use of brief interventions adapted from motivational interviewing across behavioral domains: a systematic review. *Addiction*. 2001; **96**: 1725–42.

8 Heather N. Development, evaluation and implementation of alcohol brief intervention in Europe. *Drug and Alcohol Review*. Forthcoming.

9 Russell MA, Wilson C, Taylor C, *et al.* Effect of general practitioners' advice against smoking. *British Medical Journal*. 1979; **2**: 231–5.

10 Heather N, Campion PD, Neville RG, *et al.* Evaluation of a controlled drinking minimal intervention for problem drinkers in general practice (the DRAMS scheme). *Journal of the Royal College of General Practitioners*. 1987; **37**: 358–63.

11 Bandura A. *Social Foundations of Thought and Action: a social cognitive theory*. Englewood Cliffs, NJ: Prentice Hall; 1986.

12 McAvoy B, Kaner E, Haighton C, *et al.* Drink-Less – marketing a brief intervention package in UK general practice. *Family Practice*. 1997; **14**: 427–8.

13 Hester R. Behavioural self-control training. In: Hester R, Miller WR, editors. *Handbook of Alcoholism Treatment Approaches: effective alternatives*. 2nd ed. Needham Heights, MA: Allyn & Bacon; 1995. pp. 148–59.

14 Miller WR, Rollnick S. *Motivational Interviewing: preparing people for change*. New York: Guilford Press; 2002.

15 Rollnick S, Heather N, Bell A. Negotiating behaviour change in medical settings: the development of brief motivational interviewing. *Journal of Mental Health*. 1992; **1**: 25–37.

16 Prochaska JO, DiClemente CC, Velicer WF, *et al.* Predicting change in smoking status for self-changers. *Addictive Behaviors*. 1985; **10**: 395–406.

17 West R. Time for a change: putting the Transtheoretical (Stages of Change) Model to rest. *Addiction*. 2005; **100**: 1036–9.

18 Babor TF, McRee BG, Kassebaum PA, *et al.* Screening, Brief Intervention, and Referral to Treatment (SBIRT): toward a public health approach to the management of substance abuse. *Substance Abuse*. 2007; **28**: 7–30.

19 Freemantle N, Gill P, Godfrey C, *et al.* Brief interventions and alcohol use. *Quality in Health Care*. 1993; **2**: 267–73.

20 Bien TH, Miller WR, Tonigan JS. Brief interventions for alcohol problems: a review. *Addiction*. 1993; **88**: 315–35.

21 Agosti V. The efficacy of treatments in reducing alcohol consumption: a meta-analysis. *International Journal of the Addictions*. 1995; **30**: 1067–77.

22 Kahan M, Wilson L, Becker L. Effectiveness of physician-based interventions with problem drinkers: a review. *Canadian Medical Association Journal*. 1995; **152**: 851–9.

23 Wilk AI, Jensen NM, Havighurst TC. Meta-analysis of randomized control trials addressing brief interventions in heavy alcohol drinkers. *Journal of General Internal Medicine*. 1997; **12**: 274–83.

24 Poikolainen K. Effectiveness of brief interventions to reduce alcohol intake in primary health care populations: a meta-analysis. *Preventive Medicine.* 1999; **28**: 503–9.

25 Moyer A, Finney JW, Swearingen CE, *et al.* Brief interventions for alcohol problems: a meta-analytic review of controlled investigations in treatment-seeking and non-treatment-seeking populations. *Addiction.* 2002; **97**: 279–92.

26 Ballesteros J, Duffy JC, Querejeta I, *et al.* Efficacy of brief interventions for hazardous drinkers in primary care: systematic review and meta-analyses. *Alcoholism: Clinical and Experimental Research.* 2004; **28**: 608–18.

27 Whitlock EP, Polen MR, Green CA, *et al.* Behavioral counseling interventions in primary care to reduce risky/harmful alcohol use by adults: a summary of the evidence for the US Preventive Services Task Force. *Annals of Internal Medicine.* 2004; **140**: 557–68.

28 Bertholet N, Daeppen J-B, Wietlisbach V, *et al.* Reduction of alcohol consumption by brief alcohol intervention in primary care: systematic review and meta-analysis. *Archives of Internal Medicine.* 2005; **165**: 986–95.

29 Hulse GK, Tait RJ. Six-month outcomes associated with a brief alcohol intervention for adult in-patients with psychiatric disorders. *Drug and Alcohol Review.* 2002; **21**: 105–12.

30 Graeber DA, Moyers TB, Griffith G, *et al.* A pilot study comparing motivational interviewing and an educational intervention in patients with schizophrenia and alcohol use disorders. *Community Mental Health Journal.* 2003; **39**: 189–202.

31 Kaner E, Brown N, Jackson K. A systematic review of the impact of brief interventions on substance use and co-morbid physical and mental health conditions. *Mental Health and Substance Use: dual diagnosis.* Forthcoming (2011; **4**).

32 Stead LF, Bergson G, Lancaster T. Physician advice for smoking cessation. *Cochrane Database of Systematic Reviews.* 2008; **2**: CD000165.

33 National Institute for Health and Clinical Excellence. Brief interventions and referral for smoking cessation in primary care and other settings: Public health guidance PH1. NIHCE; 2006. Available at: www.nice.org.uk/PHI001 (accessed 4 August 2010).

34 Russell MA, Merriman R, Stapleton J, *et al.* Effect of nicotine chewing gum as an adjunct to general practitioner's advice against smoking. *British Medical Journal (Clinical Research ed).* 1983; **287**: 1782–5.

35 Silagy C, Ketteridge S. The effectiveness of physician advice to aid smoking cessation. In: Lancaster T, Silagy C, editors. Tobacco Addiction module of the *Cochrane Database of Systematic Reviews.* London: British Medical Journal; 1996.

36 McNeill A. *Smoking and Mental Health: a review of the literature.* London: Smokefree London Programme; 2001.

37 Brown RA, Ramsey SE, Strong DR, *et al.* Effects of motivational interviewing on smoking cessation in adolescents with psychiatric disorders. *Tobacco Control.* 2003; **12**(Suppl. 4): SV3–10.

38 Baker A, Richmond R, Haile M, *et al.* A randomized controlled trial of a smoking cessation intervention among people with a psychotic disorder. *American Journal of Psychiatry.* 2006; **163**: 1934–42.

39 McRae AL, Budney AJ, Brady KT. Treatment of marijuana dependence: a review of the literature. *Journal of Substance Abuse Treatment.* 2003; **24**: 369–76.

40 Copeland J. Developments in the treatment of cannabis use disorder. *Current Opinion in Psychiatry.* 2004; **17**: 161–7.

41 Martin G, Copeland J, Swift W. The adolescent cannabis check-up: feasibility of a brief intervention for young cannabis users. *Journal of Substance Abuse Treatment.* 2005; **29**: 207–13.

42 Martin G, Copeland J. The adolescent cannabis check-up: randomized trial of a brief intervention for young cannabis users. *Journal of Substance Abuse Treatment*. 2008; **34**: 407–14.

43 Edwards J, Elkins K, Hinton M, *et al*. Randomized controlled trial of a cannabis-focused intervention for young people with first-episode psychosis. *Acta Psychiatrica Scandinavica*. 2006; **114**: 109–17.

44 Baker A, Lee NK. A review of psychosocial interventions for amphetamine use. *Drug and Alcohol Review*. 2003; **22**(3): 323–35.

45 Baker A, Boggs TG, Lewin TJ. Randomized controlled trial of brief cognitive-behavioural interventions among regular users of amphetamine. *Addiction*. 2001; **96**(9): 1279–87.

46 Baker A, Lee NK, Claire M, *et al*. Brief cognitive behavioural interventions for regular amphetamine users: a step in the right direction. *Addiction*. 2005; **100**: 367–78.

47 Srisurapanont M, Sombatmai S, Boripuntakul T. Brief intervention for students with methamphetamine use disorders: a randomized controlled trial. *American Journal on Addictions*. 2007; **16**: 111–16.

48 Bernstein J, Bernstein E, Tassiopoulos K, *et al*. Brief motivational intervention at a clinic visit reduces cocaine and heroin use. *Drug and Alcohol Dependence*. 2005; **77**: 49–59.

49 Marsden J, Stillwell G, Barlow H, *et al*. An evaluation of a brief motivational intervention among young ecstasy and cocaine users: no effect on substance and alcohol use outcomes. *Addiction*. 2006; **101**: 1014–26.

50 Cormack MA, Sweeney KG, Hughes-Jones H, *et al*. Evaluation of an easy, cost-effective strategy for cutting benzodiazepine use in general practice. *British Journal of General Practice*. 1994; **44**: 5–8.

51 Bashir K, King M, Ashworth M. Controlled evaluation of brief intervention by general practitioners to reduce chronic use of benzodiazepines. *British Journal of General Practice*. 1994; **44**: 408–12.

52 Heather N, Bowie A, Ashton H, *et al*. Randomised controlled trial of two brief interventions against long-term benzodiazepine use: outcome of intervention. *Addiction Research and Theory*. 2004; **12**: 141–54.

53 Gorgels WJMJ, Oude Voshaar RC, Mol AJJ, *et al*. Discontinuation of long-term benzodiazepine use by sending a letter to users in family practice: a prospective controlled intervention study. *Drug and Alcohol Dependence*. 2005; **78**: 49–56.

54 Niessen WJM, Stewart RE, Broer J, *et al*. Reduction in the consumption of benzodiazepines due to a letter to chronic users from their own general practitioner. *Nederlands Tijdschrift voor Geneeskunde*. 2005; **149**: 356–61.

55 Vicens C, Fiol F, Llobera J, *et al*. Withdrawal from long-term benzodiazepine use: randomised trial in family practice. *British Journal of General Practice*. 2006; **56**: 958–63.

56 Oude Voshaar RC, Couvee JE, van Balkom AJLM, *et al*. Strategies for discontinuing long-term benzodiazepine use: meta-analysis. *British Journal of Psychiatry*. 2006; **189**: 213–20.

57 Parr JM, Kavanagh DJ, Cahill L, *et al*. Effectiveness of current treatment approaches for benzodiazepine discontinuation: a meta-analysis. *Addiction*. 2009; **104**: 13–24.

58 Saunders B, Wilkinson C, Phillips M. The impact of a brief motivational intervention with opiate users attending a methadone programme. *Addiction*. 1995; **90**: 415–24.

59 Tait RJ, Hulse GK. A systematic review of the effectiveness of brief interventions with substance using adolescents by type of drug. *Drug and Alcohol Review*. 2003; **22**: 337–46.

60 McCambridge J, Strang J. The efficacy of single-session motivational interviewing in reducing drug consumption and perceptions of drug-related risk and harm among young people: results from a multi-site cluster randomized trial. *Addiction*. 2004; **99**: 39–52.

61 McCambridge J, Strang J. Deterioration over time in effect of Motivational Interviewing in

reducing drug consumption and related risk among young people. *Addiction*. 2005; **100**: 470–8.

62 Toumbourou JW, Stockwell T, Neighbors C, *et al*. Interventions to reduce harm associated with adolescent substance use. *Lancet*. 2007; **369**: 1391–401.

63 Cleary M, Hunt G, Matheson S, *et al*. Psychosocial interventions for people with both severe mental illness and substance misuse. *Cochrane Database of Systematic Reviews*. 2008; **1**: CD001088.

TO LEARN MORE

- Alcohol Learning Centre. Available at: www.alcohollearningcentre.org.uk/
- Help: for a life without tobacco. Available at: www.help-eu.com/
- Miller P. *Evidence-based Addiction Treatment*. San Diego, CA: Academic Press; 2009.
- National Institute for Health and Clinical Excellence. Brief interventions and referral for smoking cessation: public health guidance PH1. NIHCE; 2006. Available at: http://guidance.nice.org.uk/PH1
- National Institute for Health and Clinical Excellence. Drug misuse: psychosocial interventions: NICE guideline 51. London: NIHCE; 2009. Available at: http://guidance.nice.org.uk/CG51
- National Institute for Health and Clinical Excellence. Guidelines in Development. Psychosis with substance misuse. Available at: http://guidance.nice.org.uk/CG/Wave15/8
- National Institute for Health and Clinical Excellence. Public Health Guidance in Development. Alcohol-use disorders (prevention). Available at: http://guidance.nice.org.uk/PHG/Wave15/1
- Screening and brief alcohol intervention (SBI) materials. Available at: www.ncl.ac.uk/ihs/enterprise/

Integrated group treatment for people experiencing mental health–substance use problems

Kathleen Sciacca

INTRODUCTION

The simultaneous treatment of mental health–substance use problems is an essential service that necessitates integration of services and interventions within mental health–substance use and allied professions. When treating people who experience mental health–substance use disorders, integrated treatment has been found to be more effective than non-integrated care.[1] Integrated treatment has been shown to improve substance use outcomes including abstinence or harm reduction in the majority of people.[2] The group treatment approach outlined here can be integrated into a variety of programme models across services and systems of care.[3] This consensus-based model and integrative properties includes evidence-based interventions for people who have varying profiles of mental health–substance problems.[4,5] Discussion will be based in part on the author's consulting experience across systems of care, programme models and state-wide initiatives,[6-11] and will include: theme-centred interaction, stages of change, and client-centred reflective listening.

DEVELOPING INTEGRATED GROUP TREATMENT

The first treatment groups designed specifically for people experiencing mental health–substance use disorders began in 1984, in the New York State psychiatric care system.[4,7,12] People attending a psychiatric day treatment programme had diagnosed mental health disorders and many had undiagnosed substance use problems. They had been falling out of the system for years and continued to do so as new interventions got under way. Treatment systems remained unresponsive. In 1984, it became clear that developing interventions required that professionals:

➤ accept people 'where they were', all of their symptoms and conditions
➤ accept each person's level of readiness to address symptoms or engage in a process of change.

Interventions were 'non-confrontational' and included a phase-by-phase model that identified the individual's movement along a continuum delineated by group treatment phases and correlating objectives. Engaging and working with individuals experiencing mental health–substance use problems at various levels of readiness were later corroborated through consensus in the US SAMHSA-CMHS[13] Standards of Care, Practice Guidelines, Workforce Competencies and Training Curricula[8] and report,[13] where phase and stage-specific models of intervention are recommended when working with people who are experiencing mental health–substance use disorders. Engaging the individual at various levels of treatment readiness, including denial of symptoms, represented a clear departure from traditional substance use treatment. Individuals who were physically dependent, active users and who had active mental health symptoms were engaged into inpatient and outpatient group treatment. Individuals maintained their beliefs. Interventions were adapted to needs and responses. There was no prior theoretical basis for this work. As various hypotheses emerged, they were tested and successful outcomes guided the development of the treatment process. Psychoeducation emerged as a central component. This group treatment approach was integrated into mental health programmes and soon after into substance use programmes, services for the homeless and criminal justice services.[7,12]

PRE-GROUP INTERVIEW: ENGAGEMENT INTO GROUPS

A programme track for integrated groups begins with *screening instruments administered during the intake process*.[5,14] Individuals who screen positively are brought to the attention of the designated group leader. The individual is then included on the disposition form.[15] This roster comprises potential group members to be interviewed as groups are formed or spaces open.

With the majority starting out in denial about their mental health–substance use disorders, it is necessary to determine an alternative purpose for their participation in this group. The pre-group interview was developed for this purpose. Topics go beyond mental health and substance disorders to areas such as relationships, goal setting, stress, and change. The interview is also designed as an engagement strategy and a means of orientation to the group. Reasons other than mental health–substance use are readily identified as reasons to participate. This brief meeting (about half an hour) takes place prior to group attendance. Reasons to participate include contributions as well as benefits. There are four areas of the interview, including:[4,5,14]

1 **Support**: will the individual be supportive of others?
2 **Education**: of the many topic areas, what might be useful to the individual?
3 **Outside speakers**: does the individual have an interest in outside speakers?
4 **Openness to learning**: regardless of the readiness level, is the individual open to learning from the information and group members?

At the end of this interview, the leader measures the individual's readiness to address various symptoms. This documents a starting point and the ability to track advancement through the readiness levels.

In 1984, readiness scales were developed for this purpose.[5,14] People are frequently at different levels of readiness to address different symptoms or behaviours. Interventions match the individual's readiness to address each treatment goal.

PHASES OF GROUP TREATMENT

The initial response from the majority of individuals was rejection of any suggestion that they had a mental health–substance use disorder. After an initial attempt to conduct mental health–substance use groups where substance disorders were discussed with individuals in mental health treatment, it became necessary to adjust interventions and objectives. The *first premise* is that individuals may engage in discussion groups where they do not have to acknowledge any symptoms or disorders. Frequently, the basis for the individuals' rejection of co-occurring symptoms is the belief in related stigma, judgements and morality (*see* Book 1, Chapters 4, 5, 7 and 8). These beliefs result in shame, blame and guilt, with individuals lacking information. Mental health–substance use groups do not initially focus on individuals; group process is designed to be impersonal. The use of written materials, videos and outside speakers keeps the focus on the topics and off personal issues. This proves to be effective; individuals express their opinions and consider the relevance of the information to themselves or others. As participants engage in interactive discussion, a *second premise* emerges. Exposing individuals to the real properties of mental health–substance use disorders through valid information, psychoeducation and empathic interventions dispel beliefs in stigma, judgement and morality. This leads to some degree of acceptance of symptoms and the ability to discuss related behaviours. Each topic is discussed through a combination of didactic information and experiential feedback. Individuals give their opinions, and discuss related experiences of themselves or others. They are critics rather than students. It is repeatedly noted that experiential interaction with the information, and the opinions expressed through personal knowledge, advance individuals to self-disclosure. This is phase one.

Phase one

Objectives of phase one include:
➤ exposing the individual to the real properties of substance use disorders, mental illness and interaction effects
➤ dispelling stigma, shame, morality and self-blame
➤ facilitating movement along a continuum from denial to acknowledgement of symptoms and from precontemplation to contemplation
➤ developing a trusting atmosphere that is respectful of each group member
➤ discussing related topics, such as relationships, social networks, stressors, goals, aspirations and values.

Phase one yields movement from denial or guarded participation to self-disclosure. It usually lasts about three months of weekly group sessions. When a safe, trusting and empathic group atmosphere is established and people understand the true properties of various symptoms, in particular, physiology, genetics, loss of control and situational vulnerabilities, they begin to discuss their own behaviours or symptoms.

Phase two

This transition to self-disclosure is identified as 'phase two' of the group treatment process. In phase two interventions are more personal. Groups begin with the leader checking in with each member. The leader intervenes in a non-judgemental way to explore interaction effects between mental health and substance use. The objective is to facilitate the identification of interaction effects, risks and consequences and resulting problems of symptoms.

Phase two lasts about three months. It includes a variety of topics about interaction effects, recovery, symptom remission, decision-making and considerations for change. Clinical assessment focusing exclusively upon mental health–substance use disorders and interaction effects[14] is administered by the group leader in an individual session. New insights or information is discussed. The objectives in *phase two* include:

➤ facilitating the exploration of each person's risks, consequences and benefits of change
➤ understanding how people change
➤ facilitating advancement to problem recognition and decision-making
➤ assisting individuals in attaining the confidence and hope that change is possible.

Phase three

When people decide to make a change they move into 'phase three'. Phase three includes specific planning for change and implementing a plan. Programmes and services outside of the agency may be included as needed or recommended. Coping skills training is included as well as a relapse prevention plan (*see* Chapter 13; and Book 6, Chapters 15 and 16). The leader and the group continue to follow the individual's progress and provide support. This includes assisting the person to make adjustments and revise the plan when necessary.

When full remission for a symptom is reached, confidence usually results in targeting another area. The objective is to bring all symptoms into remission with a maintenance plan in place to prevent relapse.

PERSON-CENTRED INTERVENTIONS: ESSENTIAL AND EFFECTIVE

From the beginning the mental health–substance use model practised and underscored a **collaborative approach** between the professional and individual. The person's ideas, beliefs, feelings, experiences, aspirations and disappointments are the focus of discussion. Upon practising the formal approach to collaboration, namely person-centred reflective listening,[16] the powerful benefits of this well-articulated intervention became apparent. In 1992, person-centred reflective listening was included in mental health–substance use problems treatment and in the training curriculum. This approach is essential and extremely beneficial to both professional and individuals. People are listened to, understood and communicated with directly and beyond their clinical symptoms. This rapport-building approach fosters alliances, it is engaging versus disengaging. Communicating with professionals who are accepting and respectful, who are empathic and who allow the individual's process of change to unfold is invaluable. For professionals, collaborative explorations provide insight into many areas of the individual's situation and perspective including the behaviour change process.

Open questions,[19] such as 'What brings you here today?', provide an opportunity for people to present their point of view and for the professional to follow and understand the person's perspectives and respond with reflections. Reflections are always statements not questions (*see* Chapter 7). This approach entails following the person's thoughts for a while, and conveying, through empathic, reflective listening, that the listener understands the individual's perspectives, thoughts and feelings.

Example

> *Individual: This medication helps me with the voices but it drains my energy, I can't take it any more.*
> *Reflection: So you can see that medication is helpful, it is the side-effects that bother you.*

The experience of having a good listener, one who conveys respect and understanding, can help to build valuable rapport. Person-centred interventions and open questions are practised throughout the phases in individual and group interactions.

> If the client feels that he is actually communicating his present attitudes, superficial, confused, or conflicted as they may be, and that his communication is understood rather than evaluated in any way, then he is freed to communicate more deeply.[16]

THE PROFESSIONALS PREPARATION TO LEAD GROUPS

Professionals with various levels of clinical expertise can conduct mental health–substance use groups. A group leader without clinical training may utilise this model as an educational intervention. A skilled professional, experienced in leading therapy groups, may conduct groups that span the range of denial through recovery[4] and precontemplation through maintenance including relapse.[20] It is optimal for the group leader to be experienced in working with one area of the person's symptoms, either substance use problems or mental illness.

Education and training for all leaders includes understanding each disorder as a symptom that requires treatment. For the professional, this knowledge aids in assessing symptom severity, which will lead to effective interventions and recommendations. For group leaders with varying levels of clinical skills, knowledge of the physiological aspects of both mental illness and substance disorders provides a basis for understanding each discrete disorder and interaction effects. This is necessary if the leader is to educate people who are experiencing mental health–substance use disorders, and for the development of appropriate empathy.

THEME-CENTRED INTERACTION (TCI) GROUP PROCESS PSYCHOEDUCATION AND STAGES OF CHANGE

Overview of TCI principles[18]

Theme-centred interactional group process enhances mental health–substance use treatment groups. Theme-centred interaction applies to many kinds of groups, including organisational development and education.

Setting the theme

Theme-centred groups always include an explicit or implicit theme. One may state the theme in a formal way: Today, our theme is 'Learning about the stages of change'. A less formal way: 'Today, as part of our meeting we are going to be learning about the stages of change.'

The theme must be specific to the group's needs or interests. The group atmosphere has to be accepting and non-critical. If the group climate is basically negative, especially in the beginning, participants will have a hard time working on any other theme than their hurt feelings, taking sides, etc. It is preferable that a group leader react to every statement, including hostility towards himself/herself, in a receptive way.

INCORRECT WAYS TO SET THEMES

➤ **Do not set themes in negative terms**: when themes evolve around problems, it is best to state them in a positive way, such as 'Finding solutions for networking', rather than, 'The problems with networking'.

➤ **Do not set themes in the form of question**: questions fall flat and do not generate discussion. Theme 'How can I make new friends?' may cause participants to ponder. The alternative, 'Developing new social networks', includes an action that will generate discussion in a positive direction.

PRINCIPLES FOR SETTING THEMES

➤ **Always include an active verb**: active verbs generate discussion and are directed towards an activity, e.g. learning, exploring, finding, developing, coping, and understanding.

➤ **Always set themes in positive terms**: e.g. solving, creating, sharing, and helping.

➤ **Identifying emerging themes**: while discussing a stated theme, new themes may emerge. Learning about cocaine as a drug may shift to the discussion that one's friends and neighbours use this drug. The theme has shifted to the need to develop new social networks. Acknowledge that the theme has shifted and ask the group how they would like to proceed: finish with the learning theme, or go on to the new theme and return to the learning theme at a later date? Do not ignore the fact that the theme has shifted.

Dynamic balancing

The TCI group can be seen graphically as a triangle within a circle (*see* Figure 9.1).
The circle is referred to as *the globe*, and may include:

➤ why participants are there
➤ the physical environment, including setting, space and comfort
➤ time of day and day of the week, etc.

Each of these impacts the group experience. A group held in a mental health clinic
may be experienced differently from a group held in a church basement. One wants
to strive for an optimal globe. When it is not possible, adversities should be openly
discussed. Example: 'This space is tight and somewhat noisy; let's try to keep our
focus on our group's discussion.'

TCI gives equal importance to the three basic points of the *triangle* and their
relationships, keeping the 'globe' in mind. The triangle is defined by its three points:
'I', 'We', and 'It' (*see* Figure 9.1).

➤ 'I' refers to each individual in the group. It assures that each individual is
attended to and has the opportunity to express needs, thoughts and feelings.
➤ 'We' refers to the group as a whole, the interrelatedness of the group's
members, and group cohesiveness.
➤ 'It' refers to the group's theme, goal or purpose. This entails shifting to the
theme, goal and/or purpose of the group and relatedness of the *I* and *We*.

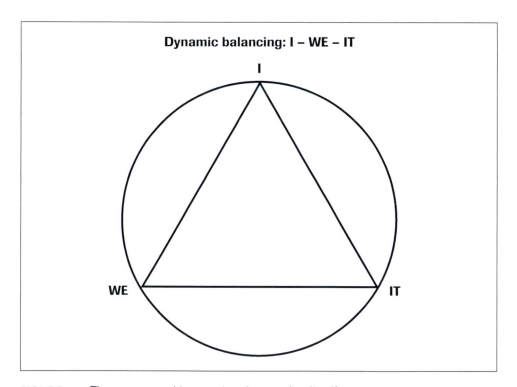

FIGURE 9.1 Theme-centred interactional group leading[18]

Balancing these factors is referred to as *Dynamic Balancing*. Equal time and attention are given to:

➤ the individual (I)
➤ the group as a whole (We)
➤ the theme (It).

Dynamic balancing is the responsibility of the group leader. The leader shifts gears from a particular individual to the group as a whole and to the theme, particularly when the process may be going out of balance. In mental health–substance use groups this process is also *used strategically and can be directive*. When an individual 'I' discusses a risk, or consequence, the leader may shift to the group 'We', and ask if other group members have had similar experiences. This may elicit the identification of risks or consequences from other members. The leader may also shift to the 'We' and ask other members to provide feedback. This may generate elaboration – a strategy that yields a more detailed discussion of adversities. The leader may also build in participation from each group member by asking a silent member for his/her input. The balance between '*I*', '*We*', and '*It*' is never perfect, but it must shift in a dynamic forward direction. The group leader's job is to employ her/his weight towards the unused pedal. That is, from 'I' to 'We', from the theme to 'I', from 'We' to the theme. Timing is important. Also important is whether the leader neglects or overprotects an individual, goes along with unrelated group interaction, or remains with a theme when group cohesion is lost. Maintaining group cohesion is critical. This is established when all participants, in their unique individual ways, are rallying around a sub-theme.

Dynamic balancing also means observing the correct timing with regard to the emotional and intellectual needs of individuals, the total group and their willingness to work with the theme.

Be your own chairperson

Group members are encouraged and empowered to make decisions about how their time and the group's time will be spent, and to speak up in the discussions. This is in keeping with the person-centred approach. The group leader is geared towards sensitising participants' recognition of their autonomy and interdependence.

Disturbances take precedence

Group and individual disturbances are encouraged to the foreground, to be dealt with as briefly as possible, until the full group is relating to the theme. Disturbances are not a central focus of the group. The leader may identify an issue, such as a hostile participant. One-on-one lengthy interventions in groups are discouraged; rather, the leader might ask the group to decide if they want to address this. An example might be: a participant complains that he/she does not want to participate in a planned group activity. The leader asks other group members if they would like to spend the first 10 minutes of their session discussing this. Group members agree or disagree; an exploration may ensue, or the complaining group member might decide to stay or to skip that meeting.

SYMPTOMS VERSUS DISTURBANCES

When working with individuals experiencing mental health–substance use problems, mental health symptoms are not considered disturbances unless they are so acute as to yield the individual out of control. This is the same for people who are intoxicated. When participation is not possible, professionals follow a procedure just as they would with any other person in crisis. However, if an individual cycles through transient symptoms as a part of her/his mental illness and is having thought disorders while the group is learning about a topic, this is not considered a disturbance or cause for a group decision. Symptoms need to be normalised. The group leader might simply acknowledge that the member is having difficulty focusing and suggest returning to the individual later on. Here, the group is learning first-hand about various symptoms and disabilities, and they are treated as such and accepted into the group process.

Focused discussion

Themes can be explored exclusively through discussion, or media may be used to sub-focus themes to a deeper level. In mental health–substance use, educational sessions sub-focusing may be done with literature, an exercise, a video or a speaker. In exploring the stages of change, the stage of change wheel or ruler may be distributed. Exclusively verbal themes are also sub-focused. Example of the verbal model (without materials) are as follows. (Note: this particular sub-focusing process – (b) and (c) – would be used with advanced, well-motivated, cohesive groups.

THEME: 'DEVELOPING NEW SOCIAL NETWORKS'

SUB-FOCUS

a **Leader**: 'I would like everyone to think about a friend you have had. How did you meet that person? What made that person special or different from other people you have met?' Members may focus with eyes open or closed and then are asked to discuss.
b **Leader**: 'Be aware of your experiences of yourself and others in the group right now.' Discuss.
c **Leader-Task**: 'Now look around the room. Who in this group do you experience to be most like your special friend.' Discuss.
d Replies may illuminate that everyone has had a friend in their life (the realm of possibility for most, if not all participants); people meet their good friends in many different ways, i.e. at the soda machine, at school, at work, etc. Some of the special qualities they find in common include ease in communication, trust, admiration, similarities and endurance.

Note: one can use the sub-themes in (a) alone and not proceed to (b) and (c).

The theme has now moved from abstract to personal and can go deeper depending on the group's strengths and the judgment of the leader. Replies to (b) essentially include how the person feels right now, what she/he is experiencing. Replies to (c) brings the theme to life, 'living-learning' in the here and now.

Speak for I

It is less risky to speak for 'we' and more risky to speak for 'I'. Participants are reminded to speak for 'I'.

Statements behind questions

Behind every question there is a statement. Questions are less risky than statements. A group member may ask a series of questions, the leader would encourage the participant to make the statement in an effort to foster direct communication.

Selective authenticity

'Selective authenticity' refers to a leader's self-disclosure. Self-disclosure is kept at a minimum except in instances where it may foster group movement. If the theme 'developing new social networks' is presented and no one speaks, the leader may give a short, selectively authentic snapshot of his/her friend as a means of conveying what an appropriate response might be.

If the leader experiences something intuitively, a sad feeling in the group, he may check this out with the group to see if this is a shared experience. Example, 'There seems to be a sad feeling in our group right now. Are others experiencing that?'

BENEFITS OF THEMED-CENTRED INTERACTION

Applying TCI group-leading principles assures that the group remains focused, and that each individual and the group as a whole are attended to. Theme-centred interaction can be used as a structural method for group leadership or as a therapeutic intervention. This is contingent upon the clinical expertise of the leader. Eventually, the TCI method was acclaimed as a form of therapy in itself.

Theme-centred interaction provides the skills and timing that allow group leaders to identify important aspects of group process and to bring them into balance. If dynamic balancing is practised, theme-centred groups provide an opportunity for group members to focus on a topic for the entire session. This permits deepening the exploration of the didactic and experiential elements of the theme. Group time is used productively, group members are empowered and intrinsic learning is afforded.[4,18,20]

MENTAL HEALTH–SUBSTANCE USE PSYCHOEDUCATION AND THEME-CENTRED INTERACTIONS

Members at the inception of the group may decide an overall theme for the group. Example: helping others, helping myself to explore alternatives. There are unlimited sub-themes that can be explored in different sessions.

For example, the theme is 'Learning about cocaine'; the handout is a fact sheet with 15 facts. Three or four predetermined facts will be read aloud by various group members who volunteer. Each fact is discussed. Educational materials do not comprise a curriculum; they serve as a catalyst for focused discussion. It may be that reading one fact will generate discussion that continues for the entire session. Recommended areas include:

➤ properties of the drug
➤ addiction properties

> physical health risks
> mental health risks
> adverse effects.

Passages are followed by open questions, 'What do people think about this?' Direct the discussion towards experiential responses. 'Does anyone know anyone this has happened to?' Individuals will likely validate the information. If so, reiterate that the literature appears to be correct because a number of individuals have witnessed or experienced this.

Dynamic balancing is used to elicit discussion of reasons to change, acknowledgement of risks, consequences, adversity and benefits of change. A group member responds to a passage: 'That happened to me. I went over the edge and I could not get back any more.' Ask for elaboration: 'Tell us more about that.' Using dynamic balancing, the leader may now shift from 'I' to 'We'. 'Has that ever happened to anyone else?' Or 'Does anyone know anyone that has happened to?' This may elicit acknowledgement of adversity from other group members.

The focus remains on learning about cocaine throughout the session. This may include effects upon brain chemistry, evoking acute symptoms or physical addiction and withdrawal effects. Information provided via handouts, videos and the like is deemed accurate when individuals validate it, and they usually do.

Everyone's opinion is respected. The leader may provide her/his opinion at the end of the meeting and address facts that may not have been highlighted by the group. Leaders do not present themselves as experts. They acknowledge what they have learned from the materials and from the group members.

The use of video in groups entails a topic, i.e. 'Women in treatment'. In a one-hour session, 15 minutes of a video will be viewed. Video segments are followed up with open questions: 'What stood out for you in this video?' Discuss. The remainder of the video can be viewed in segments in subsequent meetings.

The inclusion of outside speakers: an outside speaker may be another professional – a nurse who may discuss nutrition; a doctor who may discuss interactions between medication and illicit substances – speakers from the community, and so forth. The speaker's topic is followed by discussion. Group members must consent to the participation of an outsider or opt not to attend the session.

THEME-CENTRED GROUPS THAT ARE NOT LABELLED MENTAL HEALTH–SUBSTANCE USE BUT ADDRESS MENTAL HEALTH–SUBSTANCE USE DISORDERS

Theme: 'Coping with stress'

This theme could be the title for the group or the theme for one session. Individuals discuss areas in their present life that result in stress. Stress is normalised, everyone has stress limits. Facilitate explorations of the individuals' emotional reactions to the stressors, sadness, isolation, anger, fear and the relationship of these emotions to substance use, abstinence and mental health symptoms. Learning new coping strategies flows easily and other participants may be included in role plays, etc. The objectives and benefits of this theme include:

➤ providing an opportunity to discuss one's emotional life without being labelled mentally ill
➤ an opportunity to identify interaction effects between emotional experiences (or lack of experiencing) and substance use or abstinence.

Here the leader has the opportunity to normalise emotions, yielding them comfortable to discuss, while evaluating emotional experiences as situational versus representative of a mental health problem. As the group progresses and is more accepting of emotional issues, the leader may offer education and information that is comprehensive and related to specific symptoms and disorders; for example, depression. This will deepen the learning experience and assist individuals to determine whether or not recovery from substance use disorders is hindered by mental health issues or lack of coping skills and the potential benefits of additional help.

Theme: 'Understanding relationships'

This theme can be used as a title of a group or an individual session. It is beneficial for individuals with a history of trauma, abusive relationships, poor family histories, etc.

Participants begin this exploration in the here and now and consider their present relationships, i.e. with their child, partner, probation officer, parent, counsellor, etc.

➤ What are the emotional responses to positive and negative experiences within these relationships?
➤ How do these emotions interact with substance use, sobriety or mental health?

As the group progresses into a supportive, trusting, cohesive group, the leader takes this to a deeper level. The focus could include looking back at similar past relationships and comparing them to present relationships. Participants may identify the origins of their experiences in relationships, their emotional responses, and their choices. Formal information regarding trauma could be provided as sub-themes and be explored in more depth. Topics such as behaviours and symptoms resulting from abuse, low self-esteem, communication, etc. can be clarified. New responses and coping strategies can be practised. Individuals may move into action by including additional treatment, medication and alternative living situations.

The leader has an opportunity to evaluate the individuals' emotional experiences to determine whether they are situational and transient or enduring mental health symptoms.

Theme: 'Understanding how people change'

It is important for individuals to understand that change is 'incremental'. The stages of change can be reviewed experientially.[20] Emphasise that each stage is normal and not indicative of uncooperativeness or weakness.

CONCLUSION

The broader impact of integrated treatment and stages of change

Integrated treatment for individuals experiencing mental health–substance use disorders permits the individual to access services within the system and programme that they are most comfortable or identified with. The individual is not sent to another programme or system to address the mental health–substance use problem. This is particularly important in the early stages of change. The individual who is in the precontemplation stage regarding symptoms is not likely to attend another programme to address them. Stage and phase interventions provide the opportunity to explore and recognise the need for additional help by advancing through the stages of change and readiness levels. Without stage-matched interventions, it would be unlikely that the individual would progress to recognition of symptoms and the need for treatment.

When success is measured only in 'action' stage terms we declare failure when there may be success. This leaves no opportunity to commend the individual for his/her progress and support confidence and hope. Incremental change provides the opportunity to chart success on a number of criteria, each one representing movement and change versus stagnation and failure. This includes the success of the individual, professional and organisation, etc. Change is viewed as a process and 'intrinsic' change is the goal. Change that rests on a foundation of thorough exploration and personal decision-making rather than coercion or bribery is far more likely to be sustained.

REFERENCES

1 McHugo GJ, Drake RE, Teague GB, *et al.* Fidelity of assertive community treatment and outcome in the New Hampshire Dual Disorders Study. *Psychiatric Services.* 1999; **50**: 818–24.
2 Drake RE, McHugo GL, Xie H, *et al.* Ten-year recovery outcomes for clients with severe mental illness. *Schizophrenia Bulletin.* 2006; **32**: 464–73.
3 Sciacca K, Thompson CM. Program development and integrated treatment across systems for dual diagnosis: Mental illness, drug addiction and alcoholism, MIDAA. *The Journal of Mental Health Administration.* 1996; **23**(3): 288–97.
4 Sciacca K. An integrated treatment approach for severely mentally ill individuals with substance disorders. In: Minkoff K, Drake R, editors. *New Directions for Mental Health Services, Dual Diagnosis of Major Mental Illness and Substance Disorders.* New York: Jossey-Bass; 1991.
5 Sciacca K. Best practices for dual diagnosis treatment and program development: co-occurring mental illness and substance disorders in various combinations. *The Praeger International Collection on Addictions.* 2009; **3**: 161–88.
6 Sciacca K. GA seeks statewide implementation of dual-diagnosis strategy. *Alcoholism and Drug Abuse Weekly.* 2003; **15**(17): 1, 6–7.
7 Sciacca K. Removing barriers: dual diagnosis treatment and motivational interviewing. *Professional Counselor.* 1997; **12**(1): 41–6.
8 Sciacca K. Curriculum for MICAA and CAMI direct care providers: Mental Illness, Drug Addiction and Alcoholism MIDAA(R): training, cross-training and program development. In: SAMHSA-CMHS. *Managed Care Initiative Co-Occurring Disorder Report: co-occurring psychiatric and substance disorders in managed care systems: standards of care, practice*

guidelines, workforce competencies and training curricula. Rockville, MD: Center for Mental Health Services, 1998.

9 Sciacca K. Tennessee initiates state-wide dual diagnosis program development. *Alcoholism and Drug Abuse Weekly.* 1998; **10**(7): 5.

10 Sciacca K. DC reports progress with dual diagnosis integration initiative. *Alcoholism and Drug Abuse Weekly.* 1999; **11**(41): 5.

11 Sciacca K. Theme-Centered Interactional (TCI) Group Leading and the Workshop Institute for Living-Learning WILL, an overview. *MINT Bulletin.* 2001; **8**: 5–11.

12 Sciacca K. On co-occurring addictive and mental disorders: a brief history of the origins of dual diagnosis treatment and program development. [Invited Response.] *American Journal of Orthopsychiatry.* 1996; **66**: 474–5.

13 SAMHSA, CMHS. *Managed Care Initiative Co-Occurring Disorder Panel Report: co-occurring psychiatric and substance disorders in managed care systems: standards of care, practice guidelines, workforce competencies and training curricula.* Rockville, MD: Center for Mental Health Services, 1998.

14 Sciacca K. *MIDAA Service Manual: a step by step guide to program implementation and comprehensive services for dual/multiple disorders.* New York: Sciacca Comprehensive Service Development for MIDAA; 2008.

15 Sciacca K. Client disposition form. In: *MIDAA Service Manual.* 2nd ed. New York: Sciacca Comprehensive Service Development for MIDAA; forthcoming 2011.

16 Rogers CR, Significant aspects of client-centered therapy. *American Psychologist.* 1946; **1**: 415–22.

17 Sciacca K. Dual diagnosis treatment and motivational interviewing for co-occurring disorders. *National Council Magazine.* 2007; **2**: 22–3.

18 Cohn RC. The theme-centered interactional method: group therapists as group educators. *The Journal of Group Psychoanalysis and Process.* 1969; **2**(2): 19–36.

19 Miller WR, Rollnick S. *Motivational Interviewing: preparing people to change addictive behavior.* New York: Guilford Press; 1991.

20 Prochaska JO, DiClemente CC. *Transtheoretical Approach: crossing traditional boundaries of therapy.* Homewood, IL: Dorsey Press; 1984.

21 Sciacca K, Dobbins KR. Kentucky dual diagnosis residence yields remarkable outcome. *Mental Health Weekly.* 2001; **11**(7): 5.

TO LEARN MORE

- Educational resources. Available at: www.scribd.com/people/documents/13909546?from_badge_documents_inline=1
- Education and training events. Available at: http://users.erols.com/ksciacca/upcom.htm
- Motivational interviewing training seminars. Available at: http://users.erols.com/ksciacca/ordmot.htm

CHAPTER 10

Cognitive behavioural therapy: mental health–substance use

Anne Garland

INTRODUCTION

This chapter aims to describe the fundamental principles of cognitive behavioural therapy (CBT) theory, its basic treatment rationale and process for making psychological sense of a person's problems. The model described places most emphasis on the cognitive therapy of Beck[1,2] and the British scientist-practitioners who have over the last 20 years significantly advanced the evidence base of CBT treatments for anxiety disorders[3-6] and depression.[7-11] It is the work of Beck[1,2] and these mainly British scientist-practitioners that has greatly influenced the author's clinical work and research, and thus forms the basis of the theory and practice described in this chapter. However, it is also important to acknowledge the significant contribution the behavioural psychotherapy tradition has made to CBT literature, research and clinical practice. Behaviour therapy would undoubtedly have been a central aspect of the clinical training of the scientist-practitioners named previously and was the initial psychotherapy training undertaken by the author.[12-16] This chapter aims to encourage the reader to approach CBT in the spirit of the scientist-practitioner.[17,18] This model encourages the professional to approach their work with an enquiring mind and not only to use treatments that have been empirically validated using the scientific method, but to generate further research data by investigating the efficacy of their own clinical practice using the scientific method. In the author's view, the scientist-practitioner model is fundamental to how CBT is defined as a treatment modality.

WHAT IS COGNITIVE BEHAVIOURAL THERAPY?

KEY POINT 10.1

Cognitive behavioural therapy (CBT) is a structured, problem-solving treatment that has a strong evidence base[19,20] in the treatment and management of anxiety disorders and depression.

Cognitive behavioural therapy is a structured, problem-solving treatment that has a strong evidence base[19,20] in the treatment and management of anxiety disorders and depression. The clinical focus of CBT is on the individual's current problems, with the aim of equipping the person with practical skills to tackle problems that interfere with her/his day-to-day functioning. The treatment is goal-orientated, in that goals are agreed between the individual and professional, usually in terms of improving current problems in three domains, namely:

1   practical day-to-day problems
2   intrapersonal problems
3   interpersonal problems.[21]

Each step of the CBT assessment and treatment process is explicitly shared with the individual and the foundation of the therapeutic relationship (*see* Chapter 2) is collaborative empiricism. In this paradigm the individual and professional work together to make psychological sense within a CBT model of what factors are maintaining the person's problems. This is referred to as a maintenance formulation[22] and is shared with the person as a hypothesis to be tested during treatment. Thus, a central aspect of treatment is the use of what is referred to as behavioural experiments[23] to test out hypotheses in order to collect evidence to validate or refute these hypotheses. The evidence collected is then used to devise further behavioural experiments in order to solve problems and to develop different ways of experiencing self and others and new ways of acting in the world.

A word of caution

It needs to be acknowledged that there are a many different 'schools' of cognitive behavioural therapy. Gilbert[24] identified at least 16 schools of CBT each of which place different emphases on behavioural and/or cognitive elements and/or interpersonal factors within CBT theory and practice. For example, if the reader compares the work of Marks and colleagues[25] with that of Barlow and colleagues,[26] and Clark and colleagues,[27] in the treatment of panic and agoraphobia, the treatment methods, while sharing some commonalities, also contain some divergent theoretical principles and interventions. In addition, some CBT models are more evidence based than others and it is a mistake to assume that the acronym CBT is synonymous with the idea of its treatments being evidence based. For example Young's Schema-Focused Cognitive Therapy,[28] while drawing on some of Beck's[1,2] original theory and treatment methods has also introduced new interventions and has only limited empirical data supporting its efficacy. Similarly, the Rational-Emotive Behaviour Therapy developed by Ellis[29] and developed by Dryden[30] and associates in the UK has less supporting evidence.

KEY ELEMENTS OF CBT

Some authors describe the key elements of CBT as follows:[31]

➤   The importance of a shared psychological understanding of the problem. In the CBT literature this is referred to as formulation[32,33] or conceptualisation.[34,35]

➤   The emphasis on the individual's distinct experience.

➤ The collaborative nature of the therapeutic relationship (more recently the interpersonal dynamics between individual and professional has been emphasised[36]).

➤ Active involvement of the individual, particularly in devising homework tasks.

➤ The use of Socratic questioning.[37] Essentially, this means asking different types of questions within a specific structure in such a way that a dialogue occurs that promotes self-understanding, which is then used as a basis for taking action.

➤ Explicitness of the professional – usually little or nothing should be kept back from the individual.

➤ The emphasis on empiricism, which means gaining knowledge from experience, and to use this to guide future action.

➤ The importance placed upon what happens outside the session.

TREATMENT RATIONALE

Central to the cognitive behavioural model is the idea of a normalising treatment rationale. Thus, the emotional responses that characterise anxious and depressive states are seen to exist on a continuum with normal emotional reactions that we experience every day. Thus, when looking at the evidence base for CBT treatments, there is a wealth of research data that demonstrates many of the cognitive and behavioural features of anxiety disorders and depression present in non-clinical populations. Examples include:

➤ the frequency of reported intrusions (a feature of obsessive–compulsive disorder and generalised anxiety disorder) in the general population

➤ experiments in mood induction demonstrating a link between low mood and negative thoughts in both depressed and non-depressed individuals and the tendency for all humans when anxious to pay more attention to the object or event which is the focus of our fear, as demonstrated in threat cue detection experiments.

For comprehensive reviews of this literature *see* Williams, Watts, MacLeod *et al.*[11] and Harvey, Watkins, Mansell *et al.*[38]

REFLECTIVE PRACTICE EXERCISE 10.1

Time: 5 minutes
What is the difference between a normal human response to distress and the nature of the response that is seen in emotional disorders?

The difference between a normal human response to distress and the nature of the response seen in emotional disorders is that in emotional disorders these emotional responses are seen as more intense, persistent and out of proportion with our usual responses.

SHARING A BASIC CBT FORMULATION WITH THE INDIVIDUAL: THE VICIOUS CIRCLE METAPHOR

The most basic formulation and treatment rationale in CBT looks at the interrelationship between five elements:

1 environment
2 thoughts
3 feelings
4 physical sensations
5 behaviour.

This is referred to as a generic vicious circle maintenance formulation. This is usually described as a vicious circle and it is this metaphor that is used as a basic treatment rationale when first introducing individuals to CBT as a model (*see* Figure 10.1[37,38]).

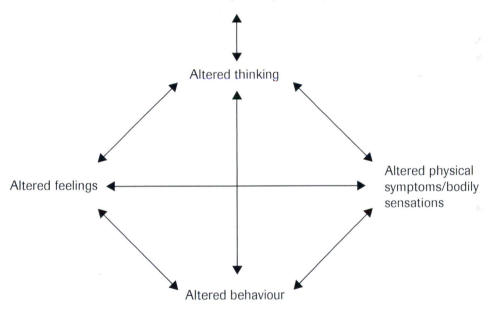

Life situation, relationships and practical problems

Altered thinking

Altered feelings

Altered physical symptoms/bodily sensations

Altered behaviour

FIGURE 10.1 Williams' generic vicious circle maintenance formulation using the Five Areas Approach[39,40]

Examples of this in the CBT literature are Williams,[39,40] and Greenberger and Padesky.[41] Typically, this model is shared collaboratively with the individual using an example from the individual's own experience. The basic message in the rationale is one of aiming to break the vicious circle by making an intervention at any one of the five elements in the circle.

The evidence base for CBT interventions is derived from research trials that use disorder-specific treatment protocols for a range of anxiety disorders and depression.[22] In CBT each disorder-specific models for anxiety such as panic disorder,[3] or social phobia[42] is presented as a vicious circle with each element (environment, thoughts, feelings, physical sensations and behaviour) represented but tailored to the clinical features defining the anxiety disorder in question.[22,42] The scientist-practitioner model would encourage the professional, wherever possible, to use a disorder-specific model to introduce the individual to the CBT treatment rationale. However, there is no disorder-specific model for depression and this generic vicious circle is the standard format for presenting a maintenance formulation to the individual who is experiencing depression. Moreover, it is often helpful to substitute the phrase physical sensations for biological symptoms.[43]

MAKING PSYCHOLOGICAL SENSE OF INDIVIDUALS' PROBLEMS WITHIN THE CBT MODEL

Within the CBT model, the individual and professional work in collaboration to make psychological sense of the individual's problems. There are two stages to this process in CBT.

1 Maintenance formulation (as described above), which refers to a generic or disorder-specific vicious circle formulation
2 Longitudinal formulation, where links are made between beliefs, attitudes and values from childhood experiences, critical incidents that precipitate current problems and the maintenance formulation in the form of the disorder-specific model or the generic vicious circle model.

Central to the Beckian model described here is the role of cognition, and different levels of thinking are represented in the formulation. These different levels of thinking are described below.

THE THREE LEVELS OF THINKING IN CBT

Within the CBT model there are three levels of thinking or cognition, which over the last 30 years have been defined, described and elaborated in a variety of ways.[1,2,22,41,44] The language used to describe these levels of thinking varies among texts and can seem complex and confusing to both the professional and the individual. Therefore, in order to simplify the language and bring clarity, the following terms have been chosen to label the three levels of thinking. After each term are the terms that are used in the broader CBT literature to describe each level of thinking. These specific labels have been chosen for their ease of use which makes the treatment much more accessible. The three levels of thinking in CBT are:

1 **Negative automatic thoughts** (NATS) – negative thoughts; automatic negative thoughts
2 **Rules for living** – dysfunctional assumptions; conditional beliefs
3 **Core beliefs** – schemas; schemata; unconditional beliefs.

From a theoretical perspective these three levels are connected, and this is best explained using a metaphor. If we were to consider the three levels in terms of a tree, the core beliefs would represent the roots that secure the tree in the ground and feed the tree with nutrients to maintain its growth (level 3). The rules for living would represent the trunk and branches that give the tree its structure and form (level 2). Finally, the negative automatic thoughts (NATS) would represent the leaves that cover the tree (level 1) and require the roots, trunk and branches to survive while reciprocally the leaves take in sunlight to sustain the branches, trunk and roots.

Level 3: core beliefs – the root of the problem

Expressed in psychological terms the core beliefs are seen as being formed in early childhood and adolescence and are viewed as being tacitly held as unquestionable truths about self, others, self in relation to others and the world. They are associated with high levels of emotional arousal. These beliefs represent our sense of self or how we experience ourselves as individuals. They are usually formulated as statements as follows: 'I am . . .', 'others are . . .', 'world is . . .'. For example, typically in depression, the following themes to core beliefs can be formulated: 'I am a failure, other people are better than me, and the world is hostile.'

Within the CBT model core beliefs are viewed as mechanisms through which an individual processes information and it is this information-processing mechanism that is viewed as driving the psychological component of emotional disorders, of which the rules for living are a related process and NATS are a product. From the perspective of an anxiety disorder or depression, core beliefs are seen to have built into them a selective bias in terms of how information is processed.

Case study 10.1 Part I: Angela – generalised anxiety disorder (GAD)

Angela (35) has a 15-year history of generalised anxiety disorder. She is the elder of two children with a sister four years younger than she is. Her father died suddenly when Angela was 10 years old. Her mother was unable to cope with the loss of her husband and became depressed and anxious. She managed this initially with alcohol and then cannabis and heroin. Angela became the main carer for both her sister and her mother. At 13, her school attendance had become irregular as she would worry about her mother's well-being and would stay at home to take care of her and try to limit her mother's drug and alcohol intake. Angela took responsibility for managing the house on a day-to-day basis. She would often return home to find men she did not know in the house and, at age 15, she witnessed a man die from a heroin overdose in the living room of the family home. On a number of occasions these men, whom her mother brought to the house, would make sexual advances towards Angela.

Core beliefs formulated in treatment are:
➤ I am vulnerable.
➤ People take advantage.
➤ The world is unpredictable.

Beckian theory holds that core beliefs are formed in childhood and adolescence because of experiences in our lives. While traumatic events such as abuse or bereavement in childhood can clearly lead to the development of strongly held core beliefs regarding self, others and the world, most people's beliefs at this level are a product of their general environment during childhood, which will be a range of different experiences. Young[28] describes core beliefs as being the product of a general noxious environment rather than the result of any one-off traumatic events. According to Beckian theory,[1,2,41] it is our rules for living and core beliefs that represent the individual's psychological vulnerability to depression and anxiety. Thus, these beliefs may lay dormant but are activated by critical incidents that in some way mirror the circumstances in childhood which led to the development of the core belief(s) and rule(s) for living.

SELF-ASSESSMENT EXERCISE 10.1

> **Time: 10 minutes**
> ● Consider the key events in Angela's childhood.
> ● Make notes of your identified findings.

Level 2: rules for living: the trunk and the branches – how the core beliefs are expressed in action

Rules for living are defined as principles that guide a person's behaviour. A defining feature of rules for living is that they operate across situations, and then they tend to exert an influence over several areas of a person's life. The behaviours an individual does and does not engage in are useful markers for identifying the themes in rules for living.

Rules for living are usually formulated in two ways as follows:

1   Those formulated as conditional *statements*: 'If . . . then . . .' or 'Unless . . . then . . .'.
2   This relates to rules for living formulated as *'demand' statements*. For example, 'I should; I must; I ought'. Rules, which are phrased as demand statements, are often associated with a strong sense of duty and morality and are often harder to tackle in treatment.

These rules for living are directly linked to the behaviours in which we engage (or avoid) in order to maintain our self-esteem and our sense of safety and security and prevent the core beliefs from being activated. Thus, provided we can meet the conditions or demand laid out for us by our rules, our self-esteem and sense of safety and security remains intact, the core beliefs are not activated and we function well. However, if for any reason our ability to keep to the conditions or demand within our rules is compromised, according to Beckian theory, this triggers our psychological vulnerability in that the core beliefs are activated, making us vulnerable to anxiety and depression. In addition, the childhood circumstances that lead to the development of these rules can mean that the demands of our rules are ultimately unrealistic and increase our vulnerability further.

In keeping with the normalisation rationale described previously, the CBT model would say we all have rules for living that guide our behavioural choices. Indeed Beckian theory holds that these rules are directly derived from our upbringing, and often reflect culturally shared values from family, school, religion, social class and the like. A defining feature of such rules is that the person holds them rigidly, often with a high degree of conviction, and often it is this inflexibility that is problematic rather than the content of the rule itself.

How do we identify rules for living?

The limited scope of this text means an in-depth discussion of methods for identifying core beliefs, rules and NATS cannot be undertaken. A useful starting point for identifying rules for living is to consider the following three themes:

1 PERFECTION/HIGH OR UNRELENTING STANDARDS/DOING THINGS PROPERLY/LIVING UP TO IDEALS

For example:

➤ 'If I can't do something properly, there is no point in doing it at all.'
➤ 'If I can't finish something, there is no point in starting.'
➤ 'If I make a mistake, I am a failure.'
➤ 'I should always strive to live up to my potential.'
➤ 'If I push myself really hard, I can achieve anything.'
➤ 'If I am perfect, people will love me.'

KEY POINT 10.2

The key is to always use the person's own language.

In considering the differences between these themes, what is key is to always use the person's language and to try to identify the specific meanings for each individual. For example, many people recognise a tendency in wanting to complete a task to a high standard. Indeed this information is often spontaneously offered, closely followed by the statement 'I'm not a perfectionist you know'. This is often a reflection of the fact the person recognises it is not possible to do things perfectly but does not recognise the possibility that they are striving towards an unrealistic cherished ideal of things being perfect. This often results in the perception of a performance gap between how they complete a task and the cherished ideal. This can lead the individual to avoid or put off certain activities or conversely drive the person hard to strive to live up to his/her unrealistic cherished ideal. Similarly, with the idea of 'doing something properly', the person may have in their mind a predetermined method and unrealistic set of standards by which a task needs to be completed and if they are not achieved it leads to frustration and disappointment.

REFLECTIVE PRACTICE EXERCISE 10.2

Time: 15 minutes
- Reflect on how many times a parent or teacher said to you as a child or you yourself have said to a partner or child, 'You are not doing it properly!'
- What does this actually mean?
- What is the standard that is being requested?

- Do you think it is realistic?
- Do you agree?

When an individual pushes themselves to meet unrelenting standards[28,45] they can have difficulty recognising this as a problem, often because they are very successful. Such individuals are often continually active, achieving one goal only to move onto the next without savouring the success of the achievement, and any sense of pleasure is often derived from working hard. Their unrelenting standards will be applied to everything they do, work, sporting activities, hobbies and relationships.

Clinical experience tells us these themes are common in depression but may also be significant in relation to feelings of frustration and anger.

2 APPROVAL/SUBJUGATION

For example:
➤ 'If I don't do what others want, they will reject me.'
➤ 'If I don't put others needs first, I will be punished.'
➤ 'If I put myself first, then I am selfish.'
➤ 'I should think of others before myself.'
➤ 'If someone has a problem, it is up to me to sort it out.'

In considering the distinction between approval and subjugation, it is useful to think of these on a continuum, as a way of providing guidance as to how difficult it may be to work with rules formulated within this theme. Someone who has a need for approval usually recognises that they have needs, rights and wants but have difficulty getting these met, often for fear of disapproval or criticism. This is very common in the general population. Meanwhile someone with a subjugation-based rule usually is unable to recognise that they are entitled to have needs, rights and wants and are unable to say what these are when asked. This is often present in therapy with either excessive passivity and deference or on occasion guardedness and hostility. This is usually a result of being raised in environments where their relationships with adults were based on putting the adults' needs first. This may have been in a role as caretaker for a parent or younger siblings. As adults, such individuals frequently pursue careers in the caring professions and enter relationships where they take high levels of responsibility for others' well-being. In the case of physical and emotional abuse, subjugating self usually helps the child stay safe from harm and, as adults, individuals who have experienced such treatment may have difficulty trusting others, anticipating exploitation, hostility or punishment, and they may be highly avoidant of conflict or expressing their own opinion for fear of reprisal. The theme of subjugation is especially important in relation to sexual abuse where the child is usually forced both to a physical and psychological subjugation position in order to meet the sexual needs of adults. This often results in extreme mistrust, passivity and powerlessness.[28,45] The need for approval is associated with onset of depression and clinical practice tells us approval and subjugation are also associated with high levels of anxiety, shame and guilt.

3 CONTROL

For example:

➤ 'If I'm not in control, something bad will happen.'
➤ 'If I'm not in control, it is a sign of weakness.'
➤ 'If I don't control my thoughts and feelings, I will go mad.'
➤ 'I should be in control at all times.'

This theme is common in the anxiety disorders and anxiety is the most commonly occurring emotional state in relation to this theme. It often arises in more chronic mental health presentations where the symptoms of the illness itself may be experienced as out of control. Examples include:

➤ psychosis
➤ mania
➤ chronic depression (characterised by rumination)
➤ chronic worry
➤ suicidality
➤ obsessive–compulsive disorder (OCD – where there is a high frequency of intrusive thoughts)
➤ borderline personality disorder.

When this theme is present individuals often put a great deal of mental and behavioural effort into strategies that they perceive help them maintain a sense of being in control. This may include:

➤ monitoring their thought processes for perceived unacceptable thoughts (OCD; psychosis)
➤ monitoring their bodily sensations for signs of danger (panic disorder, health anxiety)
➤ always keeping active in order to avoid focusing on thoughts and feelings (chronic depression)
➤ maintaining a very tidy home environment (OCD; chronic depression).

It is important to note that for ease of understanding, these themes are presented as discrete categories. The reality of clinical practice is somewhat different. Thus, when working with the individual, the critical skill to develop is the ability to define and describe rules for living, using the person's own language. Only by doing this will you capture the idiosyncratic meaning of each individual's experience. Identifying and working with this idiosyncratic meaning is important because it is this that taps into the key emotions that need to be active for CBT strategies to be effective.

Case study 10.1 Part II

Angela and her therapist identified two rules for living as follows:

1 'If I am not in control at all times, something bad will happen.'
2 'I should be responsible at all times.'

In considering the interrelationship between core beliefs and rules for living, Beckian theory holds that it is these beliefs, which form the psychological vulnerability to anxiety disorders and depression, specifically where a life event mirrors the circumstances in which the belief system was developed and elaborated. Thus, for Angela, key events in her childhood were:

- father dying at age 10
- mother unable to cope and using drugs and alcohol to cope with her own grief
- loss of parenting from mother and Angela taking on role of carer for mother and younger sister
- loss of usual structure and routine at home, school and socially
- witnessing man dying from drug overdose in own home
- from age 15, sexual harassment from unknown men whom her mother brought to the house.

The triggering event for the onset of Angela's difficulties at age 20 was becoming a mother. She has two daughters with her husband David, Julie (15) and Susan (10). David is a caring and supportive husband and they have been together since Angela was 17. Angela has always worried about the children's safety since they were born and has a tendency to be overprotective, trying to meet their physical and emotional needs to a high standard, restricting the children's activities outside of the home, taking and collecting them from school and insisting on knowing their whereabouts at all times, asking them to telephone her two or three times per day to check they are safe. Over the last two years, this has caused frequent arguments between Angela and her eldest daughter Julie. Angela recently came into contact with mental health services when she discovered Susan had been truanting from school, smoking cannabis and mixing with a group of 18-year-old boys. As a result Angela became extremely anxious, unable to sleep and worrying excessively on a daily basis. Within the CBT model it was hypothesised that the psychological triggers to the exacerbation of her predisposing anxiety difficulties was the activation of the belief system in which the conditions and demands of her rules for living were compromised, thus activating the core beliefs.

Rules for living compromised:
- 'If I am not in control at all times, something bad will happen.'
- 'I should be responsible.'

Core beliefs activated:
- 'I am vulnerable'
- 'People take advantage'
- 'The world is unpredictable'

It is possible to see the unrealistic and excessive nature of Angela's rules for living in that as children get older parents have less control over their activities. In addition, it could be hypothesised that Angela's over-control of the children's activities may lead to either overt rebellion on the part of the children or for them to be ill-prepared for surviving in the world, both of which may make them more vulnerable to the types of experiences Angela herself experienced in childhood and which she is seeking to protect them from.

Level 1: negative automatic thoughts (NATS): the leaves on the tree

Negative automatic thoughts are the direct product of both our core beliefs and rules for living, and there are two areas to consider in relation to these:

1 **content** of thinking
2 **process** of thinking.

These will be considered in turn as follows:
- ➤ thought **content** that is, *what* we think
- ➤ thought **processes**, that is, *how* we think.

What we think: thought content

In Beck's[1,2] model NATS are defined as an individual's appraisal of a specific situation or event. As such, this level of cognition represents what is going through an individual's mind in a particular situation and may be associated with pleasant, unpleasant or neutral emotional states. Within the CBT model the NATS that the professional is most interested in are those that are most closely associated with high levels of negative emotion such as anxiety, low mood, guilt, shame and anger and the like, hence the use of the label negative automatic thoughts. The content component of NATS can occur in two forms:

1 words
2 images or pictures in the mind's eye.

Each disorder-specific CBT model identifies different themes in terms of the content of NATS (and rules for living). Thus, for example, in panic disorder[3] the content theme in NATS is *a catastrophic misinterpretation of bodily sensations* and typical NATS are:

- ➤ *verbal or words*: for example, 'I'm going to faint', 'I'm going crazy'
- ➤ *an image or picture in the mind's eye*: for example, image of self flailing one's arms uncontrollably and running around the streets shouting and screaming. Imagery is a key cognitive component of anxiety disorders.

How we think: information-processing biases

In Beck's[1,2] original model these information-processing biases are referred to as 'thinking errors' or 'cognitive distortions'. Within Beck's clinical model the content of each NAT is said to contain information-processing biases and particular types of information-processing bias can be identified in relation to depression and anxiety. These are as follows:

- ➤ catastrophising
- ➤ jumping to conclusions

- mind reading
- black and white thinking
- personalisation
- should statements
- mental filter
- overgeneralisation
- labelling
- disqualifying the positive
- emotional reasoning.

Current clinical practice tends to now refer to these as *information-processing biases*. The categories defined by Beck[1,2] in his original work are derived from clinical observation. Over the last 30 years ongoing research in the field of cognitive science has developed evidence to support Beck's clinical observations of these information-processing biases and further elaborate how they maintain mental health problems. Examples of this research evidence exists[11,38] to support the idea that, in anxiety and depression, *how* information is processed is biased in a way that means only certain types of information is taken on board or given more attention and weight. These processing biases are viewed as central to the maintenance of emotional disorders by keeping the focus of attention on negative or threat-related information, and not attending to or discounting contrary information.

For example, staying with the cognitive model of panic disorder[3] there is research evidence (for an interesting discussion see Barlow[46]) to show that people experiencing panic disorder more readily detect and pay attention to changes in bodily sensations than non-anxious controls. Thus, if the panic-prone individual experiences a sensation of light-headedness, they not only detect this more quickly than non-panic-prone individuals, but they are more likely to appraise this as dangerous and threatening and they will conclude: 'I'm going to faint.' They are more likely to do this than ignoring the sensation or ascribing a more benign explanation to the sensation, such as: 'It's just a feeling; it will pass.' In the literature this is referred to as threat cue detection.[11,38,46] Similarly in depression, research evidence shows that not only is the content of thought negative but also a key processing bias that is central to the maintenance of depression is black-and-white thinking.[11,38]

These information-processing biases in common mental health problems can be briefly summarised as follows.

ANXIETY DISORDERS
- Worry – generalised anxiety disorder.
- Anxious intrusions – generalised anxiety disorder/obsessive–compulsive disorder/post-traumatic stress disorder/health anxiety/social phobia.
- Anxious rumination – generalised anxiety disorder/obsessive–compulsive disorder.

DEPRESSION
- Depressive rumination
- Intrusive memories of past unpleasant events

➤ Autobiographical memory
➤ Over general memory.

For sake of clarity, these are presented here as distinct categories. However, in the reality of clinical practice where individuals frequently present with comorbid anxiety and/or depression, people may experience a combination of the above.

There are two important distinctions to be made between NATS and rules for living, as follows:

1   While NATS represent our *appraisal of a specific situation or event*, rules for living operate *across situations*.
2   While NATS are *biased in terms of content and process*, rules for living are *value judgements*, which rather than being inherently right or wrong are to a greater or lesser degree helpful or unhelpful.

Case study 10.1 Part III

Angela's presenting problem is generalised anxiety disorder (GAD). The CBT model for this disorder is formulated as follows:[22]

Content of thinking

- Negative predictions about future events in which the person perceives there is an increased perception of risk combined with a decreased perception of their ability to cope. In other words, the person believes something bad is going to happen and they have neither the internal nor external resources to cope with it. For example, for Angela, verbal NATS form content of worry: 'What if Julie becomes a drug addict/is raped/gets murdered? It will be my fault. Susan will be taken into care, David will leave me.' Images within the worry: image of Julie lying dead with a needle in her arm, and Angela as her mother tries to revive her.
- The themes of unpredictability, unreliability and uncontrollability, for example 'I must take control', 'I must stop Julie doing these things.'

Process of thinking

Worry is a future-orientated ruminative process in which the above content is turned over and over in Angela's mind, repeatedly re-intruding as Angela tries to suppress these NATS (words and images) and push them from her mind, thus fuelling her anxiety.

In terms of the evidence base there is equivocal empirical data to support Beck's original hypothesis that rules for living and core beliefs represent a trait cognitive vulnerability to depression and anxiety disorder.[1,2] What data does exist supports the idea that such constructs are mood-dependent phenomena that dissipate once anxiety and depression lifts.[11,38] There is currently much debate regarding the implications of such data for the practice of CBT. It is the author's view that working with rules for living in relation to the maintenance of current distress has clinical validity.

HOW IS CBT APPLIED IN PRACTICE?

The overall aim of CBT is to modify each level of thinking. There is an assumption that work always starts at the level of NATS, working with both content (*what* a person thinks) and process (*how* a person thinks). This is based on the idea that content and process are:

➤ central to the maintenance of current problems
➤ the most readily accessible aspect of thinking
➤ the ones that can most readily be tackled, resulting in the most rapid symptom relief.

A further reason for not tackling rules for living and core beliefs in the first instance is that they are more closely associated with our sense of self-esteem and ourselves and tackling them is likely to give rise to high levels of emotion, which may worsen rather than alleviate distress. Thus, the individual needs to be equipped with skills to manage such emotion. These skills are acquired from work carried out at the level of NATS. The skills learned at this point in treatment are crucial if the individual and professional take the decision to carry out work on modifying rules for living and core beliefs. Any attempt to work on them will lead to a temporary exacerbation of low mood and anxiety. This is normal and necessary for this work to take place. However, the individual needs to have good grasp of the CBT skills taught at level one in order to use them while tackling levels two and three. Importantly, there is an assumption in CBT that each level of thinking is interconnected. As such, modifying NATS leads to increased flexibility in the rules for living and in turn direct work on these rules makes the processing mechanisms in core beliefs more flexible and adaptive. Thus, in short-term cognitive therapy (6–18 sessions) there is an assumption that the processing mechanisms in core beliefs are sufficiently adaptive, and that no direct work needs to be carried out on this level of thinking. However, as rules for living can play a key role in the maintenance of unhelpful behaviours that also maintain anxiety and depression, work at this level is required in order to reap lasting gains for the individual receiving treatment. It is a common mistake for people beginning to use CBT to think that CBT is 'about' verbally disputing some of the person's NATS. Although this is an element of CBT, it is really about identifying, understanding and breaking the vicious circle that is established between events in the individuals environment, the person's cognition (NATS generated by rules and beliefs), emotions, physiological symptoms and behaviours.[39,40]

CONCLUSION

What type of problems will best respond to CBT interventions?

An important consideration in deciding which individuals will benefit most from treatment is the evidence base for CBT. The CBT model has a long tradition of evaluating its efficacy and there is a robust set of research evidence demonstrating its utility in the treatment of a variety of psychological disorders. The strongest evidence base is for anxiety disorders and depression.[19,20]

Increasingly, cognitive behavioural interventions are being used to manage severe and enduring mental health problems such as bipolar disorder,[47] schizophrenia and psychosis,[48] and borderline personality disorder,[49] and is also applied in treating drug and alcohol problems[50] and chronic physical illnesses.

KEY POINT 10.3

It is vital that cognitive behavioural interventions are not seen as a panacea for tackling all psychological problems.

An important consideration is the goal of the intervention to be made. Namely, is the goal to treat the individual so that they become largely symptom free, or is it to help the individual to better manage a chronic and enduring illness? For many individuals and professionals the latter is often a more realistic goal.

The CBT assessment process can be applied to any individual presenting. The same is not necessarily true for CBT interventions. Decisions regarding which individuals will benefit from a CBT intervention can be complex and a number of factors play a role. These include:

➤ the nature of the presenting problem and its chronicity
➤ the degree to which the individual accepts the CBT rationale and can work within its principles
➤ personality factors
➤ hopelessness and pessimism.

A pragmatic discussion for the clinical implications of such factors can be found in Safran and Segal.[36] In addition, factors such as the level of the professional's adherence to the CBT model, the quality of CBT training undertaken, and the level of skill in delivering the intervention,[51,52] and the professional's optimism/pessimism regarding the individual also exert significant impact on treatment response.[11] There is much research still to be done in order to increase further the effectiveness of CBT interventions. In the spirit of the scientist-practitioner model,[17,18] this ongoing commitment to developing the evidence base of interventions and examining our own clinical practice lies at the heart of the CBT model. Equally, the dissemination of the existing interventions and skilling each professional in their implementation is still in its infancy.

REFERENCES

1 Beck T. *Cognitive Therapy and the Emotional Disorders*. New York: International Universities Press; 1976.

2 Beck AT, Rush AJ, Shaw BF, *et al. Cognitive Therapy for Depression*. New York: Guilford Press; 1979.

3 Clark DM. A cognitive approach to panic. *Behaviour Research and Therapy*. 1986; **24**: 461–70.

4 Salkovskis PM. Somatic problems. In: Hawton K, Salkovskis PM, Kirk J, *et al.*, editors. *Cognitive Behaviour Therapy for Psychiatric Problems: a practical guide*. Oxford: Oxford University Press; 1989.

5 Wells A. *Cognitive Therapy for Anxiety Disorders: a practical manual.* Chichester: Wiley; 1997.

6 Freeston MH, Rheaume J, Ladouceur R. Correcting faulty appraisals of obsessional thoughts. *Behaviour, Research and Therapy.* 1996; **34**: 433–46.

7 Scott J. Chronic depression: can cognitive therapy succeed where other treatments fail? *Behavioural and Cognitive Psychotherapy.* 1992; **20**: 25–36.

8 Fennell MJV. Low self-esteem: a cognitive perspective. *Behavioural and Cognitive Psychotherapy.* 1997; **25**: 1–26.

9 Gilbert P, editor. *Compassion: conceptualisations, research and use in psychotherapy.* Hove: Routledge; 2005.

10 Teasdale JD. Emotional processing, three modes of mind and prevention of relapse in depression. *Behaviour, Research and Therapy.* 1999; **37**: 53–77.

11 Williams JMG, Watts FN, MacLeod C, *et al. Cognitive Psychology and Emotional Disorders.* 2nd ed. Chichester: Wiley; 1997.

12 Gelder MG, Marks IM. Desensitisation and phobias: a crossover study. *British Journal of Psychiatry.* 1968; **114**: 323–8.

13 Marks IM. *Fears, Phobias and Rituals: panic, anxiety and their disorders.* New York: Oxford University Press; 1987.

14 Rachman SJ. Emotional processing. *Behaviour, Research and Therapy.* 1980; **18**: 51–60.

15 Ost LG. A maintenance programme for behavioural treatment for anxiety disorders. *Behaviour, Research and Therapy.* 1989; **27**: 123–30.

16 Davey GCL. Classical conditioning and the acquisition of human fears and phobias: a review and synthesis of the literature. *Advances in Behaviour, Research and Therapy.* 1992; **14**: 29–66.

17 Barlow DH, Hayes SC, Nelson RO. *The Scientist-Practitioner: research and accountability in clinical and educational settings.* New York: Pergamon Press; 1984.

18 Salkovskis PM. Empirically grounded clinical interventions: cognitive behavioural therapy progresses through a multi-dimensional approach to clinical science. *Behavioural and Cognitive Psychotherapy.* 2002; **30**: 3–9.

19 National Institute for Health and Clinical Excellence. *Depression: the treatment and management of depression in adults.* NICE guideline 90. London: NIHCE; 2009. Available at: http://guidance.nice.org.uk/CG90/NICEGuidance/pdf/English (accessed 12 September 2010).

20 National Institute for Health and Clinical Excellence. *Anxiety (amended): management of anxiety (panic disorder with or without agoraphobia and generalised anxiety disorder in adults in primary, secondary and community care.* NICE guideline 22. London: NIHCE; 2007. Available at: www.nice.org.uk/nicemedia/pdf/CG022NICEguidelineamended.pdf (accessed 12 September 2010).

21 Padeskey CA. Personal communication; 1994.

22 Kinsella P, Garland A. *Cognitive Behavioural Therapy for Mental Health Workers: a beginners guide.* Hove: Routledge; 2003.

23 Beenett-Levy J, Butler G, Fennell MJV, *et al. Oxford Guide to Behavioural Experiments in Cognitive Therapy.* Oxford: Oxford University Press; 2004.

24 Gilbert P. Personal communication; 1996.

25 Marks IM, Grey S, Cohen SD, *et al.* Imipramine and brief therapist aided exposure in agoraphobics having self-exposure homework: a controlled trial. *Archives of General Psychiatry.* 1983; **40**: 153–62.

26 Barlow DH, Craske MG, Cerny JA, *et al.* Behavioural treatment of panic disorder. *Behaviour Therapy.* 1989; **20**: 261–82.

27 Clark DM, Salkovskis PM, Hackmann A, *et al*. Brief cognitive therapy for panic disorder: a randomised controlled trial. *Journal of Consulting and Clinical Psychology*. 1999; **67**: 583–9.

28 Young JE. *Cognitive Therapy for Personality Disorder: a schema-focused approach*. Sarasota, FL: Professional Resources Press; 1994.

29 Ellis A. *Reason and Emotion in Psychotherapy*. Secaucas, NJ: Lyle Stuart; 1962.

30 Dryden W. *The Incredible Sulk*. London: Sheldon; 1992.

31 Blackburn IM, Twaddle V. *Cognitive Therapy in Action*. London: Souvenir Press; 1996.

32 Butler G. Clinical formulation. In: Bellack AS, Hersen M, editors. *Comprehensive Clinical Psychology*. Oxford: Pergamon Press; 1998.

33 Padesky CA, Kuyken W, Dudley R. *Collaborative Case Conceptualisation: working effectively with clients in cognitive behaviour therapy*. New York: Guilford Press; 2009.

34 Persons JB. *Cognitive Therapy in Practice: a case formulation approach*. New York: Norton; 1989.

35 Persons JB. *The Case Formulation Approach to Cognitive-Behaviour Therapy*. New York: Guilford Press; 2008.

36 Safran JD, Segal ZV. *Interpersonal Processes in Cognitive Therapy*. New York: Basic Books; 1996.

37 Padesky CA. Socratic questioning: changing minds or guided discovery? Keynote address. *European Congress of Behavioural and Cognitive Psychotherapies*. London; September, 1993.

38 Harvey AG, Watkins E, Mansell W, *et al*. *Cognitive-behavioural Processes across Psychological Disorders: a trans-diagnostic approach to research and treatment*. Oxford: Oxford University Press; 2004.

39 Williams CJ. *Overcoming Depression: a five areas approach*. 2nd ed. London: Hodder Arnold; 2006.

40 Williams CJ. *Overcoming Anxiety: a five areas approach*. London: Hodder Arnold; 2003.

41 Greenberger D, Padesky CA. *Mind over Mood: a cognitive therapy treatment manual for clients*. New York: Guilford Press; 1995.

42 Wells A, Clark DM. Social phobia: a cognitive approach. In: Davey GLC, editor. *Phobias: a handbook of description, treatment and theory*. Chichester: Wiley; 1997.

43 Moore RG, Garland A. *Cognitive Therapy for Chronic and Persistent Depression*. Chichester: Wiley; 2003.

44 Beck J. *Cognitive Therapy: basics and beyond*. New York: Guilford Press; 1995.

45 Young JE, Klosko J, Weishaar ME. *Schema Therapy: a practitioners guide*. New York: Guilford Press; 2003.

46 Barlow DH. The nature of anxious apprehension. In Barlow DH, editor. *Anxiety and its Disorders: the nature and treatment of anxiety and panic*. 2nd ed. New York: Guilford Press; 2004.

47 Scott J, Garland A, Moorhead S. A pilot study of cognitive therapy in bipolar disorder. *Psychological Medicine*. 2001; **31**(3): 459–67.

48 Chadwick PD, Birchwood MJ, Trower P. *Cognitive Therapy for Delusions, Voices and Paranoia*. Chichester: Wiley; 1996.

49 Linehan MM, Armstrong HE, Saurez A, *et al*. Cognitive-behavioural treatment of chronically parasuicidal borderline patients. *Archives of General Psychiatry*. 1991; **48**: 1060–4.

50 Liese BS, Franz RA. Treating substance use disorders with cognitive therapy; lessons learned and implications for the future. In: Salkovskis PM, editor. *Frontiers of Cognitive Therapy*. New York: Guilford; 1996.

51 DeRubeis RJ, Feeleey M. Detriments of change in cognitive therapy for depression. *Cognitive Therapy and Research*. 1991; **14**(5): 469–82.

52 Burns DD, Nolen-Hoeksema S. Therapeutic empathy and recovery from depression in cognitive behavioural therapy: a structural equation model. *Journal of Consulting and Clinical Psychology*. 1992; **60**: 441–9.

TO LEARN MORE

- Harvey AG, Watkins E, Mansell W, *et al. Cognitive-behavioural Processes across Psychological Disorders: a trans-diagnostic approach to research and treatment.* Oxford: Oxford University Press; 2004.
- Kinsella P, Garland A. *Cognitive Behavioural Therapy for Mental Health Workers: a beginners guide.* Hove: Routledge; 2003.
- Moore RG, Garland A. *Cognitive Therapy for Chronic and Persistent Depression.* Chichester, England: Wiley; 2003.
- Williams JMG, Watts FN, MacLeod C, *et al. Cognitive Psychology and Emotional Disorders.* 2nd ed. Chichester: Wiley; 1997.

CHAPTER 11

Dialectical behaviour therapy: mental health–substance use

Alexander L Chapman, Katherine L Dixon-Gordon
and Brianna J Turner

PRE-READING EXERCISE 11.1 (ANSWERS ON P. 163)

Time: 10 minutes

1 Dialectical behaviour produces more improvement in which of the following outcomes for individuals experiencing borderline personality disorder-substance use disorders, compared to treatment as usual:
   a reductions in alcohol use
   b reductions in drug use
   c reductions in parasuicidal behaviour
   d increased treatment retention?
2 According to the biosocial perspective, the individual is blamed for his/her drug use. True or false?
3 What four types of skill are taught in dialectical behaviour therapy skills training groups?

INTRODUCTION

Originally developed to treat highly suicidal women, dialectical behaviour therapy (DBT)[1] has evolved into an efficacious treatment for borderline personality disorder (BPD) and related problems, such as substance use disorders (SUDs), suicidality and self-injury. The frequent co-occurrence of BPD and SUD suggested the need to adapt and apply DBT to people who struggle with both of these clinical problems.[2,3] Indeed, more than half (57.4%) of individuals with BPD also meet criteria for a SUD,[4] and between 5% and 32% of those who struggle with SUDs meet criteria for BPD.[5,6] Within this chapter, we provide practical information on the evidence for DBT in the treatment of SUDs as well as suggestions on how to incorporate DBT into the treatment of people experiencing SUDs.

CHALLENGES IN THE TREATMENT OF BORDERLINE PERSONALITY DISORDER-SUBSTANCE USE DISORDER (BPD-SUD)

The presence of borderline personality disorders among individuals experiencing substance use disorder produces a particularly challenging clinical presentation. For instance, BPD is often characterised by emotional instability, cognitive dysregulation, impulsive, self-damaging behaviour, self-harm, suicide attempts, interpersonal discord, and identity disturbances.[7] Compared with non-BPD substance users, individuals experiencing BPD-SUDs begin using substances at a younger age, have a more chronic course of substance problems[8] and are more likely to experience adverse social, emotional and legal consequences of substance use.[9] Individuals experiencing BPD-SUDs are also more likely than individuals with SUD alone to attempt suicide and engage in self-harming behaviours.[10]

Some of the problems associated with BPD can directly interfere with the progress of therapy. Individuals with BPD often have difficulty maintaining stable relationships and, as a result, they experience frequent crises. Difficulties with sensitivity to rejection, fears of abandonment and dichotomous views of others (e.g. viewing the therapist as either 'wonderful' or 'terrible') can also interfere with the working therapeutic alliance. Furthermore, high proportions of patients with BPD prematurely drop out of therapy (67%–93%[11]) and research indicates that BPD and SUD both independently predict early termination of therapy.[12] Therefore, both the clinical severity and treatment-interfering behaviours of people experiencing BPD-SUDs present unique challenges in treatment.

SNAPSHOT OF THE RESEARCH ON DIALECTICAL BEHAVIOUR THERAPY FOR SUBSTANCE USE DISORDERS

Dialectical behaviour therapy, a comprehensive, cognitive behavioural treatment, includes several practical intervention strategies designed to manage the clinical challenges inherent in the treatment of individuals experiencing BPD-SUDs. Ten published randomised clinical trials and several uncontrolled trials have indicated that DBT is efficacious in reducing many clinical problems associated with BPD, including suicidal behaviour, self-harm, psychiatric hospitalisations, emergency room visits and treatment dropouts.[13] Moreover, many of the improvements achieved during DBT persist for at least one year following the end of treatment.[2,3] Currently, DBT is the only therapy that meets criteria for a 'well-established' treatment for BPD.[14,15]

Accumulating evidence has also indicated that DBT is useful in the treatment of persons experiencing BPD-SUD. The first published study[2] compared DBT with SUD treatment as usual in the community for people experiencing BPD-SUD. DBT patients showed significantly greater reductions in drug use, had lower dropout rates (36% versus 73%), and showed greater increases in global and social adjustment. In a second study, Linehan and colleagues[16] compared DBT to Comprehensive Validation Therapy (a manualised approach) plus 12-step groups (CVT+12S) for opioid-dependent women with BPD. Patients in the DBT group had fewer parasuicidal behaviours and less alcohol use than patients in CVT+12S, but both treatments demonstrated reductions in substance use at the end of therapy and at four-month follow-up. CVT+12S had a higher retention rate, compared with DBT.

Other research teams have also examined DBT in the treatment of people experiencing SUDs. One study compared standard DBT and treatment as usual (TAU) for women with BPD, 53% of whom had co-occurring substance use problems.[17,18] Across 12 months of therapy, individuals receiving DBT showed greater reductions in their parasuicidal behaviours and were less likely to switch therapists. At the six-month follow-up, DBT patients continued to show significantly fewer parasuicidal acts, fewer impulsive behaviours, and lower alcohol use.[18] Similarly, researchers in Canada found that, among females experiencing BPD-SUD, DBT patients showed greater reductions in parasuicidal behaviours and alcohol use compared with individuals who received TAU.[19] In both of these studies, DBT patients did not show greater reductions in drug use compared with controls. A recent study compared DBT to community treatment by experts in the treatment of co-occurring SUDs among suicidal women with BPD.[20] The DBT patients spent more time in *partial remission* (i.e. only met some criteria for SUD) and had a larger proportion of days abstinent from alcohol or drugs during and one year after treatment.[20]

In summary, the findings indicate the following.

➤ In some studies, individuals experiencing BPD-SUDs have shown greater reductions in DBT for both alcohol and drug use, compared with TAU.

➤ In other studies, findings have indicated greater reductions in alcohol use in DBT, but not drug use.

➤ DBT appears to be better than treatment by community experts at helping individuals experiencing BPD achieve remission from SUDs and at increasing their proportion of days abstinent from alcohol and drugs.

Why does DBT seem to be useful for people experiencing BPD-SUDs? One possibility is that, in DBT, the therapists directly tackle one of the main problems in the treatment of SUD, where people exit treatment. DBT includes several strategies to prevent dropout, often referred to as 'retention-enhancing strategies'.[21]

KEY POINT 11.1

From the beginning of treatment, DBT therapists place a strong emphasis on commitment to therapy.

The therapist engages in outreach efforts when the individual misses sessions. In addition, the availability of therapists for between-session phone calls and the systematic use of acceptance and validation of the individual likely enhance the therapy relationship (*see* Chapter 2) and attachment to treatment. Finally, the skills-training group provides practical skills that the individual can use and immediately experience the benefits of treatment. Illustrating these and other aspects of DBT, below, we provide guidance on what professionals can include in a DBT-oriented treatment for people experiencing BPD-SUD.

The case example below is an amalgam of hypothetical and real cases that we have seen, representing some of the presenting issues of persons experiencing BPD-SUDs. All identifying information has been disguised.

Case study 11.1: Vivian

Vivian (26) is an Asian female who was referred by her primary physician for treatment. She reported that her life has been getting increasingly out of control over the past few years. Vivian reported that she has a pattern of entering relationships that are chaotic and often end up 'ruining her life'. Vivian began using alcohol at age 11, marijuana and mushrooms at the age of 13, and at 15 she began using cocaine. After graduating from high school, Vivian attended a local college to pursue a general science degree. She began working as an escort in her sophomore year, and she reported a dramatic increase in her cocaine use at this time. While she was in college, she had several relationships that were extremely rocky. Vivian would go to extreme lengths to try to prevent these relationships from ending, often begging and threatening boyfriends if they tried to leave her. She also stated that she often 'loses it' when she is angry, and has become physically aggressive on several occasions. After graduating from university, Vivian had difficulty finding work, and continued to work intermittently in the sex trade. Around this time, she began living with a friend who frequently used crystal meth. Vivian first tried methamphetamine about a year ago, and since then has steadily increased her use. Recently, she has noticed increased withdrawal symptoms when she is not using. She has not worked for the past four months and relies on her current boyfriend for financial support. Her boyfriend knows that she has a history of substance use, but did not know about her current substance use until recently, which exacerbated current relationship difficulties. Vivian has no history of non-suicidal self-injury, and has made two suicide attempts, one involving hanging at age 12, and another involving an overdose of Tylenol three months ago. Vivian has tried several times to reduce her methamphetamine use on her own but, so far, she has been unsuccessful.

USING DBT WITH INDIVIDUALS EXPERIENCING BPD-SUDS

When treating individuals experiencing substance use disorders from a dialectical behaviour therapy framework, there are several essential treatment considerations. At minimum, the therapist must ensure that all of the key components of DBT are in place, including weekly individual therapy, telephone consultation, weekly out-patient group skills training, and a weekly therapist consultation team meeting. As other authors have discussed and described many of these treatment components in detail, we have elected to distil some of the most important guidelines from the DBT treatment package and discuss them below with the help of some illustrative examples from Vivian's treatment. These guidelines include the following.

1 Use the biosocial theory to guide treatment.
2 Adopt and use a dialectical world view.
3 Target substance use behaviour directly.
4 Improve motivation to change.
5 Teach skills.
6 Help the individual generalise skills to the natural environment.

1 Use the biosocial theory to guide treatment

The aims of DBT are guided by the *biosocial theory* of the development of BPD. According to this model, BPD is the result of a transaction between biologically based emotional vulnerability and childhood experiences of invalidation.[1] This theory posits that individuals with BPD have a biological propensity to react to low-threshold emotional stimuli, experiencing intense and long-lasting emotional responses. An invalidating rearing environment is one that communicates to the child that his/her emotional reactions are not warranted, justified or valid. Many caregivers do not know how to respond to children with such emotional temperaments, or may experience extreme emotional distress or lose control of their own behaviour when interacting with the emotional child. As a result, caregivers may punish, ignore or trivialise the child's emotional reactions. Over time, the emotionally vulnerable individual learns to mistrust and fear emotions, does not learn how to regulate emotions, and may come to rely on maladaptive ways of managing emotions.

Although developed as a model of BPD, the biosocial theory is consistent with much of what we know about SUDs. Researchers have long suggested that SUDs may have biological underpinnings.[22] Research also suggests that invalidating family environments can contribute to substance use, particularly among adolescents.[23,24] Recently, a neurodevelopmental model was advanced which suggests that adverse childhood experiences interact with brain development, leading to increased vulnerability for SUDs.[25] Substance use, in particular, may be a means for coping with distress.

Applying the biosocial model to the treatment of individuals experiencing SUD is helpful because it guides therapists towards two important overarching treatment goals:

1 The therapy should teach the individual to identify and accept the presence of his or her emotions.
2 The therapy should assist the individual in developing skills for managing emotional distress.

Dialectical behaviour therapy is well equipped to address these goals.

KEY POINT 11.2

DBT focuses on highlighting the validity of emotional responses, while simultaneously helping people to manage their emotion-dependent behaviours (such as substance use).

The therapist should help the individual to understand the biosocial model. By framing the individual's present difficulties within this model, the therapist and individual can take a non-judgemental stance towards treatment. Rather than being viewed as an intractable character flaw or personal failure, this model views substance use as a maladaptive but understandable way of coping. The biosocial model thus allows both the therapist and the individual to take the blame away from the individual, and to focus instead on learning more effective ways to cope with overwhelming emotions.

A biosocial case conceptualisation can be used to understand the case of Vivian presented earlier. Box 11.1 presents an example of an interaction between the therapist and Vivian that illustrates these points.

BOX 11.1 Vignette 1: sharing the biosocial model

> **Therapist**: The idea behind this treatment is that some people simply grow up being more emotional than others do. Even as a child, some people may have strong emotional reactions, or get upset or happy about things other people don't. Do you think this fits for you?
>
> **Vivian**: Yeah! I just remember freaking out a lot, like having a lot of tantrums and stuff. I remember one time when I just lay down in the driveway, screaming, and refused to move when my dad told me I couldn't go to my friend's house.
>
> **Therapist**: Did you feel like the black sheep?
>
> **Vivian**: Yes, I did! I mean, everyone else was just calm all the time, and nobody seemed to take the time to help me out when I was upset. They just avoided me or told me to get over it.
>
> **Therapist**: Now, sometimes, when you don't get the help you need to deal with your really strong emotions, you can end up like a powerful car with no breaks. It's like, once you get going, you have no way to stop.
>
> **Vivian**: Yeah, it's definitely that. That's what all the meth is about. I have no clue what else to do, and I feel like I'm going to just drown in all the hurt and sadness.
>
> **Therapist**: That's another thing that can happen. Meth has probably been really useful for you in helping you to cope with these overwhelming emotions. That's why it's so hard to quit!
>
> **Vivian**: Exactly – without meth, I don't think I could survive all these ups and downs.
>
> **Therapist**: It might feel like there's no other way – in fact, for you, meth really has been the only thing you found that actually worked! But that's what this treatment is about. We are going to teach you other ways to put the brakes on your emotions when you feel like you're out of control. Can you imagine giving up meth if you had some other ways of managing your emotions?
>
> **Vivian**: That's why I'm here. If I had something else – and it worked – I think I could stop.

2 Adopt and use a dialectical world view

Another essential ingredient of DBT for individuals experiencing BPD-SUD is a dialectical world view.[26] From this perspective, the universe consists of a continuous and dynamic interaction between opposites (i.e. **thesis** and **antithesis**). A 'dialectic' is tension between opposites. Much like thesis and antithesis, for every idea there is an equally valid opposite idea. In DBT, the primary dialectic is between acceptance and change. On the one hand, adopting an approach that constantly pushes the individual to change dysfunctional thoughts and behaviours is likely to be met with resistance. The more the therapist pushes the individual to change, the more the individual wants the therapist to understand and accept her. On the other hand, if the therapist simply adopts a purely accepting stance, the individual may feel invalidated as well; individuals experiencing BPD-SUD have serious problems that require change.

KEY POINT 11.3

Based on dialectics, DBT therapists react to opposing forces within the session by focusing on what is missing, and working towards a synthesis of these polarised views.

For example, Vivian understood the problems with drug use and wanted to stop, but she insisted on keeping a steady supply of methamphetamines on hand 'just in case'. The therapist, of course, was attuned to the downsides of keeping temptations so close by, but taking a dialectical approach, the therapist also validated Vivian's perspective and worked to find common ground (*see* Box 11.2).

BOX 11.2 Vignette 2: dialectical approach in session

> **Therapist**: It makes perfect sense that you would want to keep drugs around – they are your safety net if things get too bad. And, I have to say, the skills you're learning will help, but they probably won't give you that immediate relief. I could imagine having a hard time wanting to bother with all this skills stuff if I had an easier fix just sitting right in front of me . . .
>
> **Vivian**: But what if the skills don't work? I still need something. It's kind of a big leap to just give them up and hope for the best [*appearing agitated*].
>
> **Therapist**: It's true, it's a huge leap. I know I'm asking for a lot, maybe even too much. It seems to me that you want those around to calm your fears about what might happen if you really lose control. Is that right?
>
> **Vivian**: Yes [*crying*].
>
> **Therapist**: I wonder if there's a way that we can do both. If you keep the drugs around, and one skill doesn't work, I think you're way less likely to try another one. So, let's agree that that's true, OK? It seems to me that we need to find a way to settle your mind that maybe doesn't involve having meth around. Are you willing to work on that?

Drawing from Zen practice, mindfulness strategies and skills were incorporated into DBT as a counterpoint to the change-oriented strategies of traditional cognitive behavioural treatments (such as cognitive restructuring and behavioural skills training). Mindfulness practice promotes acceptance of reality as it is, including aversive thoughts and emotions. The acceptance of negative emotions and cognitions, in contrast to trying to keep these experiences from mind, actually serves to reduce the distress associated with such experiences. Further, encouraging people to focus on the present moment increases their ability to control their attention and move it away from potentially emotion-eliciting cues in the environment. For these reasons, mindfulness skills are the core component of DBT skills training.

3 Enhance motivation to change

In DBT for SUDs (DBT-SUD), there is increased emphasis on increasing motivation to engage in treatment and decrease substance use. During the orientation to therapy, individuals in standard DBT are asked to make explicit commitments to stay alive, work on therapy-interfering behaviours, and to participate in DBT for the duration of treatment. In DBT-SUD, people are asked to commit to working on substance use as well.

Several strategies are used to obtain commitments. For example, therapists may use 'foot in the door' to obtain commitment, which is the process of beginning with a small request, and progressively raising the stakes. Alternatively, therapists may use 'door in the face', which involves making such a large request that is very likely to be rejected. At this point, a more reasonable request is made, which seems relatively small by comparison. Therapists may also use 'devil's advocate' strategies to strengthen a commitment, once it has been elicited. This involves taking the opposite position, and highlighting some of the difficulties with maintaining the commitment. This prompts the person to identify reasons for the initial position. All of these strategies rely on the individual voicing commitment, or expressing reasons to cease the behaviour, which have been associated with better outcomes in substance use reduction (*see* Box 11.3).[27]

BOX 11.3 Vignette 3: commitment

Therapist: OK, we've got 10 minutes left. Let me just check in – do you think you can go the rest of the day without using? [*Foot in the door*]

Vivian: Yes, I feel like this plan's gonna work for today.

Therapist: Now, what if you used this plan to get through until Friday?

Vivian: That sounds harder. . . . My boyfriend gets back tomorrow. I know he's gonna say something.

Therapist: Oh, I can't believe we missed that! Well, what if we spend a few minutes planning how to deal with your boyfriend and not use drugs. What do you think?

Vivian: That sounds like a good idea . . .

Therapist: OK, but why does it sound like a good idea? I'm starting to think, 'If I were Vivian, I don't know . . .' I mean, your boyfriend says such hurtful things to you. And, the drugs work so well when stuff happens between you two. Wouldn't it be easier just to say you won't use till he comes back, and then all bets are off? [*Devil's advocate*]

Vivian: But I can't keep doing that. I know he says hurtful stuff, but I love him, and he'll leave me if I don't stop using. I just don't know what I'd do if that happened.

Therapist: Sounds like you want to work on this, even though it's going to be hard. You really don't have to, but I agree with you that things will probably get worse pretty fast without finding a way through conflict with him without using drugs. [*Freedom to choose and Absence of alternatives*] Do you really want to do this?

Vivian: Yeah, let's figure out what I can do.

REFLECTIVE PRACTICE EXERCISE 11.1

- Reflect on your own working environment.
- Have you ever used the above strategies in order to engage?
- If yes: Did they work? What do you think made them work?
- If you have not used these strategies, would you consider doing so?
- Consider why you may, or may not, use them.
- Can you think of other strategies that may be helpful?

In addition to commitment strategies, a DBT therapist may use other strategies, such as validation and cheerleading (giving each individual the message that he/she is capable of change), to provide encouragement and motivation for change. Using these techniques, the therapist might communicate that Vivian is doing the best she can, express hope that she can change, and focus on her capabilities and strengths.

Occasionally, a person's commitment may waver. In cases such as this, DBT-SUD therapists pay particular attention to helping people not 'fall out' of therapy. This requires a certain degree of flexibility on the part of the professional. If a person comes to therapy late, a DBT-SUD therapist may do their best to accommodate seeing the individual. Occasionally, therapists may rely upon various outreach or attachment strategies. If a person does not come to session at all, the therapist might call or send a note, encouraging a return to therapy. The goal is to focus on getting the individual to session, so that commitment to therapy can be assessed, and strengthened using the strategies above.

4 Target substance use behaviour directly

The philosophy of treatment in DBT-SUD is perhaps most similar to that of relapse prevention and harm reduction,[28,29] where the focus is on abstinence, but the therapist also implements harm reduction strategies (*see* Book 3, Chapter 15; Book 6, Chapters 15 and 16). One strategy used in DBT is *dialectical abstinence*, which involves focusing on lengthening the time between using. When taking a DBT approach to the treatment of SUDs, the therapist directly targets SUD, with an emphasis on reducing substance use as well as the harm caused by substance use. Some of these direct-targeting strategies include:

➤ regular monitoring of substance use and other behaviours using a DBT Diary Card
➤ highlighting and assessing the behaviour in session, and
➤ using problem-solving strategies to determine alternatives to substance use.

One of the major struggles in the treatment of people experiencing BPD or SUDs is the presence of multiple problems. In Vivian's case, she might arrive to session having used methamphetamines twice over the past week. In addition, she might have active suicidal ideation, be considering hoarding her medications so she would have the means to overdose, and have just received an eviction notice. Vivian's therapist might struggle with knowing which behaviour to focus on within the session.

In order to determine when and how to target the myriad difficulties, the DBT therapist uses the DBT hierarchy of treatment targets. Within this hierarchy, the therapist gives highest priority to behaviours that are life-threatening (e.g. suicide attempts, self-harm), followed by behaviours that interfere with therapy (e.g. absence, tardiness, anger at the therapist), and those that interfere with the individual's quality of life (e.g. substance use problems, instability in finances or housing, interpersonal discord). Each session, the person brings in a DBT Diary Card, and a collaborative decision is made on what to focus on during that particular session.

Dialectical Behavior Therapy — Skills Diary Card
Initials: Vivian ID #
Filled out in Session? Y N (Circle)
How often did you fill out this side? Daily ✓ 2-3x 4-6x Once
Started: Date July 17

Circle Start Day — Day Of Week	Highest Urge To:			Highest Rating For Each Day			Drugs/Medications							Actions				
	Commit Suicide 0-5	Self Harm 0-5	Use Drugs 0-5	Emotion. Misery 0-5	Physical Misery 0-5	Joy 0-5	Alcohol #	What?	Illicit Drugs #	What?	Meds. As Prescribed Y/N	PRN/Over the Counter #	What?	Self Harm Y/N	Lied #	Skills 0-7	Rein-force ✓	
MON	2	0	2	2	1	2	1	beer	0		y			N	0	4		
TUE	5	0	5	5	2	0	2	beer	0		y	1	Ativan	N		4		
WED	4	0	5	4	1	0	0		1	meth	y			N	2	1		
THUR	4	0	3	4	2	1	0		0		y			N	1	3		
FRI	2	0	2	2	3	2	3	beer	0		y			N	0	5		
SAT	3	0	2	1	1	3	1	wine	0		y			N	0	5		
SUN	2	0	3	2	1	2	0		0		y			N	0	3		

Chain Analysis Notes

Med Changes/Other.

* USED SKILLS:
0 = Not thought about or used
1 = Thought about, not used, didn't want to
2 = Thought about, not used, wanted to
3 = Tried but couldn't use them
4 = Tried, could do them but they didn't help
5 = Tried, could use them, helped
6 = Didn't try, used them, didn't help
7 = Didn't try, used them, helped

Urge to:	Coming into Session (0-5)	Ability to self-regulate self-control	Coming into Session (0-5)
Quit Therapy	2	Emotions:	2
Use Drugs	5	Action:	2
Commit Suicide	4	Thoughts:	0

© Behavioral Research and Training Clinic, University of Washington; NIMH4 2004

DBT Skills Diary Card Filled out this side? Daily ✓ 2-3x 4-6x Once In session — Check skills; circle days skill was practiced

1. Wise mind		MON	TUE	WED	THUR	FRI	SAT	SUN
2. Observe: just notice		MON	TUE	WED	THUR	FRI	SAT	SUN
3. Describe: put words on, just the facts		MON	TUE	WED	THUR	FRI	SAT	SUN
4. Participate: enter into the experience		MON	TUE	WED	THUR	FRI	SAT	SUN
5. Non-judgmental stance		MON	TUE	WED	THUR	FRI	SAT	SUN
6. One-mindfully: present moment		MON	TUE	WED	THUR	FRI	SAT	SUN
7. Effectiveness: focus on what works		MON	TUE	WED	THUR	FRI	SAT	SUN
8. Describe__ Express__ Assert__ Reinforce__	DEAR	MON	TUE	WED	THUR	FRI	SAT	SUN
9. Mindful: Broken record__ Ignore attacks__	MAN	MON	TUE	WED	THUR	FRI	SAT	SUN
10. Appear confident__ Negotiate__		MON	TUE	WED	THUR	FRI	SAT	SUN
11. Gentle__ Interested__ Validate__ Easy manner__	GIVE	MON	TUE	WED	THUR	FRI	SAT	SUN
12. Fair__ no-Apologies__ Stick to values__ Truthful__	FAST	MON	TUE	WED	THUR	FRI	SAT	SUN
13. Attend to relationships		MON	TUE	WED	THUR	FRI	SAT	SUN
14. Figure out interpersonal goals and priorities		MON	TUE	WED	THUR	FRI	SAT	SUN
15. Opposite-to-emotion action		MON	TUE	WED	THUR	FRI	SAT	SUN
16. Temperature__ Intense exercise__ Progressive relaxation__		MON	TUE	WED	THUR	FRI	SAT	SUN
17. Mindfulness of Current Emotion		MON	TUE	WED	THUR	FRI	SAT	SUN
18. Problem solving: Checked facts__ Brainstormed__ Acted__		MON	TUE	WED	THUR	FRI	SAT	SUN
19. Accumulate positives__ Build mastery__ Cope ahead__	ABC	MON	TUE	WED	THUR	FRI	SAT	SUN
20. Care: Physical ills__ Eating__ Avoid drugs__ Sleep__ Exercise__	PLEASE	MON	TUE	WED	THUR	FRI	SAT	SUN
21. Troubleshoot emotion regulation		MON	TUE	WED	THUR	FRI	SAT	SUN
22. Distract		MON	TUE	WED	THUR	FRI	SAT	SUN
23. Self-Soothe__ Improve the moment__	CRISIS SURVIVAL	MON	TUE	WED	THUR	FRI	SAT	SUN
24. Pros and Cons		MON	TUE	WED	THUR	FRI	SAT	SUN
25. Turn the mind__ Radical acceptance__		MON	TUE	WED	THUR	FRI	SAT	SUN
26. Willingness	REALITY ACCEPT	MON	TUE	WED	THUR	FRI	SAT	SUN
27. Mindfulness of current thoughts		MON	TUE	WED	THUR	FRI	SAT	SUN
28. Half-smiling__ Observing breath__ Awareness exercises__		MON	TUE	WED	THUR	FRI	SAT	SUN

FIGURE 11.1 DBT Skills Diary Card: Vivian

For example, Vivian's diary card (*see* Figure 11.1) indicated that high priorities for the session would include a recent increase in suicidal ideation two days ago as well as the use of methamphetamines yesterday.

The basic approach in DBT is for the therapist to highlight the problematic behaviour, conduct a thorough assessment, and help the individual engage in problem-solving to prevent the recurrence of problem behaviours. In terms of assessment, one of the primary DBT strategies is the chain analysis. A chain analysis is a detailed discussion of the chain of events that led to and followed a problem behaviour. The therapist, for example, might ask questions such as:

➤ How is it that you ended up using meth yesterday?
➤ At what moment did it occur to you that you were going to use meth?
➤ Where were you when you first noticed the urge?
➤ What were you doing?
➤ What were you thinking or feeling before you used?
➤ How did meth influence your mood?

The goal of a chain analysis is to obtain information that will help both therapist and individual to identify all the points at which solutions might be implemented. For example, if a chain analysis revealed that Vivian used methamphetamines in response to feeling worthless and hopeless after a particularly stressful day of job hunting, the therapist might suggest that Vivian delete her dealer's number from her cell phone, practise alternative ways of tolerating her distress (such as practising mindfulness of her current emotion), or use stress management or emotion regulation strategies. These analyses of behaviours also assist the individual to identify 'apparently irrelevant behaviours', actions which unknowingly predispose substance usage. In the example above, Vivian maintaining her dealer's phone number was an apparently irrelevant behaviour.

Finally, often-ancillary care plays a role in combination with DBT. In certain cases of substance use, pharmacotherapy may play an important role. Therapists should consider the use of medication to address substance dependence, and work with individuals, ensuring that they are communicating with other treatment providers regarding these needs.

5 Teach skills

As noted earlier, the biosocial model points to difficulties with managing emotions as one of the core problems associated with BPD-SUD. Many people turn to substance use in an attempt to avoid emotional suffering. Therefore, one important aim within DBT is to provide individuals with alternative, adaptive skills to regulate or manage emotions. These skills are taught within a separate skills training group.

DBT skills training group involves a weekly group meeting, usually lasting 1.5 to 2 hours each week. Two co-leaders, in a format much like a class, run this group. Typically, the first half of group therapy involves homework review, while the second half consists of new skills training. These skills include strategies at improving mindfulness, interpersonal effectiveness, emotion regulation and distress tolerance. Each of these skills is relevant not only to the problems of those with BPD, but also to the difficulties experienced by persons who struggle with SUDs.

Group skills training in DBT-SUD incorporates several additional skills that target problems specific to individuals experiencing substance use difficulties. Other skills, present in standard DBT, are modified to apply to difficulties commonly encountered among people experiencing substance use disorders. Together, the treatment techniques tailored to address substance use difficulties constitute the 'path to clear mind'.[30]

The mindfulness skills taught in standard DBT are particularly useful for individuals experiencing DBT-SUD. In standard DBT, Linehan[1] described the three states of mind as:
1 emotion mind
2 reasonable mind
3 wise mind.

In DBT-SUD, the following characterisations of states of mind were added:
4 **clear mind** – the state of mind which predisposes the individual to abstain from substance use
5 **addict mind** – the state of mind focused on using drugs
6 **clean mind** – the state of mind which naively overlooks potential risks of drug use.

People are also taught the skill of *urge surfing,* which consists of observing urges to use drugs come and go, much like ocean waves.[28] This frequently reminds individuals that urges will abate, and allows them to notice urges without acting on them. Further, acceptance-oriented strategies can be used to help people manage symptoms associated with withdrawal.

Interpersonal effectiveness skills are crucial for reducing substance use, as substance use is often maintained by social support. For people whose substance use is reinforced by a specific peer group, DBT-SUD may assist development of alternative social supports. Also, the **DEAR** skill provides a framework for helping people practise how to make a request, or say no:
➤ **D**escribe
➤ **E**xpress
➤ **A**ssert
➤ **R**einforce.

Coping ahead is taught for situations which are likely to be stressful or elicit urges to engage in unwanted behaviours, such as substance use, and planning alternative behaviours. In DBT-SUD, *coping ahead* can be useful for relapse prevention.

Another adaptation of DBT for SUDs involves teaching distress tolerance skills that are particular to substance use. In standard DBT, individuals are taught to temporarily use the skill of *pushing away* distressing thoughts during times of crisis. In DBT-SUD, these skills are distilled to the concept of *adaptive denial.* This skill involves pushing away or blocking distressing thoughts which may lead the individual down the path of drug use.[31,32] For example, a person may essentially 'deny' that she/he is working towards abstinence from drugs or alcohol. In the case of Vivian, she might say to herself, 'I might be able to fit methamphetamines into my life in the future. So, I don't have to stop forever.' Individuals are also encouraged to *burn bridges* with all access to substances. This might involve deleting the phone numbers of drug-using friends or drug dealers, changing social groups, or taking a different route to work to avoid people or places associated with drug use. Thus, individuals are coached to use their newly acquired skills to structure their environment (*see* Table 11.1).

TABLE 11.1 Dialectical behaviour therapy skills modules

The dialectical behaviour therapy skills modules and their associated behavioural targets

Module	Target
Mindfulness	• Increase attentional control
	• Decrease worrying, ruminating
	• Notice judgemental thoughts
Emotion Regulation	• Understand functions of emotions
	• Identify specific emotions
	• Decrease emotional vulnerability
	• Increase ability to manage aversive emotions in the moment
Distress Tolerance	• Provide with alternative strategies to cope with crises
	• Acknowledge and accept distress
Interpersonal Effectiveness	• Increase skills in making requests or saying no
	• Increase relationship-enhancing skills
	• Increase skills in maintaining self-respect.

6 Help the individual generalise skills to the natural environment

Once adaptive skills have been learned it is necessary to assist the individual in applying these skills effectively in his/her everyday life. In DBT, there are several components to help generalise the use of skills to natural environments. This is accomplished through a combination of homework assignments, diary cards and phone calls.

In both individual therapy and group skills training, people receive individualised homework assignments. Often, these assignments involve finding opportunities to practise specific skills. A skills training group provides an opportunity for collaborative problem-solving regarding how to help people effectively complete homework practice. Further, the DBT diary card serves as a portable reminder of DBT skills.

Intersession phone calls also facilitate the translation of skills learning to the real world. These phone calls typically last up to 10 minutes. Therapists should orient people to their particular availability for phone calls, when they check their voicemail, or expect to be able to return phone calls. Individuals are instructed to call therapists prior to engaging in any self-harm, suicidal or substance use behaviours. Telephone consultation provides therapists with the opportunity to help in reducing risk and to use distress tolerance strategies instead. Individuals may also call therapists for coaching with use of any other skills (*see* Box 11.4).

BOX 11.4 Vignette 4: skills-coaching phone call

> *Therapist*: Hi Vivian. I saw you called a few hours ago. What's going on?
>
> *Vivian*: I'm having a hell of a time – I saw my ex earlier – I don't think he saw me, but it just got me thinking about all this stuff, I was so upset. I wanted to use so bad – I still do. I keep trying to calm down, but now I just can't keep using out of my head, and then I'm pissed about that – I was actually just thinking about heading out a second ago to see him and tell him some things.
>
> *Therapist*: Well, I am glad you called! It sounds like you've been able to keep yourself from using so far – how have you managed to do that?
>
> *Vivian*: I just didn't have cash – that was the thing, we decided I shouldn't keep too much cash around or I'd buy.
>
> *Therapist*: Looks like your plan has worked so far – have you tried any other skills yet?
>
> *Vivian*: No – and I have cash now, I needed to have some to pay for some pizza anyway so . . .
>
> *Therapist*: OK, so you have cash now, and you were planning on going out. Do you think these may be some of those apparently irrelevant behaviours we were talking about?
>
> *Vivian*: Not really – well, probably. So what am I supposed to do? I am so mad about all the crap he put me through!
>
> *Therapist*: This might be a perfect opportunity to use some of your distress tolerance skills to help you coast through these emotions without doing anything to make the situation worse! What skills could you try?
>
> *Vivian*: I guess I could take a hot shower.
>
> *Therapist*: That might work – using temperature to help regulate your emotions. What else did you learn in group?
>
> *Vivian*: Well, I could do some progressive muscle relaxation – that worked last time. Or I could distract by calling a friend . . .
>
> *Therapist*: Great! You've just named several skills which could help you get through this moment. Now, I know these skills are short term, and they won't fix this situation. But they will help you avoid making things worse by using drugs. And, that's one of the things you really want, right, to move away from using drugs whenever you're upset?
>
> *Vivian*: I don't know, I guess. I'll give it a shot, though.
>
> *Therapist*: OK, why don't you give those a try and see how they work for you?

CONCLUSION

Dialectical behaviour therapy is a comprehensive cognitive behavioural treatment designed to manage the behavioural and emotional problems of persons who struggle with BPD and related difficulties. DBT has been adapted for individuals experiencing SUD, with some noteworthy success. For instance, the research suggests that DBT is efficacious at treating substance use problems among persons with BPD. The data also indicate that DBT is at least as good, and in some cases, better, than control treatments (often including treatment as usual) at reducing alcohol use and, in some cases, drug use. Within a DBT approach to SUDs, there are six primary considerations:

1 Use the biosocial theory to guide treatment.
2 Adopt and use a dialectical world view.
3 Enhance motivation to change.
4 Target substance use directly.
5 Teach skills.
6 Enhance generalisation to the natural environment.

Amid the numerous obstacles present in treating individuals experiencing BPD-SUD, there is a risk that both individual and professional may lose sight of treatment goals and motivation. These DBT guidelines provide a compass for navigating this terrain. The shared, non-judgemental conceptualisation of the person's difficulties demonstrated within the biosocial theory orients the person to the rationale for treatment. Often, this model resonates with the individual, thereby enhancing motivation to engage in therapy. The dialectical balance of acceptance and change within DBT models the validation of emotional experience that many individuals lack in their environments, while also developing new skill sets. Although research on DBT for SUD alone is in its infancy, it is likely that several aspects of DBT will lend themselves to the compassionate and effective treatment of individuals experiencing difficulties with emotion regulation and other out of control behaviours.

POST-READING EXERCISE 11.1 (ANSWERS ON P. 164)

Time: 10 minutes
1 An individual receiving therapy arrives late, having used alcohol and considered suicide over the past week. Which of these issues do you prioritise in your session?
2 What techniques might you use if an individual indicates they cannot commit to abstaining from substance use?
3 According to the biosocial perspective, how might you conceptualise an individual's drug use?

REFERENCES

1 Linehan MM. *Cognitive Behavioural Therapy of Borderline Personality Disorder*. New York: Guilford Press; 1993.
2 Linehan MM, Schmidt H, Dimeff LA, *et al*. Dialectical behaviour therapy for patients with borderline personality disorder and drug-dependence. *American Journal of Addictions*. 1999; **8**: 279–92.
3 Linehan MM, Comtois KA, Murray AM, *et al*. Two-year randomized controlled trial and follow-up of Dialectical Behaviour Therapy vs. Therapy by Experts for suicidal behaviours and borderline personality disorder. *Archives of General Psychiatry*. 2006; **63**: 757–66.
4 Trull TJ, Sher KJ, Minks-Brown C, *et al*. Borderline personality disorder and substance use disorders: a review and integration. *Clinical Psychology Review*. 2000; **20**: 235–53.

5 Brooner RK, King VL, Kidorf M, *et al*. Psychiatric and substance use comorbidity among treatment-seeking opioid abusers. *Archives of General Psychiatry.* 1997; **54**: 71–80.

6 Weiss RD, Mirin SM, Griffin ML, *et al*. Personality-disorders in cocaine dependence. *Comprehensive Psychiatry.* 1993; **34**: 145–9.

7 American Psychiatric Association. *Diagnostic and Statistical Manual of Mental Disorders.* 4th ed. Text version. Washington, DC: American Psychiatric Association; 2000.

8 Ross S, Dermatis H, Levounis P, *et al*. A comparison between dually diagnosed inpatients with and without Axis II comorbidity and the relationship to treatment outcome. *The American Journal of Drug and Alcohol Abuse.* 2002; **29**: 263–79.

9 Links PS, Heslegrave RJ, Mitton JE, *et al*. Characteristics of borderline personality disorder. *Canadian Journal of Psychiatry.* 1995; **33**: 336–54.

10 Kosten TA, Kosten TR, Rousaville BJ. Personality-disorder in opiate addicts show prognostic specificity. *Journal of Substance Abuse Treatment.* 1989; **6**: 163–8.

11 Skodol AE, Buckley P, Charles E. Is there a characteristic pattern to the treatment history of clinic outpatients with borderline personality? *Journal of Nervous and Mental Disease.* 1983; **171**: 405–10.

12 Martinez-Raga J, Marshall EJ, Keaney F, *et al*. Unplanned versus planned discharges from in-patient alcohol detoxification: retrospective analysis of first-episode admissions. *Alcohol and Alcoholism.* 2002; **37**: 277–81.

13 Lynch TR, Trost WT, Salsman N, *et al*. Dialectical behaviour therapy for borderline personality disorder. *Annual Review of Clinical Psychology.* 2007; **3**: 181–205.

14 Chambless DL, Hollon SD. Defining empirically supported therapies. *Journal of Consulting and Clinical Psychology.* 1998; **66**: 7–18.

15 Chambless DL, Ollendick TH. Empirically supported psychological interventions: controversies and evidence. *Annual Review of Psychology.* 2001; **52**: 685–716.

16 Linehan MM, Dimeff LA, Reynolds SK, *et al*. Dialectical behaviour therapy versus comprehensive validation therapy plus 12-step for the treatment of opioid dependent women meeting criteria for borderline personality disorder. *Drug and Alcohol Dependence.* 2002; **67**: 13–26.

17 Van den Bosch LMC, Verheul R, Schippers GM, *et al*. Dialectical behaviour therapy of borderline patients with and without substance use problems: implementation and long-term effects. *Addictive Behaviors.* 2005; **27**: 911–23.

18 Van den Bosch LMC, Koeter MWJ, Stijnen T, *et al*. Sustained efficacy of dialectical behaviour therapy for borderline personality disorder. *Behaviour Research and Therapy.* 2005; **43**: 1231–41.

19 McMain S. Dialectical behaviour therapy for individuals with borderline personality disorder and substance abuse: a randomized, controlled pilot study. *Proceedings of the Association for the Advancement of Behavior Therapy Conference*; 2004 Nov. 18–21; New Orleans, LA.

20 Harned MS, Chapman AL, Dexter-Mazza ET, *et al*. Treating co-occurring Axis I disorders in recurrently suicidal women with borderline personality disorder: a 2-year randomized trial of dialectical behavior therapy versus community treatment by experts. *Personality Disorders: theory, research and treatment.* 2009; (Suppl. 1): S33–45.

21 Bornovalova MA, Daughters SB. How does dialectical behavior therapy facilitate treatment retention among individuals with comorbid borderline personality disorder and substance use disorders? *Clinical Psychology Review.* 2007; **27**: 923–43.

22 Ball D, Collier D. Substance misuse. In: McGuffin P, Owen, MJ, Gottesman I, editors. *Psychiatric Genetics and Genomics.* Oxford: Oxford University Press; 2002. pp. 267–302.

23 Feldstein SW, Miller WR. Substance use and risktaking among adolescents. *Journal of Mental Health.* 2006; **15**: 633–43.

24 Hersh MA, Hussong AM. The association between observed parental emotion socialization and adolescent self-medication. *Journal of Abnormal Child Psychology.* 2009; **37**: 493–506.

25 Andersen SL, Teicher MH. Desperately driven and no brakes: developmental stress exposure and subsequent risk for substance abuse. *Neuroscience and Biobehavioral Reviews.* 2009; **33**: 516–24.

26 Marx K, Engels F. *Selected Works*, vol. 3. New York: International Publishers; 1970.

27 Amrhein PC, Miller WR, Yahne CE, *et al.* Client commitment language during motivational interviewing predicts drug use outcomes. *Journal of Consulting and Clinical Psychology.* 2003; **71**: 862–78.

28 Marlatt GA, Gordon JR. *Relapse Prevention: maintenance strategies in the treatment of addictive behaviours.* New York: Guilford Press; 1995.

29 Marlatt GA, Witkiewitz K. Harm reduction approaches to alcohol use: health promotion, prevention, and treatment. *Addictive Behaviours.* 2002; **27**: 867–6.

30 Rosenthal MZ, Lynch TR, Linehan MM. Dialectical behaviour therapy for individuals with borderline personality disorder and substance use disorders. In: Frances RJ, Miller SI, Mack AH, editors. *Clinical Textbook of Addictive Disorders.* New York: Guilford Press; 2005. pp. 615–36.

31 Dimeff L, Rizvi SL, Brown M, *et al.* Dialectical behaviour therapy for substance abuse: a pilot application to methamphetamine-dependent women with borderline personality disorder. *Cognitive and Behavioral Practice.* 2000; **7**: 457–68.

32 Linehan MM, Dimeff LA. *Dialectical Behaviour Therapy Manual of Treatment Interventions for Drug Abusers with Borderline Personality Disorder.* Seattle: University of Washington; 1997.

TO LEARN MORE

- American Psychiatric Association. Practice guideline for the treatment of patients with borderline personality disorder. *American Journal of Psychiatry.* 2001; **158**: 1–52.
- Behavioural Tech, LLC: Available at: www.behavioraltech.com
- Chapman AL, Glatz KL. *The Borderline Personality Disorder Survival Guide: everything you need to know about living with BPD.* Oakland, CA: New Harbinger Publications; 2007.
- Linehan MM. *Cognitive-behavioural Treatment of Borderline Personality Disorder.* New York: Guilford Press; 1993.
- Linehan MM. *Skills Training Manual for Treating Borderline Personality Disorder.* New York: Guilford Press; 1993.

ANSWERS TO PRE-READING EXERCISE 11.1

1 Dialectical behaviour therapy has been shown to produce greater efficacy in reducing alcohol use, in reducing parasuicidal behaviour and in improving treatment retention, compared to treatment as usual. Although some studies have found that DBT produces greater reductions in drug use, other studies have not found differences between DBT and treatment as usual in reducing drug use.

2 False. Although the individual is not to blame for using drugs, he/she is ultimately responsible for changing this behaviour.

3 Mindfulness skills, emotion regulation skills, distress tolerance skills and interpersonal effectiveness skills.

ANSWERS TO POST-READING EXERCISE 11.1

1 A DBT therapist would first address life-threatening behaviours (i.e. suicidal thoughts), then address therapy-interfering behaviours (i.e. arriving late for session), and then address quality of life-interfering behaviours (i.e. alcohol use).

2 A DBT therapist might use *foot in the door*, *door in the face*, *devil's advocate*, *validation* or *cheerleading* to enhance commitment.

3 The biosocial perspective suggests that drug use functions primarily as a maladaptive way to regulate overwhelming emotions that result from the interaction between:

a a biological vulnerability to intense, reactive emotions and

b an invalidating environment which punishes, ignores or trivialises emotions.

Eye movement desensitisation and reprocessing (EMDR): mental health–substance use

Susan H Brown, Julie E Stowasser and Francine Shapiro

INTRODUCTION

Substance use disorders remain a persistent social and medical problem. According to a recent report,[1] addiction is the number one health problem in the United States. The report notes that when one considers the direct costs of drug-induced health problems, deaths due to accidents, human immunodeficiency virus (HIV), or drug-related acts of violent crime, there are '*more deaths, illnesses and disabilities from substance use than from any other preventable health condition*'.[1]

Most experts today agree that substance use disorders are a complex interaction between genetics, environment and experience.

> Substance dependence is not a failure of will or of strength of character,
> but a medical disorder that could affect any human being. Dependence is
> a chronic and relapsing disorder, often co-occurring with other physical
> and mental conditions.[2]

The question remains: why has it been that over the course of human history, where people and cultures have had access to alcohol and potent mind-altering substances, only some become addicted while the rest are able to regulate their use?

The drugs that people experiencing substance use disorders select are not chosen randomly but are a result of an interaction between the psychopharmacologic action of the drug and the dominant painful feelings with which they struggle. Edward Khantzian[3] observed that opiates are often preferred because of their powerful numbing action on the affects of rage and aggression. Cocaine has its appeal because of its ability to relieve distress associated with depression. Although ill-fated, '*addicts discover that the short-term effects of their drugs of choice help them cope with distressful subjective states and an external reality otherwise experienced as unmanageable or overwhelming*'.[3] Thus emerges a compelling hypothesis which proposes that people use psychoactive substances in an attempt to control painful symptoms resulting from psychological trauma. This is referred to as 'self-medication'.

Some studies in the United States show that more than 50% of people with mental disorders also suffer from substance dependence compared to 6% of the general population.[2] It is from our interest in providing integrated treatment for the complex interaction of genes, environment, trauma and psychological pain as a driving force behind mental health–substance use disorders that this chapter is written.

MENTAL HEALTH–SUBSTANCE USE

> *'No one ever died from their feelings, but millions of people have died from taking drugs, alcohol, and other toxic substances to help them avoid their feelings . . .'*[4]

Mental health–substance use disorders ignore age, gender, intellect, marital status, economic, social class, race and nationality, leaving no one immune from their impact. The prevalence of mental health–substance use disorders, and the dearth of effective treatment interventions for them, leaves individuals in a state of suffering, with impressive personal, familial, social and economic consequences.

The correlation between trauma, especially when first experienced in childhood, and co-occurring mental health and substance use disorders is strongly established in the literature.[5-8] The definition of *co-occurring disorders* (COD) states that one or more psychiatric or medical conditions coexist in addition to one or more addictive disorders. CODs do not simply have overlapping symptoms but are distinct and they are independently diagnosed from one another.[9]

Examples of diagnoses frequently co-occurring with substance use disorders include:
➤ post-traumatic stress disorder and other anxiety disorders
➤ bipolar disorder
➤ borderline personality disorder
➤ major depression
➤ attention deficit disorder.

The many possible permutations of mental health–substance use conditions lead to a complicated clinical picture that is challenging to untangle and treat effectively, particularly when the role of trauma in their development is overlooked.

Mental health–substance use disorders are associated with:
➤ poorer motivation, retention and treatment outcomes compared to individuals with a single psychiatric disorder
➤ a substance use cycle that worsens in frequency and intensity over time
➤ less social support
➤ underemployment
➤ failure at work or school
➤ poorer overall health conditions
➤ impaired family relations
➤ abuse and violence
➤ legal difficulties.[6,10-12]

Historically, these areas of mental health have separate treatment, education, training and funding avenues, creating significant barriers to receiving integrated treatment services. Currently, the development and implementation of effective, integrated treatment services is a public health challenge worldwide.

The purpose of this chapter is to:

➤ illustrate the relationship between trauma, mental disorders and the development of substance use disorders and behavioural, or process, addictions

➤ describe the connections between substance and behavioural addictions[13]

➤ describe the Adaptive Information Processing (AIP) model as the theoretical framework for case conceptualisation in eye movement desensitisation and reprocessing (EMDR)[14-17]

➤ provide a basic understanding of the principles, protocols and procedures that define EMDR[14,15]

➤ illustrate when and how to use EMDR as an integrated treatment approach for mental health–substance use disorders.

THE RELATIONSHIP BETWEEN TRAUMA AND MENTAL HEALTH–SUBSTANCE USE DISORDERS

'Nothing is predestined: The obstacles of your past can become the gateways that lead to new beginnings.'[18]

Trauma is often the crucible from which psychiatric symptoms and addictions emerge. With trauma, *the past is present*. The Adverse Childhood Experiences (ACE) Study provides retrospective and prospective analysis of over 17,000 individuals, primarily middle-class US citizens, from Kaiser Permanente's Department of Preventive Medicine in San Diego, California.[6] The study examined the effect of traumatic life experiences during the first 18 years on later well-being, social function, health risks, disease burden, healthcare costs and life expectancy.

The 10 reference categories experienced during childhood are listed in Table 12.1, with their prevalence in parentheses (*see* To learn more).

TABLE 12.1 Adverse childhood experiences (adapted[6])

Category	Behaviour	Prevalence
Abuse		
1 Emotional	● recurrent humiliation	11%
2 Physical	● beating, not spanking	28%
3 Sexual abuse	● contact sexual abuse	
● women		28%
● men		16%
● overall		22%

(continued)

Category	Behaviour	Prevalence
Household dysfunction		
4 Mother	• treated violently	13%
5 Household member	• alcohol or drug use problems	27%
6 Household member	• imprisoned	6%
7 Household member	• chronically depressed, suicidal, mentally ill, in psychiatric hospital	17%
8 Household member	• not raised by both biological parents	23%
Neglect		
9 Physical	• lack of proper food, clothing, shelter	10%
10 Emotional	• isolation, lack of interaction	15%

Scoring was simple: exposure to any one category was scored as one point. Thus, an individual reporting sexual molestation by one person would score the same as someone who experienced multiple sexual assaults by several individuals. As a result, these findings tend to be under, rather than overstated. Nevertheless, several surprising outcomes regarding the significance of early trauma and the development of later substance use problem and/or behavioural addiction were revealed. For example, the study found *'strong, proportionate relationships between the number of categories of adverse childhood experiences (ACE score) and the use of various psychoactive materials or behaviours . . . including alcoholism and intravenous drug abuse'.*[6]

Not surprisingly, childhood trauma and neglect disrupts and can dysregulate the brain's information processing systems.[19-22] Lesser-known risk factors in the development of a child's brain and quest for mastery over emotional regulation are the significant roles played by the quality of parental attunement and attention.[21] Those who are unable to manage emotional responses to everyday stressors are compelled to seek ways to control or numb their affect.[3]

Addictions and other compulsive behaviours temporarily change the experience of painful emotions and body sensations and thereby provide a transitory sense of relief. Often referred to as self-medication, this may be seen by the user as effectively managing distress, thereby promoting a vicious cycle of addictive coping strategies.[8,13,23,24] Such cycles create challenges during treatment because the individual experiencing the addiction incorrectly perceives it as being a beneficial regulator of their discomfort. An illustration of how this works can be seen in Figure 12.1.

THE LINK BETWEEN SUBSTANCE USE DISORDERS AND BEHAVIOURAL ADDICTIONS

> *'Drunkenness – that fierce rage for the slow, sure poison, that oversteps every other consideration; that casts aside wife, children, friends, happiness, and station; and hurries its victims madly on to degradation and death'*[26]

Research suggests a strong neurobiological link between chemical and behavioural, or process, addictions. However, it is the neurochemistry associated with 'reward' or

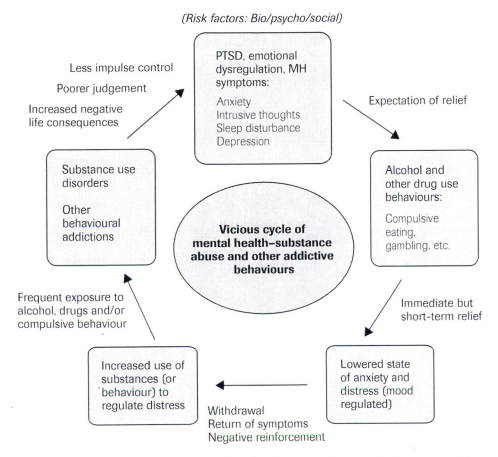

FIGURE 12.1 Vicious cycle of mental health–substance abuse and other compulsive behaviours for emotional regulation (© Illustration Copyright 2009 Brown S (adapted[25]). Used with the kind permission of Susan Brown LCSW)

'pleasure pathways'[13] to which the individual becomes addicted, not the substance or behaviour.

Impulsive behaviour seems to have an underlying predisposition that may or may not be related to existing mental health or medical conditions. Research over the past decade has stressed the substantial comorbidity of Impulse Control Disorders with mood disorders, anxiety disorders, eating disorders, substance abuse, personality disorders and with other specific impulse control disorders.[27] Addictions and compulsions are, at least in part, disorders of 'impulse control', whether they are behavioural or chemical. They follow similar symptomatic cycles[13] as can be seen in Table 12.2.

TABLE 12.2 Addictions, compulsions and the similarities between them

Addictions and compulsions	Symptoms and cycles
• Alcohol and other substance use disorders	• Preoccupation (obsession)
• Gambling	• Anticipation (craving)
• Shopping	• Mood modification (regulation)
• Pornography	• Continued use despite severe adverse life consequences (compulsion)
• Internet	• Serious impairment in major areas of life functioning
• Binge eating and food restriction	
• Compulsive exercising	• Attempts to stop the behavioural or addictive cycle
• Cutting	
• Skin picking and hair pulling	• Relapse
• Abusive or controlling interpersonal behaviour patterns	

THE EMDR APPROACH: TREATMENT OF PTSD AND TRAUMA

Eye movement desensitisation and reprocessing is a comprehensive, integrative and empirically supported treatment approach for post-traumatic stress disorder.[28-32] Seventeen clinical trials in peer-reviewed journals attest to EMDR's efficacy with PTSD and trauma. EMDR has been found equivalent to Prolonged Exposure (PE) therapy[33-35] and other cognitive behavioural therapies in reducing PTSD symptoms.[29,34,36-38] However, EMDR has also been found to be more efficient and more widely tolerated without the individual's need for one to two hours of daily homework as in PE.[36,37]

As is true for all psychotherapies, the mechanism of action responsible for EMDR's effectiveness is still unknown. Over a dozen randomised studies have examined the eye movements in EMDR and found they decrease the vividness and emotional intensity of autobiographical memories and enhance retrieval of episodic memories.[39-41] One hypothesis regarding the development of PTSD is the failure to process episodic memory, thereby leaving upsetting memories 'stuck' in the past instead of being integrated into semantic networks.[42-44] For a more complete review of the hypothesised mechanisms of action involved in EMDR see Solomon and Shapiro.[17]

The EMDR model of psychotherapy includes an eight-phase structured protocol that is compatible with elements of psychodynamic, cognitive behavioural, experiential, interpersonal, and body-oriented therapies.[15] EMDR's theoretical orientation is based on the Adaptive Information Processing model described below.[15]

THEORETICAL BASIS OF EMDR: THE ADAPTIVE INFORMATION PROCESSING MODEL[15]

> 'The burned child fears the flame' (Anon.)

The Adaptive Information Processing model (AIP) explains clinical phenomena, predicts successful treatment effects and guides the overall practice of EMDR across its wide range of therapeutic applications.[14,15] It asserts that the brain possesses an intrinsic ability to process information in the moment, interpreting and integrating current perceptions within the existing memory networks. The brain also processes distressing memories to an adaptive resolution. It is posited that unresolved trauma can interfere with the brain's natural information-processing capabilities.

According to the AIP, symptoms result from dysfunctional, physiologically stored, unresolved memories. Some, or all, parts of the memory (imagery, body sensations, thoughts, beliefs, attitudes and perceptions) remain encoded as they were originally experienced and are therefore fragmented, and unassimilated into the more adaptive memory networks. These maladaptively stored memories result in distortions that can negatively influence an individual's thoughts, feelings and behaviours until they are reprocessed and integrated into a more fluid and adaptive whole.

A current situation can contain triggers to these earlier memories, causing the individual to experience the disturbing affects and perspectives encoded at the time of the original event. This in turn can influence the individual's perceptions of the present event. Externally, a trigger can be a sight, sound, smell, person, activity or event. Internally, it can be an emotion, body sensation, mood or dream. The purpose of EMDR is to **access** the disturbing material, **activate** the information-processing system and allow the brain to **move** it into a more adaptive state.

EMDR theory sensitises professionals to recognise that even ubiquitous events can have the same debilitating effects as major trauma. To that end, the terms 'big-T' and 'small-t' traumas are often used. When diagnosing PTSD, big-T traumas are those designated as Criterion A events.[9] Examples that might cause intense fear, helplessness or horror include experiencing, witnessing or hearing about something that is an immediate threat to one's own or a loved one's life or safety, such as: physical, emotional or sexual abuse or assault, domestic violence, vehicular accident, combat, terrorism or natural disaster. However, a person can also be severely affected by more common, small-t life events, such as attachment or attunement problems with parents, and/or siblings, bullying in school, peer problems, the death of a pet, parent's divorce or the breakup of a romance.

Recent research supports this concept. A survey of 832 'general population' people reported that more PTSD symptoms were related to common distressing life events, such as chronic illness, marital discord or unemployment (small-t) than to Criterion A (big-T) events.[45] A subsequent study[46] examined three groups of exposure in 1190 adults, aged 18–26:

1 individuals experiencing traumatic events (e.g. combat, rape, assault) in the past year
2 individuals experiencing only significant stressful events (e.g. divorce, relational problems, expected death of a loved one) in the past year
3 individuals who experienced both.

The researchers arrived at the same conclusion as the previous report, finding that all three groups experienced similar PTSD symptoms across clusters, suggesting that the type of events that cause symptoms of PTSD may be broader than current diagnostic criteria designates.

In EMDR, these common distressing events are referred to as small-t traumas not because they are less traumatic, but because they are normalised in our experience and are frequently overlooked as a cause of later problems.[14-16]

MENTAL HEALTH–SUBSTANCE USE DISORDERS THROUGH THE LENS OF THE AIP MODEL
Case conceptualisation

Most of the current randomised controlled research on EMDR focuses on the treatment of PTSD.[32] However, a growing body of case studies using EMDR for other mental disorders and addictions reveals a history of trauma as a contributing factor in their development.

Examples of disorders other than PTSD that were treated with EMDR include:
- body dysmorphic disorder[47]
- borderline personality disorder[48]
- choking phobia[49,50]
- deliberate self-harm[51]
- domestic violence perpetration and victimisation[52]
- eating disorders[53,54]
- obsessive–compulsive disorder[55]
- phantom limb pain[56-59]
- phobias[60,61]
- panic disorder[62,63]
- pathological gambling[64]
- sex offender treatment[65,66]
- social phobia[67]
- substance use disorder.[68-71]

Controlled research is needed in all these areas to further determine the efficacy of EMDR with these diagnoses that are implicated as causal or related to substance use and other addictive behaviours. However, based on this emerging literature, it does not seem to be a matter of whether to consider using EMDR to treat complex disorders with a basis in trauma, but rather when, how and with whom.

EMDR GENERAL PRINCIPLES, PROTOCOLS AND PROCEDURES

'Man is made by his belief. As he believes, so he is.'[72]

EMDR is taught to licensed clinicians at Eye Movement Desensitisation and Reprocessing International Association (EMDRIA) and EMDR-Europe approved trainings worldwide. These trainings tend to be a minimum of six full days of instruction and practicum with an additional 10 hours of consultation, and are considered to be a basic training.

EMDR uses a three-pronged protocol within an eight-phase approach to sequentially target:
1 **Past** experiential contributors that laid the groundwork for the current symptoms.
2 **Present**-day triggers that activate cognitive, affective, and/or somatic symptoms.
3 **Future** templates of desired states and behaviours (*see* Table 12.3).[73]

TABLE 12.3 Overview of EMDR Phases (adapted[73]) (Used with the kind permission of Francine Shapiro)

Phase	Purpose	Procedures
1 Client history	• Collect background information	• Standard history taking, keeping the AIP in mind
	• Assess suitability for EMDR	• Review EMDR inclusions/exclusions/client resources
	• Identify specific treatment targets from history	• Elicit: (1) past events related to symptoms, (2) present-day triggers, and (3) future desired outcomes
2 Preparation	• Prepare the individual for EMDR processing	• Educate about symptom development
	• Stabilise and increase access to positive affects	• Teach stabilisation techniques such as a 'safe/calm place'
3 Assessment	• Activate the chosen targets for reprocessing	• Elicit the following:
		— distressing image
		— negative belief currently held (assess SUD 0–10*)
		— desired positive belief (assess VOC 1–7**)
		— current emotions
		— current physical sensations
4 Desensitisation	• Process past experiences and current triggers to an adaptive resolution (SUD of 0)	• Process past, present, future
		• Standardised EMDR protocols, including sets of bilateral stimulation, allow for spontaneous emergence of insights, emotions, sensations and other memories
	• Fully desensitise all channels	
	• Incorporate positive future templates	• If processing becomes blocked, use Cognitive Interweave to activate more adaptive information
		• 'Stay out of the way' of the individual's natural processing
5 Installation	• Increase connections to positive cognitive networks	• Have individual identify the best positive cognition (initial or emergent)
	• Increase generalisation effects within associated memories	• Continue processing until positive cognition is a 7 on the VOC scale
6 Body scan	• Complete processing of any residual distress associated with target	• Concentration on physical sensations and processing any residual distress

(continued)

Phase	Purpose	Procedures
7 Closure	• Ensure individual stability at the end of an EMDR session whether completely reprocessed or not	• Use relaxation or guided imagery to leave individual in comfortable state to leave office • Ask individual to monitor what happens between sessions
8 Reassessment	• Evaluation of treatment effects to ensure comprehensive reprocessing	• Explore what has emerged since last session by re-accessing the previous target • Evaluate integration after all targets processed

Notes:
* Subjective Units of Disturbance (SUD) developed by Wolpe.[88]
** Validity of Cognition (VOC) developed by Shapiro[14,15] © Reprinted with permission of the EMDR Institute, Watsonville, CA, USA.[73]

Following the principles of the AIP model, EMDR is a treatment that views false negative beliefs about oneself to result from dysfunctionally stored memories and the attendant emotions, body sensations and behavioural patterns they can generate. These negative beliefs are not the cause of the dysfunction; they are a symptom of the unprocessed memories at the root of pathology. Rather than directly challenging the beliefs, as in cognitive behavioural therapy for example, EMDR treatment identifies these core, irrational, negative beliefs and the memories that gave rise to them. It is understood that even when the individual recognises the beliefs as false at an intellectual level, insight will not necessarily stop their substance use or other behavioural addictions and compulsions. For genuine change to occur, the memories generating the incorrect belief: 'I am not good enough' must be fully reprocessed at cognitive, affective and somatic levels such that the correct belief: 'I am fine the way I am' or 'I am good enough' is integrated into the nervous system and experienced as true at a 'felt-sense' level.

The use of bilateral stimulation in EMDR

EMDR procedures incorporate alternating bilateral stimulation (BLS) of attention, also referred to as dual attention stimulation (DAS), by using eye movements, tactile taps or audio tones during which the individual is mindfully aware of imagery, thoughts, emotions and body sensations. Bilateral stimulation is also used during the preparation phase to strengthen the individual's resources and positive affective states, as in the Safe Place exercise. The resource development phase uses slow (and short) sets of BLS to avoid stimulating potentially negative material, which often occurs naturally when faster BLS is conducted.

EMDR therapy is organised around the principles of a person-centred model, meaning the individual's internal pathways for healing override the interpretations and directives of the therapist. In EMDR, professionals do not assume they know the precise way the individual needs to heal because their memories are linked in ways that are not always evident. During the reprocessing phases (3–6), the clinician utilises standardised procedures that most often follow the individual's free association of the material.

During desensitisation (Phase 4 – Table 12.3) longer and faster sets of BLS are used to access, activate, desensitise and reprocess the distressing elements of the targeted event. This type of purposeful activating, accessing and moving of the stored information liberates a person's reactions and behaviours at an unconscious level until the material is held as a coherent, adaptive narrative and integrated as a synthesised, functional whole, in present time. This resolution allows the person's own intrinsic drive towards mental, physical and spiritual health to emerge in the place of addictive patterns.

THE TREATMENT OF MENTAL HEALTH–SUBSTANCE USE DISORDERS WITH EMDR

The concept of a tri-stage model for treating complex trauma was first introduced by Pierre Janet in 1907[75] and then again by Judith Herman in 1992.[76] The tasks of this model are:

➤ safety and stabilisation
➤ trauma processing and mourning
➤ reconnection and reintegration.[75,76]

With addiction, an essential part of the third stage includes relapse prevention (*see* Chapter 13; and Book 6, Chapters 15 and 16). Please note that with complex treatment populations, neither the phases of standard EMDR therapy nor the three-stage complex trauma model are rigid or discrete, but intertwine and overlap as needed throughout treatment.

EMDR is highly effective and efficient. However, it is also emotionally evocative, which can pose an additional temporary risk of relapse with addiction in the initial phases. Therefore, attention to safety, support and resources is primary. The individual and family members need thorough education about the relationship between trauma and addiction. The therapist explains that EMDR conceptualises urges and the use of substances or other behaviours as being symptoms of unresolved trauma. Nightmares, flashbacks and hyper-arousal trigger the desire to medicate with drugs and/or alcohol.[7,25] It is proposed that once EMDR reprocesses traumatic memories, they will no longer hold any physical, emotional or cognitive distress, naturally leading to less interest in self-medication, thereby ultimately reducing the risk of relapse. Not all psychiatric disorders are life threatening, but substance use can be. Hence, it is recommended that EMDR be used as a 'staged model' within the standard eight-phase approach.

TASKS OF A PHASED, INTEGRATED MODEL OF EMDR
Stage one
(Phases 1 and 2 in EMDR: Table 12.3)
History, assessment, motivation, safety and stabilisation include:

➤ history gathering and diagnostic assessment
➤ safety and stabilisation skills[15,77]
➤ motivation.[78,79]

History: Phase 1 of EMDR

The individual's history is gathered with the AIP model in mind, using the designated three-prong protocol. It is just as important to identify the internal strengths and external resources to which the individual has access, as it is to uncover traumatic material. This ensures that the individual will be prepared for the reprocessing phases of trauma work. Reprocessing is defined as forging neurophysiological connections between the targeted memory and more adaptive networks. If the individual does not have access to positive memory networks there will be little with which to connect their dysfunctionally stored material and reprocessing would not be expected to go smoothly.[15]

Professionals are cautioned to gather information slowly when presented with a person who has a lifelong history of complex trauma in order to minimise potential triggering of negative, emotionally charged material. A gradual and paced history taking process is preferred, as 'too much too soon' can increase the risk of relapse (*see* Book 5, Chapter 9). The following guidelines are recommended.

➤ Assess for and provide any needed self-control or affect management techniques.

➤ Gather the individual's bio/psycho/social history including mental status, strengths, chronological trauma history, PTSD, anxiety and depressive symptoms.

➤ Assess for the presence of coexisting mental health–substance use disorders.

➤ Specifically access for dissociative disorders using the Dissociative Experiences Scale (DES)[80] or other appropriate screening tools for dissociation such as the Structured Clinical Interview for Dissociative Disorders (SCID-D).[81] It is important to note that the presence of a dissociative disorder is contraindicated for treatment using EMDR without both the expertise of the professional in this specialty area and readiness of the individual.[15,82]

➤ Elicit a detailed history of substance use and behavioural addiction:
  — note all substances used and pattern of use, e.g. binge, regular use, increasing amounts, maintenance
  — first use: what was happening at the time the individual first started using
  — assess current triggers and urges to use substances or other addictive behaviours
  — assess relapse patterns.

➤ Evaluate past treatment attempts and outcomes.

➤ Assess level of motivation for treatment: precontemplation, contemplation, preparation and action (*see* Chapters 6 and 7).[78,79]

➤ Educate the family about the nature of addiction as a brain disorder[24] and how untreated trauma is understood to be a contributing factor – this is considered a key to successful treatment.

➤ Assess level of support from family, friends and co-workers – each family member's role in either supporting or undermining the treatment process should be assessed, addressed and treated, whenever possible.[83]

Case study 12.1: PTSD, coexisting bipolar disorder, marijuana and alcohol abuse, compulsive use of pornography

John's wife referred her 33-year-old husband for EMDR because she had become fearful about his 'rapidly deteriorating emotional state'. She reported that during the last six months he had become increasingly more depressed, anxious, withdrawn, physically and emotionally abusive, and experienced occasional suicidal ideation. His marriage was on the line.

John reported that one year ago he had attended a family gathering where he unexpectedly saw an older cousin who molested him between the ages of 11 and 13. He had not seen that cousin in 10 years and thought he had 'already dealt with the molestation'. He was upset to find he was still powerless over his reactions. His parents dismissed his distress by asking him why something from 'such a long time ago' would bother him now.

Attempting to 'deal with' the symptoms listed below, John self-medicated with alcohol and marijuana on and off since adolescence. These behaviours and moods had escalated since seeing his cousin, and were threatening his job and marriage.

John's history: Phase 1 of EMDR (Table 12.3)

Presenting symptoms:
- sleep disturbance
- severe marital discord with emotional and physical rage outbursts
- mood swings
- self-injurious impulses and behaviours
- compulsive use of pornography
- marijuana and alcohol abuse.

Past: to be reprocessed during initial stage of the three-prong protocol:
- Family history of alcoholism, depression and suicide.
- Extreme parental mis-attunement and emotional neglect (e.g. John's isolated, unsafe conditions at home frightened and overwhelmed him. When he tried to communicate his fear to his parents, they minimised him and told him 'how easy he had it compared to them').
  - this ongoing invalidation was later revealed as the *earliest contributor* for the present-day overreactivity to wife's communications with him.
- Extended periods of isolation and loneliness.
- Sexual molestation from age 11–13 by 18-year-old male cousin.

John reported that his preoccupation with pornography and substance abuse emerged shortly after the molestation began. This is the most commonly reported temporal relationship between trauma and substance abuse.[25]

Early relational mis-attunement, poor attachment, parental neglect and extended periods of isolation would be expected to decrease John's developing ability to manage affect in childhood on into adulthood.[19-22] The AIP model would view John's symptoms, including his bipolar disorder, as being an expression of genetic, environmental and experiential factors, ultimately manifesting as diagnosable mood and substance use disorders.[6,14,84]

The sexual molestation by his older cousin, a known Criterion A event that was endured but never reported, would put him at risk for the development of PTSD.

The negative, irrational beliefs or Negative Cognitions (NCs) that often emerge from a history such as John's are a focus of treatment in EMDR. These beliefs are clustered under the headings of:
➤ responsibility
➤ safety
➤ choices.

Positive Cognitions (PCs), which the individual would prefer to feel and believe are true, are identified and measured at a 'gut level' by the Validity of Cognition scale (VOC)[14,15] and are remeasured after the reprocessing and installation phases 4–6 of EMDR. An increased felt-sense of the VOC indicates a positive treatment effect.

John's negative belief clusters related to the molestation treatment target are listed in Table 12.4. Each belief was targeted through the complete three-pronged protocol (past contributors, present day triggers, and desired future states and behaviours).

TABLE 12.4 Negative belief clusters related to the molestation treatment target

Negative cognitions (NC)	Positive cognitions (PC)	Cluster types
'I am permanently damaged'	'I am fine as I am'	Responsibility
'There's something really wrong with me'	'I'm fine as I am'	Responsibility
'I'm not safe'	'I can keep myself safe now'	Safety
'I can't trust'	'I can learn to trust'	Safety
'I am powerless'	'I have choices now'	Choices
'I can't stand it'	'I can handle it'	Choices

PRESENT TRIGGERS: TO BE PROCESSED DURING THE SECOND PHASE OF THE THREE-PRONG PROTOCOL
1 Feeling 'criticised'
2 Feeling 'misunderstood' and 'not able to be heard'
3 Feeling 'unimportant' to his wife.

Preparation: Phase 2 of EMDR
SAFETY, STABILISATION AND RESOURCE DEVELOPMENT
Readiness for EMDR reprocessing (Phases 3–6: Table 12.3) includes:
➤ the ability to access and use safe coping skills[14,15,77] to soothe high levels of distress
➤ the ability to have a dual awareness of the past traumatic material while still maintaining present-moment orientation
➤ the willingness to engage available resources such as a 12-step programme, sober living, family, and/or other personal support systems – this is especially crucial when individuals are still using substances
➤ sobriety of at least 30 days or until symptoms of withdrawal are minimised,

although this recommendation has exceptions; *see* the section 'Early trauma treatment in substance use disorders: guidelines and exceptions' later in this chapter.

Safety and stabilisation comes first with any population but because of the potentially evocative nature of EMDR, and the risk for relapse with mental health–substance use disorders, timing of the reprocessing (phases 3–6) is carefully assessed. When EMDR is used to treat single incident traumas, such as a motor vehicle accident, dog-bite or one-time assault, reprocessing with EMDR can be an exceedingly brief, effective intervention consisting of 1–3 (90-minute) reprocessing sessions.[15,85,86] There are also individuals who have strong personal strengths and resources who will not necessarily need a lengthy preparation phase. Sobriety and self-soothing are often enough to allow those individuals who have less complex histories to move forward into trauma reprocessing.

However, for those who have confounding variables of long-term, complex childhood trauma and exhibit a more severe and chronic course of symptoms, extensive preparation is *strongly recommended* to ensure the 'safest' trauma reprocessing experience. Reprocessing with EMDR has a lengthier preparation phase and reprocessing may take longer.

Additional resource development is needed when individuals are missing internal capacities that may interfere with their ability to tolerate reprocessing. For example, Resource Development and Installation (RDI)[87] can accesses, incorporate and strengthen a variety of internal positive affective states. Other grounding and self-soothing exercises may include visualisations in which people are able to imagine themselves thinking, feeling and behaving in a more positive, adaptive way. This manner of preparation for trauma treatment is a variation of the third prong, or Future Template, of EMDR.

More structured interventions may be integrated with EMDR in environments where group work or more intensive individualised preparatory experience is needed prior to individual trauma processing, for example:

➤ Seeking Safety[77]
➤ Motivational interviewing (MI)[78]
➤ Desensitisation of Triggers and Urge Reprocessing (DeTUR)[69]
➤ dialectical behaviour therapy (DBT – *see* Chapter 11; *see* To learn more).[88]

John's Preparation: Phase 2 of EMDR

Personal strengths and resources include:

➤ creative and artistic
➤ intelligent
➤ sensitive and warm
➤ long-term friendships from high school
➤ supportive wife.

Resources needed include:

➤ ability to self-soothe (Safe Place)
➤ willingness to commit to sobriety.

When John initially sought treatment he was not sober and had suicidal thoughts. Substance use disorders can confound assessments and trigger or prolong symptoms. Therefore, a psychiatrist conducted a medical evaluation and concluded, in collaboration with the treating therapist, that John required medically managed stabilisation prior to initiating any trauma processing with EMDR. John agreed to take medication and enter into a course of sobriety to allow the clinical picture to clear. He was able to remain clean for 30 days and the co-occurring disorders of bipolar, PTSD and substance use disorder were confirmed.

John was able to demonstrate his use of the Safe Place exercise,[15] along with other self-soothing techniques, which strengthened and allowed for the assessment of his ability to shift from a state of high distress to a state of calm. This, along with his sobriety and medical stabilisation, allowed us to move forward and reprocess his first EMDR target.

Stage two
Trauma reprocessing
PHASES 3 THROUGH 8 (TABLE 12.3) IN EMDR (ASSESSMENT, DESENSITISATION, INSTALLATION, BODY SCAN, CLOSURE AND RE-EVALUATION) USING THE THREE PRONGS OF PAST, PRESENT AND FUTURE

➤ Desensitise and reprocess all *past* traumas (big-T and small-t) and *present day* symptoms and triggers until they no longer cause cognitive, affective or somatic distress.
➤ Teach necessary skills and imaginarily rehearse future reactions and behaviours with BLS in order to develop *future* templates that can allow for more adaptive choices.

Assessment: Phase 3 of EMDR
John collaborated in his treatment planning and chose the molestation as his first and most distressing target.

Setting up the target includes doing the following.
➤ Identify the most disturbing image associated with the event (the first time he was held captive in a closet and molested by his older cousin).
➤ Identify the irrational negative belief (NC) related to the event ('There's something really wrong with me').
➤ Identify the desired positive, more accurate belief (PC) ('I'm fine the way I am').
➤ Assess the Validity of Cognition (VOC) when the incident is held in mind, on a gut-level scale of 1–7, where 1 feels totally false and 7 feels completely true *now* (John reported a VOC of 2).
➤ Assess the Subjective Units of Disturbance (SUD)[74] on a scale of 0–10, where 0 is no disturbance and 10 is the highest imaginable (John reported a SUD of 9).
➤ Identify where in the body the distress is noticed (John reported tightness in chest, nausea, stomach cramping and 'head spinning').

Desensitisation: Phase 4–6 (Table 12.3) of EMDR

The desensitisation and reprocessing phases initially use BLS sets of 18 to 24 passes while asking the individual to mindfully 'just notice' what is emerging during and between sets. The length of subsequent sets is based upon the individual's affective and cognitive responses. A deep breath is taken when BLS is stopped, and the individual then reports what is being experienced. The clinician then helps guide the individual to the focus of attention for the next set. After approximately 20 sets, John stated with clear conviction that he was only 11 years old, that his cousin was 'almost an adult' at 18, and that he could not imagine an 11-year-old child 'causing or being responsible for their own molestation'. He also noted that the 'absence of his parents' supervision' during much of his childhood left him at greater risk for exploitation. Clearing those networks revealed additional NCs such as 'I'm unimportant' and 'I can't trust', and then led to the insight that he managed 'feeling misunderstood or unduly criticised' by becoming explosive and abusive towards his wife.

THE TREATMENT OF PRESENT DAY TRIGGERS AND URGES TO USE

John's present day triggers and urges to use alcohol, marijuana, pornography and abuse his wife were reprocessed. It should be emphasised that it is necessary to process any early memories that set the groundwork for pathology in order to prevent relapse.

John's triggers to use can be found in Table 12.5.

TABLE 12.5 Triggers and substance of choice

Triggers	Substance of choice
Perception of being criticised	Marijuana (calming)
Feeling misunderstood	Marijuana, alcohol, and angry outburst (calming, and to relieve tension)
Social events	Marijuana and alcohol (felt more social)
Loneliness and isolation	Pornography (felt more connected)

When exploring John's triggers, they were revealed to be directly associated with the experiences and emotions he had first felt as a child in response to his parents' behaviour. Their insensitive responses frequently left him feeling misunderstood, unheard, unimportant and extremely frustrated.

In EMDR's standard three-prong protocol, triggers are identified and reprocessed as an individual EMDR target. For example, after reprocessing an earlier memory of a familiar interaction with his parents (first prong of three), his current 'feeling of being misunderstood' was set up as follows:

➤ Target image: arguing with his wife
➤ NC: 'I'm not important'
➤ PC: 'I am important and deserve to be heard'
➤ VOC: 3
➤ Emotions: extreme frustration, anger, sadness, fear
➤ SUD: 8

➤ Felt in the body: tightness in chest, stomach
➤ Reprocessed to SUD of 0 and VOC of 7 with clear body scan.

At the conclusion of reprocessing this target, John saw even more clearly that his parents were 'good people' who often communicated with criticism due to their own anxiety, not his shortcomings as he had previously thought. They also left him alone for long periods of time because they both worked long hours, not because he was unimportant, but to support him, the child they loved. These clarifications spontaneously emerged during processing and were key to John's establishing a positive, loving connection within and for himself.

As a result of reprocessing, his triggers no longer activated an urge to use substances or pornography, allowing him to enter a long-term period of sobriety for the first time in his life. His nervous system was cleared of the 'old feelings' of 'I don't matter' and quieted the overreactivity, which often resulted in the abuse of his wife.

Installation: Phase 5 (Table 12.3) of EMDR
Once a SUD of 0 (or with some ecological exceptions, a 1) is reported, installation of the PC is continued until a VOC of 7 is reached. John's original NC was 'There's something really wrong with me.' John's PC evolved into 'I am fine as I am' and was reported at a VOC of 7.

Body scan: Phase 6 (Table 12.3) of EMDR
BODY SCAN
The individual brings up the original target and the positive belief and scans their body for any remaining distress or sensation. If anything even slight is reported, reprocessing continues until no remaining discomfort or body sensations can be identified. John reported he was clear and had no remaining bodily distress.

FUTURE TEMPLATE
At this point, a future imagined rehearsal is conducted. In John's case, he was asked to think about a future time that he might run into his cousin and 'notice' whether there was any distress connected with that possibility. John was able to imagine the scene without much problem, until the therapist suggested that he visualise his cousin chatting with another young male family member. This triggered some distress and feelings of 'protectiveness'. John stated that, as an adult, he would do whatever might be necessary to keep a child safe from his cousin. The visualisation was continued until John could 'view it' calmly and assertively with no physical, emotional or cognitive disturbance.

Closure: Phase 7 (Table 12.3) of EMDR
Close down complete or incomplete sessions by using the Safe Place or any other positive resources developed and strengthened by the individual during the preparation phase of EMDR. John's session on the molestation was closed down as a complete session, as he had arrived at a SUD of 0, a VOC of 7, with a clear body scan.

Re-evaluation: Phase 8 (Table 12.3) of EMDR

Treatment targets are re-evaluated at the following session to see if any change has occurred. The individual is asked to 'bring up the memory' previously worked on and 'notice what comes up for you today'. If the individual reports any distressing thoughts, feelings or body sensations they are reprocessed until complete (SUD of 0, VOC of 7) using the same procedures noted during the assessment and desensitisation phases. When no further disturbance is reported, Phase 3 of EMDR is revisited and the next target in the treatment plan is selected.

At John's follow-up visit, the target remained at a SUD of 0, a VOC of 7, with a clear body scan. He also reported he experienced a sense of 'lightness' between sessions when he would think of the molestation, as if the weight of a boulder had been lifted from his chest.

Stage three

Reconnection, integration and relapse prevention

This occurs in all phases of EMDR, and particularly during the future template or third prong of the standard protocol.

Reconnection and reintegration takes place in all phases of EMDR and most powerfully in Phases 3–6. When traumatic memories are successfully reprocessed and one's personal strengths and resources are fully accessible, an often-reported outcome is connection with one's core spiritual self. This then allows the freedom to reconnect with family, friends, co-workers and society at a higher level of cognitive, affective, physiological and behavioural functioning.

Stage 3 of trauma treatment involves and results in the following:

➤ A felt-sense of integration with oneself, along with an enhanced ability to connect or reconnect with others that is believed to be a natural result of reprocessing and integrating distressing material more adaptively and fully.

➤ Use of the third prong of EMDR, the Future Template (a processed and encoded imaginary rehearsal): The third prong gives the individual an opportunity to systematically *imagine* the future, as if running a movie, with (potentially relapse-triggering) a variety of experiences (people, places or things) in mind. These targets are reprocessed with bilateral stimulation until they can be imagined without distress and with the self-referencing statements (e.g. 'I am deserving') feeling true at a 'felt-sense' level.

➤ It prepares the neural networks for future adaptive action without the use of substances or other self-destructive behaviours.

Future Template: third prong of the three-prong protocol

'How would you like to see yourself handling these issues in the future?' included:

➤ calm and rational communications with wife

➤ able to hear and receive feedback without interpreting it all as 'critical'

➤ clean and sober from substances and pornography

➤ able to be alone or connect with others and be comfortable either way.

Example of Future Template with John

Future Template target: remaining calm when in disagreement with his wife.

John was asked to imagine a movie scene of he and his wife disagreeing about the social plans she made without first consulting him. This triggered the belief, 'I don't matter' along with anger and tension in his chest. The image, emotion and sensation were reprocessed until he reported they were neutral and no longer disturbing. Asked if there was any level of urge to use substances or self-destructive behaviours at the thought of arguing with his wife, John said, 'No.' It is expected that successful use of the Future Template will lower the risk of relapse because it reduces or eliminates identified motivators to self-medicate.

EARLY TRAUMA TREATMENT IN SUBSTANCE USE DISORDERS: GUIDELINES AND EXCEPTIONS

Treating professionals must be experienced both as chemical dependency and EMDR therapists, or be under close supervision of someone with those qualifications. As a rule, EMDR is not recommended before a minimum 30-day period of sobriety has been established. Clearly, there are risks in treating trauma early in recovery or without sobriety. However, there are also cases where targeting a traumatic event can reduce the symptoms resulting from unprocessed trauma that interfere with attempts to attain or maintain sobriety.

Case study 12.2: Jeannie

Jeannie had a rocky childhood with adoptive parents who had decided, 'They really didn't want a child after all'. She was physically cared for but was emotionally neglected and verbally berated. Alcoholic and cocaine dependent since her teens, she was now 41, married, with a teenage son.

At 15, Jeannie's parents, who often fought with one another, seemingly about her, divorced bitterly. She blamed herself for their marital failure. Jeannie lived with her mother, who made it clear that she was not to open the door to her father if she was not present. Her father, who suffered from severe emphysema, came by one day hauling his oxygen tank behind him. He became angry and escalated into a rage when Jeannie refused to open the door. The angrier he got the more impaired his breathing became. Terrified of her mother, Jeannie did not let him in. Later that week, her father was hospitalised and died shortly thereafter. She blamed herself for his death and her mother did as well. Jeannie soon began to use substances to cope with these childhood events, and her addictions quickly spiralled out of control. She found herself unable to manage without the use of substances.

Jeannie had numerous previous attempts at counselling and sobriety but, when sober, the flashbacks and anxieties stemming from her childhood overwhelmed her. After several months of trauma treatment preparation: teaching safe coping skills, strengthening inner resources and developing emotional management skills, she was still unable to establish sobriety for more than a few days and could not maintain a serious recovery programme. While sobriety is preferable before EMDR reprocessing, in Jeannie's case the therapist and Jeannie collaboratively decided to proceed and targeted her belief that she was responsible for her father dying.

The reprocessing was successful within two sessions and freed Jeannie from her 26-year-old belief that she was at fault for her father's death. She also came to know that the way her parents treated her in childhood was not because something was 'wrong with her', but was because of her parents' own issues, which were not her fault either. With these deeply felt perceptual changes, Jeannie was finally able to enter into and sustain recovery. She said that resolving that experience had given her hope that the remainder of her traumatic past could be reprocessed as well. It took over a year to target her remaining issues with one relapse early in recovery. Jeannie is now in her fourth year of uninterrupted sobriety.

AN INTEGRATED TRAUMA TREATMENT PROGRAM (ITTP) USING EMDR AND SEEKING SAFETY[77] IN A US DRUG COURT PROGRAM

The Integrated Trauma Treatment Program (ITTP)[89] was designed for the Thurston County Drug Court Program in Olympia, Washington to treat co-occurring PTSD/trauma, and substance use disorders in non-violent felony offenders who had been arrested on drug-related charges. Between 2004 and 2007, 219 drug court participants were assessed for the ITTP that combines Seeking Safety[77] and EMDR. These two evidence-based, empirically supported treatment modalities were field tested between 2004 and 2007 as an enhancement to the existing 12–18 month Drug Court Program that offers treatment in lieu of incarceration.

Seeking Safety is a present-focused, empirically supported, manualised CBT-based treatment program for PTSD, trauma and substance abuse that has demonstrated significant treatment effects for PTSD symptom reduction[77] (*see* To learn more). Composed of 25 topics that provide education, safety, stabilisation, skill building and rehearsal in preparation for possible later-stage treatment of past trauma such as EMDR, it is now listed as a Best Practice through the Substance Abuse and Mental Health Services Administration.[90] Seeking Safety participants learn about the relationship between trauma and substance abuse, how to develop and practise safe coping skills, for example: participate in a recovery programme, ask for help, create healthy relationships, spend time with clean and sober friends, and learn about 'red flags' or triggers to use. Seeking Safety was provided in a same-gender group format and served as part of a structured Phase 2 (Preparation) of the EMDR treatment approach.

Seeking Safety facilitators need to have an empathic interest in the participants, familiarity with PTSD, trauma and substance abuse, and a willingness and ability to work with a manualised treatment protocol.[77] Completion of 15 pre-selected topics of Seeking Safety was a prerequisite to receiving individual treatment with EMDR. Sobriety was supervised via random urine drug screens throughout the entirety of the Drug Court Program.

Preliminary data analysis from the ITTP[89] indicates that of the 219 drug court participants assessed for trauma with the Clinician Administered PTSD Scale (CAPS[91]) and the Detailed Assessment of Posttraumatic Stress (DAPS[92]), 160 or 73% reported at least one Criterion A event. Of these 160 (100% of the resulting treatment sample) enrolled in the ITTP, 123 or 77% completed Seeking Safety and were offered EMDR as a voluntary supplement to the existing Drug Court Program.

Fifty completed Seeking Safety but declined EMDR. Sixty-nine completed Seeking Safety and chose to participate in EMDR (more than half of these participants designated methamphetamine as their drug of choice) and graduated from the Drug Court Program at a rate of 91%, compared to a graduation rate of 62% for those who declined EMDR. Further analysis of this data set will be reported in an article currently in preparation.[89]

Graduation required:

➤ achieving 180 consecutive days of medically substantiated sobriety
➤ obtaining a General Education Diploma (GED) or high school diploma prior to or while in the programme
➤ becoming employed full-time in a tax-paying job or enrolling full-time in school
➤ payment of all restitution and programme fees.

Drug Court Program completion and graduation are the strongest predictors of lower post-programme recidivism rates.[93]

One Drug Court participant, Tom, had been arrested 14 times for felony drug possession. He was in his third and final Drug Court Program opportunity when EMDR was introduced. His history revealed two alcoholic parents, substance abuse beginning in adolescence, and his father's death from cancer. At the age of 31, Tom and his brother were cross-country tractor-trailer truck-driving partners. While driving drunk, they engaged in a bitter argument. Tom's brother, in a fit of rage, unbuckled his seat belt and stepped out of the truck as it was going 65 mph (105 kph). He died in Tom's arms on the side of the road.

Tom blamed himself for his brother's death. His subsequent increase in addictions and arrests led to the loss of his family, business and freedom. He never had treatment for his traumatic past, nor had he known it fuelled his addictions. Successfully targeting and reprocessing the memory of the death of his brother with EMDR was the beginning of a long-lasting recovery for Tom, now seven years sober. One of the first successful participants of the ITTP, Tom has been an avid spokesperson and role model for the programme and often speaks publically to inspire other Drug Court participants.

The following case study illustrates the importance of considering small-t traumas, as well as the big-T traumas, when treating this population.

Case study 12.3: Karen – co-occurring panic and substance use disorder rooted in a small-t trauma

Karen (47) was referred for EMDR. She was nine months sober from poly-substance abuse, but was still sexually compulsive and continued to have panic attacks, which despite several trials of psychotropic medication led her to use again. She thought drugging herself was more effective than the medication, even though using only deepened her sense of guilt, shame and isolation.

She had more than 10 years of unsuccessful treatment for her panic attacks before her earliest memories of them were targeted for EMDR reprocessing. She focused on the 'fear in her body' and within a few moments connected with a memory at age four of being dropped off at a park with instructions to care for her two-year-old sister. It seemed to Karen like her parents left her there the entire day. By the time they returned, Karen was in a panic, vomiting, sobbing and unable to catch her breath. Her father screamed at her to 'knock it off and quit acting like a baby'. Her panic shifted to shame and humiliation when his rage changed to laughter about what a 'wimp' she was.

The developing brain of a child requires a certain level of attunement and safety in order to develop its emotional regulation capacities,[20,21] without which a child is potentially more vulnerable to later substance use.[88] Thus, Karen tried to regulate her emotions in the absence of supportive parenting. In less than a year, at age five, Karen took her first sip of beer at an unsupervised party of her parents and never stopped drinking thereafter. At age 12, she began smoking marijuana. She did not stop using until age 46.

More serious traumas occurred throughout her childhood, including multiple sexual molestations; however, Karen states that the park incident was the first and most overwhelming experience that set the tone for the 'rest of my life'. She reported that the feelings she experienced at age four felt just like the panic attacks she continued to experience into adulthood and attempted to medicate with drugs, alcohol and compulsive sex; but by all clinical standards, the park incident was a small-t trauma.

Karen's panic attacks diminished in intensity and frequency after the reprocessing of this pivotal memory with EMDR, thereby easing her urges to use marijuana and alcohol to medicate them. This case underscores the importance of reprocessing the memories responsible for not only the faulty cognitive beliefs one holds about themselves, but also reprocessing the body sensations that are reported, such as are evident in panic attacks, that may, or may not, have a specific negative belief associated with them. This example illuminates the importance of not only reprocessing big-T, but also all the relevant life experiences we consider to be small-t traumas.

CONCLUSION

Why use EMDR to treat mental health–substance use disorders?

'Although the world is full of suffering, it is also full of overcoming it.'[94]

As research and clinical experience suggest, the incidence of mental health–substance use disorders within the criminal justice system[90,93] and substance use treatment centres across the nation indicates the need for specialised treatment programmes designed specifically for this challenging population. The personal, familial, social, health and economic consequences that result from failing to treat these individuals has been staggering and seems remediable.

Mental health–substance use disorders are a unique treatment challenge and EMDR is a unique response to that challenge. EMDR's AIP model predicts that early trauma is a primary contributor to the emergence of clinical symptoms and disorders, often leading to the use of substances and behaviours designed to regulate distress. The eight-phase treatment approach and three-prong protocol of EMDR is ideally suited to the treatment of mental health–substance use disorders, and targets the:

> **past** experiential contributors to present day symptoms
> **present**-day triggers that activate distress
> **future** templates of desired states and behaviours.

It is the third prong in particular that gives individuals an opportunity to imagine encountering many possible relapse-triggering situations (people, places and things) in the future. These targets are then reprocessed with BLS until the future can be visualised without distress and the individual's positive self-referencing statements feel true at that 'felt-sense' level. It is believed that the treatment effects observed with EMDR offer people experiencing mental health–substance use disorders an extra measure of inoculation against future relapse with drugs, alcohol or other self-destructive behaviours intended to help the individual 'feel better'. The temporary solution of addiction eventually displaces a person's true spiritual self with powerlessness and self-loathing that impacts on the individual and the family in a vicious intergenerationally transmitted cycle. This chapter began with the observation that substance use disorders are the number one social problem in the United States and the assertion that unresolved trauma and neglect are strongly correlated with the vast majority of those who suffer from addictions. Therefore, we call to attention the hypothesis that *society's number one* problem is not substance abuse but unresolved trauma and neglect.

It is hoped that the ITTP pilot programme will be replicated using a comparison treatment, within a randomised controlled trial, in order to more rigorously illuminate the efficacy and real-world applicability of this type of treatment intervention.

The following elements highlight EMDR as a treatment of choice for mental health–substance use disorders:

> EMDR is an empirically supported clinical intervention.
> It is a comprehensive, integrative approach to the treatment of trauma-based disorders, including substance use disorders and behavioural addictions.
> The Adaptive Information Processing model predicts outcomes.
> It is applicable to individual, family[83] and programme treatment.[89]
> Progress is measurable with subjective internal scales: Validity of Cognition (VOC)[14,15] and Subjective Units of Disturbance (SUD).[74]
> Its efficacy is measurable by standardised professionally administered assessments and self-report.
> It can be used with diagnoses in addition to PTSD.
> It has high potential for significantly reduced treatment time.[85]
> It has reduced treatment dropout rates compared to other treatments and is well tolerated by the individual.[28,30,35–38,85,95]

REFERENCES

1 Schneider Institute for Health Policy, Brandeis University for the Robert Wood Johnson Foundation. *Substance Abuse: the nation's number one health problem.* Princeton, NJ; 2001.

2 World Health Organization. *Neuroscience of Psychoactive Substance Use and Dependence.* Geneva: WHO Library; 2004.

3 Khantzian EJ. The self-medication hypothesis of addictive disorders: focus on heroin and cocaine dependence. *American Journal of Psychiatry.* 1985; **142**: 1259–64.

4 Weinhold JB, Weinhold BK. *The Flight from Intimacy: healing your relationship of counter-dependence.* Novato, CA: New World Library; 2008.

5 Kessler RC, Sonnega A, Bromet E, *et al.* Posttraumatic stress disorders in the National Comorbidity Survey. *Archives of General Psychiatry.* 1995; **52**: 1048–60.

6 Felitti VJ, Anda RF, Nordenberg D, *et al.* Relationship of childhood abuse and household dysfunction to many of the leading causes of death in adults: The Adverse Childhood Experiences (ACE) Study. *American Journal of Preventive Medicine.* 1998; **14**: 245–58.

7 National Child Traumatic Stress Network (NCSTN). *Making the Connection: trauma and substance abuse; understanding the links between adolescent trauma and substance abuse; a toolkit for providers.* 2nd ed. June 2008. Available at: www.nctsnet.org/nccts/asset. do?id=1377 (accessed 13 September 2010).

8 Ouimette P, Brown P, editors. *Trauma and Substance Abuse: causes, consequences and treatment of comorbid disorders.* Washington, DC: American Psychological Association; 2003.

9 American Psychiatric Association. *Diagnostic and Statistical Manual of Mental Disorders: DSM-IV-TR.* Washington, DC: American Psychiatric Association; 2000.

10 Brady KT, Killeen T, Saladin ME, *et al.* Comorbid substance abuse and posttraumatic stress disorder: characteristics of women in treatment. *The American Journal on Addictions.* 1994; **3**: 160–4.

11 Brown PJ, Stout R, Mueller T. Post-traumatic stress disorder and substance abuse relapse among women: a pilot study. *Psychology of Addictive Behaviors.* 1996; **10**: 124–8.

12 Najavits LM, Weiss RD, Shaw SR. A clinical profile of women with PTSD and substance dependence. *Psychology of Addictive Behaviors.* 1999; **13**: 98–104.

13 Grant J, Brewer J, Potenza, M. The neurobiology of substance and behavioral addictions. *CNS Spectrum.* 2006; **11**: 924–30.

14 Shapiro F. *Eye Movement Desensitization and Reprocessing: basic principles, protocols, and procedures.* New York: Guilford Press; 1995.

15 Shapiro F. *Eye Movement Desensitization and Reprocessing: basic principles, protocols and procedures.* 2nd ed. New York: Guilford Press; 2001.

16 Shapiro F. EMDR, adaptive information processing, and case conceptualization. *Journal of EMDR Practice and Research.* 2007; **1**: 68–87.

17 Solomon R, Shapiro F. EMDR and the adaptive information processing model: potential mechanisms of change. *Journal of EMDR Practice and Research.* 2008; **2**: 315–25.

18 Ralph Blum. Available at: www.great-inspirational-quotes.com/inspirational-quotes.html (accessed 13 August 2010).

19 Perry B. Memories of fear: how the brain stores and retrieves physiologic states, feelings, behaviors and thoughts from traumatic events. In: Goodwin J, Attias R, editors. *Splintered Reflections: images of the body in trauma.* New York: Basic Books; 1999.

20 Schore A. Dysregulation of the right brain: a fundamental mechanism of traumatic attachment and the psychopathogensis of posttraumatic stress disorder. *Australian and New Zealand Journal of Psychiatry.* 2002; **36**: 9–30.

21 Siegel D. *The Developing Mind: toward a neurobiology of interpersonal experience.* New York and London: Guilford Press; 1999.

22 Van der Kolk B, Pelcovitz D, Roth S, *et al.* Dissociation, affect dysregulation and somatization:

the complex nature of adaptation to trauma. *American Journal of Psychiatry.* 1996; **153**(Festschrigt Supplement): S83–93.

23 Brown PJ, Stout RL, Gannon-Rowley J. Substance use disorder – PTSD comorbidity: patients' perceptions of symptom interplay and treatment issues. *Journal of Substance Abuse Treatment.* 1998; **15**: 445–8.

24 Volkow N. Addiction and the brain's pleasure pathway: beyond willpower. The Addiction Project; 2007. Available at: www.addictioninfo.org/articles/1376/1/Addiction-and-the-Brains-Pleasure-Pathway-Beyond-Willpower/Page1.html (accessed 12 August 2010).

25 Steward SH, Conrod PJ. Psychosocial models of functional associations between post-traumatic stress disorder and substance use disorder. In: Ouimette P, Brown P, editors. *Trauma and Substance Abuse: causes, consequences, and treatment of comorbid disorders.* Washington, DC: American Psychological Association; 2003.

26 Charles Dickens. *Sketches by Boz.* Oxford: Oxford University Press; 1956.

27 Hucker SJ. Disorders of impulse control. In: O'Donohue W, Levensky E, editors. *Forensic Psychology.* New York: Academic Press; 2004.

28 American Psychiatric Association. *Practice Guideline for the Treatment of Patients with Acute Stress Disorder and Posttraumatic Stress Disorder.* Arlington, VA: American Psychiatric Association; 2004.

29 Bisson J, Andrew M. Psychological treatment of post-traumatic stress disorder (PTSD). *Cochrane Database of Systematic Reviews.* 2007; **3**: CD003388. DOI: 10.1002/14651858. CD003388.pub3.

30 Department of Veterans Affairs and Department of Defense. *VA/DoD Clinical Practice Guideline for the Management of Post-Traumatic Stress.* Washington, DC: Department of Veterans Affairs and Department of Defense; 2004.

31 National Institute for Health and Clinical Excellence. *Post-traumatic Stress Disorder (PTSD): the management of adults and children in primary and secondary care.* NICE guideline 26. London: NIHCE; 2005.

32 Maxfield L, Hyer L. The relationship between efficacy and methodology in studies investigating EMDR treatment of PTSD. *Journal of Clinical Psychology.* 2002; **58**: 23–41.

33 Foa EB, Hembree EA, Rothbaum BO. *Prolonged Exposure Therapy for PTSD: emotional processing of traumatic experiences therapist guide (treatments that work).* Oxford: Oxford University Press; 2007.

34 Davidson PR, Parker KCH. Eye movement desensitization and reprocessing (EMDR): a meta-analysis. *Journal of Consulting and Clinical Psychology.* 2001; **69**: 305–16.

35 Ironson GI, Freund B, Strauss JL, *et al.* Comparison of two treatments for traumatic stress: a community-based study of EMDR and prolonged exposure. *Journal of Clinical Psychology.* 2002; **58**: 113–28.

36 Jaberghaderi N, Greenwald R, Rubin A, *et al.* A comparison of CBT and EMDR for sexually abused Iranian girls. *Clinical Psychology and Psychotherapy.* 2004; **11**: 358–68.

37 Lee C, Gavriel H, Drummond P, *et al.* Treatment of post-traumatic stress disorder: a comparison of stress inoculation training with prolonged exposure and eye movement desensitization and reprocessing. *Journal of Clinical Psychology.* 2002; **58**: 1071–89.

38 Power KG, McGoldrick T, Brown K, *et al.* A controlled comparison of eye movement desensitization and reprocessing versus exposure plus cognitive restructuring, versus waiting list in the treatment of post-traumatic stress disorder. *Journal of Clinical Psychology and Psychotherapy.* 2002; **9**: 299–318.

39 Andrade J, Kavanagh D, Baddeley A. Eye-movements and visual imagery: a working

memory approach to the treatment of post-traumatic stress disorder. *British Journal of Clinical Psychology.* 1997; **36**: 209–23.

40 Barrowcliff AL, Gray NS, Freeman TCA, *et al.* Eye-movements reduce the vividness, emotional valence and electrodermal arousal associated with negative autobiographical memories. *Journal of Forensic Psychiatry and Psychology.* 2004; **15**: 325–54.

41 Christman SD, Garvey KJ, Propper RE, *et al.* Bilateral eye movements enhance the retrieval of episodic memories. *Neuropsychology.* 2003; **17**: 221–9.

42 Bergmann U. Further thoughts on the neurobiology of EMDR: the role of the cerebellum in accelerated information processing. *Traumatology.* 2000; **6**: 175–200.

43 Bergmann U. The neurobiology of EMDR: exploring the thalamus and neural integration. *Journal of EMDR Practice and Research.* 2008; **2**: 300–14.

44 Stickgold R. EMDR: a putative neurobiological mechanism of action. *Journal of Clinical Psychology.* 2002; **58**: 61–75.

45 Mol S, Arntz A, Metsemakers J, *et al.* Symptoms of posttraumatic stress disorder after non-traumatic events: evidence from an open population study. *British Journal of Psychiatry.* 2005; **186**: 494–9.

46 Robinson JS, Larson C. Are traumatic events necessary to elicit symptoms of posttraumatic stress? *Psychological Trauma: theory, research, practice, and policy.* 2010; **2**: 71–6.

47 Brown KW, McGoldrick T, Buchanan R. Body dysmorphic disorder: seven cases treated with eye movement desensitization and reprocessing. *Behavioural and Cognitive Psychotherapy.* 1997; **25**: 203–7.

48 Brown S, Shapiro F. EMDR in the treatment of borderline personality disorder. *Clinical Case Studies.* 2006; **5**: 403–20.

49 de Roos C, de Jongh A. EMDR treatment of children and adolescents with a choking phobia. *Journal of EMDR Practice and Research.* 2008; **2**: 201–11.

50 Schurmans K. A clinical vignette: EMDR treatment of choking phobia. *Journal of EMDR Practice and Research.* 2007; **1**: 118–21.

51 McLaughlin D, McGowan I, Paterson M, *et al.* Cessation of deliberate self harm following eye movement desensitization and reprocessing: a case report. *Case Journal.* 2008; **1**: 177.

52 Stowasser J. EMDR and family therapy in the treatment of domestic violence. In: Kaslow F, Shapiro F, Maxfield L, editors. *The Integration of EMDR and Family Therapy Processes.* New York: Wiley; 2007.

53 Beer R. Symposium: EMDR and eating disorders – EMDR for adolescents with anorexia nervosa: evolution of conceptualization and illustration of clinical applications. EMDR European Association Conference, Brussels, Belgium; 2005, June.

54 Bloomgarden A, Calogero RM. A randomized experimental test of the efficacy of EMDR treatment on negative body image in eating disorder inpatients. *Eating Disorders.* 2008; **16**: 418–27.

55 Whisman M, Keller M. Integrating EMDR in the treatment of obsessive-compulsive disorder. *Proceedings of the EMDR International Association Annual Conference*; 1999; Las Vegas, NV.

56 Wilensky M. Eye movement desensitization and reprocessing (EMDR) as a treatment for phantom limb pain. *Journal of Brief Therapy.* 2006; **5**: 31–44.

57 Russell MC. Treating traumatic amputation-related phantom limb pain: a case study utilizing eye movement desensitization and reprocessing within the armed services. *Clinical Case Studies.* 2008; **7**: 136–53.

58 Schneider J, Hofmann A, Rost C, *et al.* EMDR and phantom limb pain: theoretical implica-

tions, case study, and treatment guidelines. *Journal of EMDR Practice and Research*, 2007; **1**: 31–45.

59 Tinker RH, Wilson SA. The phantom limb pain protocol. In: Shapiro R, editor. *EMDR Solutions: pathways to healing*. New York: WW Norton; 2005. pp. 147–59.

60 de Jongh A. Anxiety disorders – treatment of phobias with EMDR. *Proceedings of the EMDR European Association Conference*; 2003; Rome, Italy.

61 de Jongh A, ten Broeke E. Treatment of specific phobias with EMDR: conceptualization and strategies for the selection of appropriate memories. *Journal of EMDR Practice and Research*. 2007; **1**: 46–56.

62 Fernandez I, Faretta E. Eye movement desensitization and reprocessing in the treatment of panic disorder with agoraphobia. *Clinical Case Studies*. 2007; **6**: 44–63.

63 Feske U, Goldstein A. Eye movement desensitization and reprocessing treatment for panic disorder: a controlled outcome and partial dismantling study. *Journal of Consulting and Clinical Psychology*. 1997; **65**: 1026–35.

64 Henry S. Pathological gambling: etiologic considerations and treatment efficacy of eye movement desensitization/reprocessing. *Journal of Gambling Studies*. 1996; **12**: 395–405.

65 Ricci RJ. Trauma resolution using Eye Movement Desensitization and Reprocessing with an incestuous sex offender. *Clinical Case Studies*. 2006; **5**: 248–65.

66 Ricci RJ, Clayton CA, Shapiro F. Some effects of EMDR on previously abused child molesters: theoretical reviews and preliminary findings. *The Journal of Forensic Psychiatry and Psychology*. 2006; **17**: 538–62.

67 Sun TF, Chiu NM. Synergism between mindfulness meditation and eye movement desensitization and reprocessing in psychotherapy of social phobia. *Chang Gung Medical Journal*. 2006; **29**: 1–4.

68 Zweben J, Yeary J. EMDR in the treatment of addiction. *Journal of Chemical Dependency Treatment*. 2006; **8**: 115–27.

69 Popky AJ. Desensitization of triggers and urge reprocessing (DeTUR). In: Shapiro R, editor. *EMDR Solutions*. New York and London: WW Norton; 2005.

70 Shapiro F, Vogelmann-Sine S, Sine LF. Eye movement desensitization and reprocessing: treating trauma and substance abuse. *Journal of Psychoactive Drugs*. 1994; **26**: 379–91.

71 Vogelmann-Sinn S, Sine LF, Smyth NJ, *et al*. *EMDR Chemical Dependency Treatment Manual*. New Hope, PA: EMDR Humanitarian Assistance Programs; 1998.

72 Goethe. Available at: www.whale.to/a/goethe_q.html (accessed 26 August 2010).

73 Shapiro F. *Eye Movement Desensitization and Reprocessing (EMDR) Training Manual*. Watsonville, CA: EMDR Institute; 2005.

74 Wolpe J. *The Practice of Behavior Therapy*. New York: Pergamon Press; 1969.

75 Janet P. *The Major Symptoms of Hysteria*. London and New York: Macmillan; 1907.

76 Herman J. *Trauma and Recovery: the aftermath of violence – from domestic abuse to political terror*. New York: Basic Books; 1992.

77 Najavits L. *Seeking Safety: a treatment manual for PTSD and substance abuse*. New York: Guilford Press; 2002.

78 Miller WR, Rollnick S. *Motivational Interviewing: preparing people to change addictive behavior*. New York: Guildford Press; 1991.

79 Prochaska J, DiClemente C. Stages and processes of self-change of smoking: toward an integrative model of change. *Journal of Consulting and Clinical Psychology*. 1983; **51**: 390–95.

80 Bernstein, EM, Putnam, FW. Development, reliability and validity of a dissociation scale. *Journal of Nervous and Mental Disease*. 1986; **174**: 727–35.

81 Steinberg M, Rounsaville B, Cicchetti DV. The structured clinical interview for DSM-III-R

dissociative disorders: preliminary report on a new diagnostic instrument. *American Journal of Psychiatry*. 1990; **147**: 76–82.

82 Forgash C, Copeley M, editors. *Healing the Heart of Trauma and Dissociation with EMDR and Ego State Therapy*. New York: Spring Publishing; 2008.

83 Shapiro F. EMDR, Adaptive information processing, and case conceptualization. In: Shapiro F, Kaslow F, Maxfield L, editors. *Handbook of EMDR and Family Therapy Processes*. New York: Wiley; 2007.

84 National Institute of Mental Health (NIMH). *Bipolar Disorder*. NIH Publication 09-3679. Available at: www.nimh.nih.gov/health/publications/bipolar-disorder/complete-index. shtml (accessed 12 August 2010).

85 Marcus S, Marquis P, Sakai C. Controlled study of treatment of PTSD using EMDR in an HMO setting. *Psychotherapy*. 1997; **34**: 307–15.

86 Rothbaum B. A controlled study of eye movement desensitization and reprocessing in the treatment of post-traumatic stress disordered sexual assault victims. *Bulletin of the Menninger Clinic*. 1997; **61**: 317–34.

87 Korn D, Leeds A. Preliminary evidence of efficacy for EMDR resource development and installation in the stabilization phase of treatment of complex posttraumatic stress disorder. *Journal of Clinical Psychology*. 2002; **58**: 1465–87.

88 Linehan M. *Cognitive-Behavioral Treatment of Borderline Personality Disorder*. New York: Guilford Press; 1993.

89 Brown SH, Gilman SG, Fava NM, Goodman EG, Smyth NJ. Combining EMDR and Seeking Safety: a pilot study of an Integrated Trauma Treatment Program in the Thurston County Drug Court Program (in preparation).

90 Substance Abuse and Mental Health Services Administration (SAMHSA). *Treatment Improvement Protocol (TIP) 42*. Substance Abuse Treatment for Persons with Co-Occurring Disorders. SAMHSA/CSAT Treatment Improvement Protocols. Rockville, MD: Center for Substance Abuse Treatment; 2005.

91 Blake DD, Weathers FW, Nagy LM, *et al*. The development of a Clinician-Administered PTSD Scale. *Journal of Traumatic Stress*. 1995; **8**: 75–90.

92 Briere J. *Detailed Assessment of Posttraumatic Stress (DAPS)*. Odessa, FL: Psychological Assessment Resources; 2001.

93 National Institute of Justice. *Drug Courts: the second decade*. US Department of Justice, Office of Justice Programs; 2006. Available at: www.ojp.usdoj.gov/nij/pubs-sum/211081. htm (accessed 12 August 2010).

94 Helen Keller. Available at: www.brainyquote.com/quotes/authors/h/helen_keller.html (accessed 26 August 2010).

95 Edmond T, Rubin A, Wambach KG. The effectiveness of EMDR with adult female survivors of childhood sexual abuse. *Social Work Research*. 1999; **23**: 103–16.

TO LEARN MORE

- EMDR Institute: www.emdr.com
- EMDR International Association: www.emdria.org
- Seeking Safety: www.seekingsafety.org
- Adverse Childhood Experiences (ACE) Study: www.acestudy.org
- Motivational interviewing resources: www.motivationalinterview.org
- EMDR books: www.emdrsolutions.com/book.cfm
- MentalHelp.net Dialectical Behaviour Therapy: www.mentalhelp.net/poc/view_doc.php? type=doc&id=8140&cn=91

CHAPTER 13

Cue reactivity: working with cues and triggers to craving

David S Manley

PRE-READING EXERCISE 13.1

Time: 30 minutes

We all experience strong desires (craving). This can be associated with foods, drinks, cigarettes and other 'things' we enjoy or which we get benefit from. This exercise aims to stimulate thought in preparation for further reading.

- Thinking about something you crave (e.g. chocolate, nicotine, exercise, a favourite food): what triggers your desire for it (craving)?
- Identify the specifics of the situation in which you crave:
  - Think carefully and jot down some specific factors that make you think about your chosen 'substance'. Do you prefer one type of chocolate? Does your favourite food come in a particular wrapper? Do you buy from only one store? What does it look, smell, taste like?
  - What 'paraphernalia' do you need to consume it? A particular glass/plate/bowl/ashtray.
  - What environmental factors do you note that are important. Sitting in your favourite chair? Hot/cold? Time of day?
  - What is your emotional state like when you have a strong 'craving' (to eat, drink, smoke or exercise? Revved up, bored, happy, sad, stressed, contented, frustrated, relaxed?)
- Compare how these feelings or cravings are affected by the situation you find yourself in, be it environmental or emotional.
- How do these compare with cravings you perceive in others?

Thinking about cravings or a desire to have something in this way helps you begin to explore the multifaceted nature of craving and habituation.

INTRODUCTION

Case study 13.1: Andy

Andy catches the bus, feeling good, if a little worried about what the future holds. He has just left the ward in Newton after a three-month stay. He has been cocaine and alcohol free for three months, two weeks and one day . . . and counting. Not only that, Andy has been really well for ages, that old gnawing anxiety and stress seem to be a thing of ancient history. Andy can tell he's better, he's feeling much less paranoid, no sneaking a glimpse to see who's following today, no, none of that.

Twenty minutes later, he gets off the bus at his old stop just opposite the off licence, round the corner from his ma's house. As Andy turns the corner past the alleyway next to Dev's place, Donna shouts out to him, 'Hey Andy . . . where you been?' Thoughts of all the parties, good times and briefly forgotten friends flash through Andy's mind. A wave of sheer panic mixed with a warm rushing glow hits him . . . up his legs, down his fingers; his heart begins to pound, palms sweat and that taste . . . that taste. The desire for drugs and a quick slug of 'white lightning' burns in the pit of his stomach. He turns right into the old alleyway and to the drug that will make everything fine again.

Psychoactive drugs are rewarding.[1] However, this does not explain why some people become 'addicted'. Not everyone takes drugs or drinks, and not all people who use drugs or alcohol take substances all the time. Relapse happens, sometimes after only a brief period of abstinence, sometimes after much longer. It is unfortunate that relapse is a common outcome from substance use treatment! The process of helping individuals to tackle the risk of relapse, especially cues and triggers, that are associated with, and lead to, substance use is a common element of relapse prevention. Similarly, examination of relapse signatures – those circumstances and factors that can lead to crises and deterioration in mental well-being – can be used by the professional to aid the individual in learning coping strategies to avoid relapse.[2] For individuals who experience mental health–substance use concerns and dilemmas, cues and triggers experienced are likely to be similar to any other person who uses substances. However, they will almost certainly experience cues and triggers associated with the mental health problems too.

Personal practice using the principles of Cue Exposure Therapy (CET), with a number of individuals over many years, suggests that the general principles of cue reactivity benefit the person considerably. However, pure CET can be too challenging for some. Consequently, my personal view is that all professionals working with the individual experiencing mental health–substance use concerns and dilemmas need to expand their 'personal toolkit' to include some elements of cue reactivity skills. Cognitive behavioural interventions, which help the individual to substitute adaptive coping strategies by changing their cognitions, in order to cope with learned behaviours, can be of significant benefit in helping to cope with cravings and subsequently the risk of lapse into drug using or drinking. The rationale for tackling cues and triggers are twofold:

1 A number of studies indicate that alcohol and drug users experience strong physiological reactions to cues for using (i.e. cue reactivity), thereby increasing the probability of relapse after treatment.[3-5]
2 Despite substitute prescribing (e.g. methadone) and symptomatic medication to help with withdrawals, many drug users continue to take drugs or drink heavily (often on top of a substitute prescription).

The reasons for using drugs are rarely because of the need to deal with the discomfort of withdrawal and are more often a desire to get, or recapture, the 'buzz' experienced from the substance of choice. It could be argued that the 'buzz' *must* be due to learned behaviours (because the chemical 'addiction' is being adequately managed by the substitute medication) and so cognitive behavioural cue-related coping techniques are likely to be of significant benefit in helping the individual cope with the substance use.

This chapter aims to explore how cues and triggers can lead to craving and subsequent lapse and relapse into drug taking and/or drinking. The chapter will deal with some of the main principles of cue reactivity:
➤ how you can work with the individual to aid understanding of cues and triggers to craving
➤ how to elicit cravings, and the cues and triggers, associated with craving
➤ some of the techniques the professional can use to aid the individual in learning to assist in the development of coping strategies relating to cravings and increase self-efficacy (the ability, and belief in the ability, to help oneself).

SO WHY USE CUE REACTIVITY SKILLS?
Reasons for using CET include the following:
➤ CET is a relatively straightforward cognitive behavioural intervention.
➤ CET has been proven to work well for stimulant users but is effective with other drugs including alcohol.
➤ The process relies on self-efficacy and empowerment and may lead to improvements in self-esteem for individuals who are impoverished in this area.
➤ The emphasis is on change without substances, either illicit or prescribed.

The UK Department of Health (DH) produced the *Mental Health Policy Implementation Guide: dual diagnosis good practice guide* (MHPIG).[6] The MHPIG supports the National Service Framework for Mental Health[7] and clearly outlines elements of good practice in mental health–substance use. The DH highlights the need for staged interventions, including robust relapse prevention work.

> The principles and strategies of 'relapse prevention' for substance misuse and the management of relapses to psychosis are recommended for this purpose. This approach aims to identify high-risk situations for substance misuse and rehearse coping strategies proactively.[6]

One possible reason for relapse is that drug-related cues may trigger strong craving and arousal. Cue exposures, and the principles of cue reactivity, are practices that are useful in helping individuals understand habituation and learn to cope with some of the behaviours developed as part of the substance use problem.

The guide suggests, '*Flexibility and adaptation are essential skills for a workforce charged with providing treatment and care for this client group.*' It further states that training should '*raise awareness of drugs related issues and therapeutic responses . . . [and] increase staff confidence and reduce fear and anxiety in relation to working with people with complex needs.*'[6] Often, for the individual experiencing mental health–substance use concerns and dilemmas, the chosen substance of use can act as a cue triggering mental health problems. Moreover, deteriorating or fluctuating mental health may be a trigger for drug or alcohol use. Cue reactivity skills:

➤ are not complex
➤ are easily adapted
➤ can be used in clinical and home settings (in fact, the less clinical the better . . . it feels more real!)
➤ can be used formally (on a sessional basis)
➤ can be ad hoc
➤ can be used to benefit an individual's drug, alcohol and mental health problems
➤ can have the benefit of significantly empowering individuals (what we might call self-efficacy).

It has been suggested that individuals dependent on opiates, who achieved abstinence in treatment, still presented physiological arousal to drug cues 30 days after treatment completion.[3] The rationale for cue exposure, as a treatment technique, stems from results indicating that alcohol and drug users experience strong physiological reactions to cues (i.e. cue reactivity), thereby increasing the probability of relapse after treatment.

A meta-analytical review of 18 published studies of Cue Exposure Therapy (CET) suggests that 'cue exposure failed to prove efficacious in treating addiction.'[8] The authors comment that CET, as it is practised, has failed to incorporate new knowledge about extinguishing learned behaviour, and note that if the techniques were adapted to do so, they 'can be directly informed by recent animal learning research'.[14] The outcomes are supported to some degree by another study suggesting that even after participating in CET interventions, cocaine users craved and relapsed in to cocaine use when experiencing 'reminders' of drug use in the 'natural environment'.[9] The studies[8] analysed were not adequate tests of the therapy. The numbers of exposure sessions (2–3) were too low in most cases to examine the effect of CET (which typically consists of a minimum of six sessions when conducted in a therapeutic setting). Furthermore, the authors[8] have excluded some studies that demonstrate significantly positive results.[4] Other studies published after the review[5,10] have undermined the claim of the lack of evidence for positive outcomes from CET.[8] The main thrust of the argument[8] seems to rely on the concept that CET is ineffective because relapses still occur in those individuals in the studies, which they included in the meta-analysis. The study is limited by its assumptions that abstinence or absence of relapse following CET is the only positive outcome measure in the studies analysed. In stating this, the authors[8] ignore the significance of results demonstrating that, even if individuals relapse, they learn significant coping strategies from CET that reduce the severity, frequency and effect of lapses.[4] The second part of this article is more positive, in that it can be suggested that they see no reason why CET should not work.[8]

One study compared and contrasted outcomes between CET interventions and a combination of relaxation and coping skills training (CST) for people in treatment with alcohol problems.[5] Follow-up data was taken from the study after 6 and 12 months. In the first six months, individuals who received both interventions demonstrated fewer heavy drinking days than a control group who received neither. At 12 months, CET resulted in fewer heavy drinking days among those individuals who lapsed into drinking and resulted in greater reductions of individuals reporting urges to drink. In addition, the study indicated that there tended to be reports of higher use of coping strategies to cope with urges to drink and a subsequent reduction in heavy drinking days.

In one study,[5] 91 cocaine-dependent individuals were recruited to examine if there was a significant difference in cue-induced craving between groups with severe mental health problems, and those without. Participants were surveyed using a validated cocaine-craving questionnaire (VCCQ). Thirty-five participants had a confirmed diagnosis of schizophrenia under DSM-IV.[11] The authors comment that the VCCQ was useful in this instance because of the ease of use, and the recent positive experience of use with cognitively impaired individuals. A cue exposure procedure was used to raise craving in participants. Once administered, participants were asked to recomplete the VCCQ to see if they were cue reactive. This study demonstrated that craving showed a statistically significant increase, after the exposure, in individuals with schizophrenia, as opposed to those participants without mental health problems. The study makes a recommendation, which is significant: '*The preliminary results support the need to develop specialised treatments to manage craving, particularly amongst cocaine dependent persons with schizophrenia.*'[5] Part of the criticism of this study has been the reliance on subjective measures of craving, and a lack of objective physiological measures of craving and changes in craving. However, given that craving is a behaviour it is entirely reasonable that it is seen as a subjective experience. A further study[10] of CET principles applied to individuals with schizophrenia, aimed at smoking cessation, found the techniques were of significance in preventing relapse and reinforced the results of the previous study along with those results.[4]

SELF-ASSESSMENT EXERCISE 13.1

Time: 1 week
- To experience the sense of craving, stop drinking tea, coffee or another favourite drink for one week.
- Note down how you feel. What did you do to reduce the craving experience?

A study examined the acceptability to services in USA of substance misuse interventions including CET.[12] The study used a previously piloted questionnaire to gain data from 500 randomly selected substance use agencies across the USA. The study found that few services utilised CET (only 11% of responding services). Fifty-four per cent of respondents thought that CET was an acceptable intervention with substance using individuals. In those 11% of services that offered CET as an intervention, the technique was found to be both appropriate and effective in preventing or ameliorating relapse in problematic substance use.

DEVELOPING CUE REACTIVITY SKILLS

The principles of cue reactivity and cue exposure are based on the principles of classical conditioning[13] (sometimes called Pavlovian or respondent conditioning – *see* Figure 13.1). The basis of the idea is: if cravings are presented without being satiated by drugs or alcohol, then this should eventually lead to extinction of the cravings. This concept is borne out when observing individuals who have become habituated, when they experience cues but no satiation there is initially often a bewildered response, followed by a 'eureka' moment. In essence, the bond between cues, triggers, craving and drug taking are so immediate and regularly reinforced, through drug taking, that individuals lose their awareness that for them cravings can be divorced from taking drugs. The substance used disempowers the individuals, who do not see that it is possible to break the link that causes relapse.

One study noted that 'one of the largest problems in the treatment of substance abusers is the remaining, untreated or persistent reactivity to drug-related cues'.[15]

SELF-ASSESSMENT EXERCISE 13.2

Time: 10 minutes
List the coping strategies that could be used by the person experiencing craving.

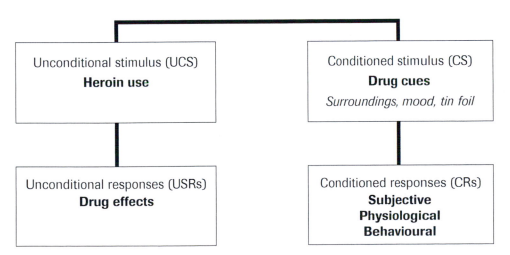

FIGURE 13.1 Classical conditioning and cue reactivity[14]

INTERVENTIONS
Avoidance of cues and triggers

One possible way of breaking the link between cues and triggers, cravings and drug using or drinking is through avoidance. Removing oneself from the vicinity of the cues or triggers, avoiding drug using or drinking friends and significant places may well have some short-term, temporary benefits. However, this is only possible when cues and triggers form physically avoidable phenomena and, even then, is not pragmatic. As an example, try telling a cigarette smoker or a 'chocoholic' to avoid cues and triggers for their substance of choice, with all those cigarette butts lying around, adverts and discarded wrappers! It is less pragmatic when we realise that cues and triggers to drug using and drinking regularly comprise emotional states often combined with physical reminders (*see* Case study 13.1: Andy, in the opening paragraph), which are much more difficult, if not impossible, to avoid. With individuals who experience mental health problems, it is impossible to avoid symptoms of the mental illness, which often form significant cues and triggers to drug or alcohol use. Mental health–substance use problems can increase the risk of relapse or interfere with effective use of coping skills. For example, in people with an affective disorder emotional situations can be associated with a higher risk of relapse. Accordingly, those individuals require an enhanced focus on the management of the emotional states.[16]

BOX 13.1 Coping strategies for use in cue reactivity skills training[16]

- Using delay as an active cognitive coping tool, i.e. the individual using drink/drugs tells himself/herself that the urge will 'go away' if he/she just 'waits it out'.
- Thinking about the negative consequences of consuming drugs/alcohol in the imagined situation.
- Thinking about the positive consequences of staying abstinent in the imagined situation.
- Using urge-reduction imagery, e.g. imagining slashing the urge with a sword, or crumpling it up like a sheet of paper.
- Using behavioural substitution, i.e. imagining engaging in an alternative activity.
- Using reward substitution, e.g. consuming favourite foods and sodas instead of drugs or alcohol.
- Employing mastery statements, e.g. 'I am strong; I can get through this without drinking', 'I'll do it for Mary'.
- Using pleasant imagery, i.e. imagining escaping to a pleasant place.

Keeping drugs and alcohol on the agenda

Simply discussing relapse, the effects of cues and triggers, subjective experience of craving, self-efficacy and high-risk situations can form a valuable face-to-face intervention with individuals who have mental health–substance misuse concerns and dilemma. However, it is important to recognise that discussing cues, triggers and craving may actually instigate the onset (*see* Box 13.1). Assessing motivation to change (*see* Chapters 5 and 6) can help give the professional and individual

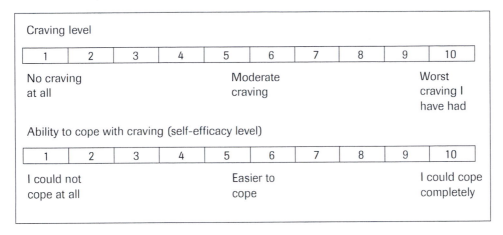

FIGURE 13.2 Craving and self-efficacy self-assessment bar

indicators of when a more active treatment phase may be warranted. At this stage, focused work on cues and triggers is an area to explore.

Self-assessment of craving and ability to cope

Throughout cue reactivity interventions the individual learns to use subjective self-assessment scales of level of craving (*see* Figure 13.2, where 0 = no craving, and 10 = the worse craving ever experienced), and scales indicating the individual's ability to cope with craving (or self-efficacy), where 0 = 'I could not cope with cravings at all', and 10 = 'I could easily cope with cravings'.

These scales can be individualised and refined to meet specific needs, cognitions and language ensuring that self-assessment is accurate and valuable. It is important that the individual learns to use these scales effectively, as they form an evaluative tool to assess learning and the effectiveness of coping strategies. Using self-assessment craving and self-efficacy scales enables the professional and individual to set a 'baseline' at the outset of interventions. Baselines are important, not only as an evaluative tool from session to session, but to ensure that craving and self-efficacy are restored to the same (or better) levels on conclusion of the session, to ensure any risk of relapse is no greater than it was prior to the session.

SELF-ASSESSMENT 13.3

Time: 10 minutes
- List what you would/could include to assess craving, cues and triggers.
- What would you focus on?

In-depth assessment

All Cue Exposure Therapy (CET) or cue reactivity interventions should begin with a specific and in-depth assessment of cravings, cues and triggers. However, before commencing assessment, it is worth teaching and using the self-assessment scales mentioned above to establish a baseline. Simply discussing cues triggers and paraphernalia can induce cravings. Box 13.2 below highlights the domains that assessment should take into account.

BOX 13.2 Assessment domains

Assessment should focus on several domains:
- coexisting biological or psychiatric conditions
- intrapersonal (emotional) and interpersonal risk factors
- specifics of paraphernalia used to take substances (including the shape, colour, size, etc.)
- environmental and situational risk factors
- overt cues and triggers to drug taking (covert cues and triggers will become apparent as interventions progress).

Each area should be assessed in depth, exploring the particular nuances of the individual's substance use. For example, when assessing cannabis smoking look for information on:

➤ what type of cigarette papers (make, colour, king-size or normal?) are used to roll the 'joints'
➤ the specific tobacco used (or indeed, whether tobacco is used at all)
➤ whether a filter tip is used
➤ whether the person rolls his/her own 'joint'
➤ the situation, under which she/he smokes
➤ the seat used (armchair or otherwise, colour, etc.)
➤ whether in company or not
➤ what music is listened to
➤ what preparation the individual goes through before smoking.

The detail of assessment may seem overly intricate but it helps the individual begin to recognise cues and triggers in things that may have previously seemed innocuous. Moreover, the detail permits the opportunity to ensure any exposure work is done as accurately as possible, recreating craving situations as authentically as is possible (which is why sessions *in vivo*, i.e. real life, elicit stronger cravings, and may eventually be preferable to clinical situations).

Teaching coping strategies

Before commencing any significant work on cue reactivity or specific CET sessions, it is important that the individual learns new coping strategies. Passive delay, sitting and waiting out the craving, eventually leads to reduction in arousal without actively intervening. However, teaching new coping strategies enable the individual to speed up desensitisation or extinction of cravings, exert control over their situation and increase feelings of self-efficacy, which in turn can increase the effectiveness of coping strategies. Individuals should try out coping strategies to see what has the 'best fit', what works best for the individual. Sometimes, physical reinforcers can work well in combination with a particular coping strategy. For example, when using the partner's or child's name in a mastery statement ('I'll do it for Mary'), a photograph of the partner or child may add weight to the efficacy of the coping strategy. Different situations, times of the day or craving experiences may demand a different approach. Practising coping strategies helps gain mastery, builds confidence and aids efficacy. It is often worth reminding the individual that she/he has probably taken many months or years to 'learn' to use drugs or alcohol, and that unlearning this habit, by using new adaptive coping strategies, may take time. Box 13.1 shows the main coping strategies that are taught to participants so that the individual can begin to refine the ability to cope with cravings and find strategies best for him/her.

Once an individual has practised and successfully used new coping strategies to desensitise himself/herself, he/she begins to use them in more challenging practice situations. Generally, when conducting formal CET sessions, exposures start with pictorial reminders of drug and alcohol use. A range of pictures and video from less pertinent to highly pertinent are used as the individual becomes more expert. For example, when working with 'Ann', a woman in her twenties who smokes cannabis, we might commence using pictures of older men smoking during the development of coping strategies. Eventually, a move is made to more relevant pictures of younger women smoking once Ann has practised, and feels comfortable with, the newly learned strategies. There is a degree of 'trial and error' with this process. The use of baseline measures of craving act as a 'safety net' to ensure the individual can always return to the original level of craving and self-efficacy.

As the individual develops and progresses through the hierarchy of exposure situations, it is important that the professional exudes optimism and reinforces this with the individual. An optimistic attitude for success through increased self-efficacy can be very powerful in helping the individual move forward and achieve their goals. However, the professional should be aware of unfounded optimism or over-eagerness to progress too quickly. Over optimism may be especially risky where the individual has yet to achieve competence in developing and effectively practising a suitable coping strategy, such as an accurate mastery statement. Moreover, at this stage, optimism goes hand in hand with rationalisation. Helping the individual recognise that she/he has managed to cope effectively, and found effective solutions to achieve chosen goals before, reinforces that this can be done again and builds optimism for positive change, transformation and progress.

KEY POINT 13.1

Exposure situations have a hierarchical effect with pictures being the least challenging, paraphernalia the next, imagined scenarios eliciting strong reactions and *in vivo* (real life) exposures eliciting the strongest arousal response.[16]

CONCLUSION

Adapting and implementing cue reactivity with individuals who have mental health problems

These skills make a useful addition to the professional working with the complex needs of individuals experiencing mental health–substance use problems. In practice, they can be adapted for use in a variety of situations, with numerous people, with differing levels of skill. Good, accurate assessment, taking adequate time to educate and model coping strategies, is vital. Brief ad hoc sessions may be a flexible way to meet the individual's needs (though structured sessions are better!), as long as the professional returns to the topic frequently (*see* 'Keeping drugs and alcohol on the agenda' earlier in the chapter), checks learning and understanding, and reinforces coping strategies using self-assessment.

KEY POINT 13.2

Remember, it has taken a long time (months and even years) to learn the process of drinking or drug taking; unlearning it may take just as long.

Assessment is a continuous process and the individual's understanding of lapse and relapse should be assessed and discussed, as well as education given on the principles of rule violation (*see* Box 13.3).[17]

BOX 13.3 Rule or abstinence violation effect (RVE/AVE)

The rule violation effect (RVE) occurs when a person, having decided to abstain from using a substance, has an initial 'lapse', i.e. the substance or behaviour is engaged in at least once. Some people go on to *full* relapse or continued uncontrolled use. The RVE occurs when the person attributes the cause of the initial lapse (the first violation of abstinence) to internal factors (e.g. lack of willpower or the underlying addiction or disease). This can often be attributed to negative self-talk such as '*I knew I couldn't do it*' or '*I always fail*', which often leads on to secondary self-talk which justifies a full relapse. '*Ah . . . what's the point of even trying to give up – I was just kidding myself.*'

The aim in relapse prevention is to minimise this effect of lapse and learn what risks were present so that effective coping strategies are learned and used in future. By recognising RVE we help the person transform their negative self-talk to positive: '*Well, I slipped this time but I've learned my lesson and the next time I'll avoid that risk.*'

Accurate, separate (for ease of access during one-to-one sessions) and descriptive-narrative notes, of all sessions working on cue reactivity, are essential and enable:

➤ reflection
➤ accessing of information
➤ summarisation and reflecting on the content of previous sessions
➤ development of discussions on areas of success and risk.

Conclude sessions with a summary of learning and reflecting an optimistic sense of progress. This is essential, and highly therapeutic. However, if individuals experience high levels of cognitive dissonance, it may be impractical to use these techniques. The skills of the professional make a difference. Providing written and visual reminders, revisiting learning frequently, evaluating and reflecting accurately, listening empathically and encouraging with a strong sense of optimism helps even the most distracted to begin to work on issues associated with substance use concerns and dilemmas.

POST-READING EXERCISE 13.1 (ANSWERS ON P. 206)

Time: 20 minutes

1 Why is taking a baseline craving and self-efficacy measure so important before commencing cue reactivity work?
2 What factors might you build in to a thorough assessment of craving, cues and triggers?
3 What is the hierarchy of cue-related arousal situations?
4 How might you adapt cue reactivity to the individual?

REFERENCES

1 Wise RA. The neurobiology of craving: implication for the understanding and treatment of addiction. *Journal of Abnormal Psychology.* 1988; **97**: 118–32.
2 Birchwood M, Spencer E, McGovern D. Schizophrenia: early warning signs. *Advances in Psychiatric Treatment.* 2000; **6**: 93–101.
3 Childress AR, McLellan AT, Ehrman R, *et al.* Classically conditioned responses in opioid and cocaine dependence: a role in relapse? *National Institute of Drug Abuse (NIDA) Research Monograph.* 1988; **84**: 25–43.
4 Rohsenow DJ, Monti PM, Rubonis AV, *et al.* Cue exposure with coping skills training and communication skills training for alcohol dependence: 6- and 12-month outcomes. *Addiction.* 2001; **96**: 1161–74.
5 Smelson DA, Losonczy MF, Kilker C, *et al.* An analysis of cue reactivity among persons with and without schizophrenia who are addicted to cocaine. *Psychiatric Services.* 2002; **53**: 1612–16.
6 Department of Health. *Mental Health Policy Implementation Guide: dual diagnosis good practice guide.* London: Department of Health; 2002.
7 Department of Health. *National Service Framework for Mental Health: modern standards and service models.* London: Department of Health; 1999.
8 Conklin CA, Tiffany ST. Applying extinction research and theory to cue-exposure addiction treatments. *Addiction.* 2002; **97**: 155–67.
9 O'Brien CP, Childress AR, McLellan T, *et al.* Integrating systematic cue exposure with standard treatment in recovering drug dependant patients. *Addictive Behaviours.* 1990; **15**: 355–65.
10 Ziedonis D, Williams JM, Smelson D. Serious mental illness and tobacco addiction: a model program to address this common but neglected issue. *American Journal of the Medical Sciences.* 2003; **326**: 223–30.

11 America Psychiatric Association. *Diagnostic and Statistical Manual of Mental Disorders [DSM-IV-TR]*. 4th ed. Washington, DC: American Psychiatric Association; 2000.

12 Rosenberg H, Phillips KT. Acceptability and availability of harm-reduction interventions for drug abuse in American substance abuse treatment agencies. *Psychology of Addictive Behaviors*. 2003; **17**(3): 203–10.

13 Pavlov, IP. *Conditioned Reflexes: an investigation of the physiological activity of the cerebral cortex*. Anrep GV, translator. London: Oxford University Press; 1927.

14 Marissen MAE, Franken IHA, Blanken P, *et al.* Cue exposure therapy for opiate dependent clients. *Journal of Substance Use*. 2005; **10**(2–3): 97–105.

15 Franken IHA, deHaan HA, van de Meer CW, *et al.* Cue reactivity and effects of cue exposure in abstinent post-treatment drug users. *Journal of Substance Abuse Treatment*. 1999; **16**: 81–5.

16 Monti PM, Rohsenow DJ. Coping skills training and Cue Exposure Therapy in the Treatment of Alcoholism. *Alcohol, Research and Health*. 1999; **23**(2): 107–115.

17 Marlatt GA, Gordon JR, editors. *Relapse Prevention: maintenance strategies in the treatment of addictive behaviors*. New York: Guilford Press. 1985.

TO LEARN MORE

- Classical Conditioning: Available at: http://psychology.about.com/od/behavioralpsychology/a/classcond.htm
- Drummond CD, Tiffany ST, Glautier S, *et al. Addictive Behaviour: cue exposure theory and practice*. Chichester: Wiley; 1995.
- Marlatt GA, Gordon JR. Determinants of relapse: implications for the maintenance of behavior change. In: Davidson PO, Davidson SM, editors. *Behavioral Medicine: changing health lifestyles*. New York: Brunner/Mazel; 1980.

ANSWERS TO POST-READING EXERCISE 13.1

1 To act as an evaluation tool and to ensure that the individual is returned to the original level of craving and self-efficacy (or better) before the completion of the session.

2 Coexisting biological or psychiatric conditions; intrapersonal (emotional) and interpersonal risk factors; specifics of paraphernalia used to take substances (including the shape, colour, size, etc.); environmental and situational risk factors; overt cues and triggers to drug taking (covert cues and triggers will become apparent as interventions progress).

3 Pictures, paraphernalia, imagined situations, and *in vivo* or real-life situations.

4 Through being aware of levels of cognitive dissonance; accurate and thorough assessment of cues triggers and mental health; applying factors flexibly and, using brief sessions, providing written information and summaries; reflecting on and revisiting understanding and modelling a sense of optimism.

CHAPTER 14

Mutual aid groups

Andrew Rosenblum, Stephen Magura,
Alexandre B Laudet and Howard Vogel

PREVALENCE OF MENTAL HEALTH–SUBSTANCE USE

Emerging recognition of mental health–substance use disorders dates back to the 1970s, when professionals became increasingly aware that a significant number of people presented with both disorders.[1] Subsequently, numerous studies of both community and patient samples have shown substantial rates of mental health–substance use disorders. A large prevalence survey (National Survey on Drug Use and Health; NSDUH) conducted annually in the United States estimates that in 2007 there were 5.4 million adults who had serious psychological distress (SPD)*[†] and a co-occurring substance use disorder (SUD).[5] The Epidemiologic Catchment Area study reported lifetime prevalence of 29% for drug dependence among those with a mental disorder and lifetime prevalence of a mental disorder of 53% among those with a drug disorder.[6] Similar rates of comorbidity in the US were also found in the National Comorbidity Study.[7] A review of several studies[8] found somewhat higher prevalences of comorbidity: in mental health settings 20%–50% of clients had a lifetime co-occurring SUD, while among substance abuse treatment clients 50%–75% had a lifetime co-occurring mental disorder. Rates of comorbidity in the UK (where serious mental illness is restricted to psychosis) are generally lower than in the US, 20%–37% in mental health settings, and 6%–15% in addiction settings.[9]

CONSEQUENCES OF MENTAL HEALTH–SUBSTANCE USE

Despite increasing recognition of the prevalence of comorbidity and the benefits of treatment, the majority of persons experiencing mental health–substance use disorders remain underserved. According to the NSDUH (and as shown in Figure 14.1[5]), more than half (53.5%) of persons experiencing SPD and a SUD did not receive

---

* The NSDUH uses a symptom-driven approach to collect data on serious psychological distress which indicates that a respondent experienced a high level of distress from any type of mental problem.[2] In contrast, serious mental illness (SMI) typically indicates functional impairment that meets the criteria for a psychiatric disorder as defined by the *Diagnostic Statistical Manual of Mental Disorders* (DSM-IV). Two national US surveys use this diagnostic approach to measure SMI: the National Epidemiologic Survey on Alcohol and Related Conditions (NESARC) and the National Comorbidity Survey-Replication.[3]

† Effectiveness of Self Help for the Dually Diagnosed (R01 DA11240); Control Trial of Self-Help for Dually-Diagnosed Persons (R01 DA015912); (http://projectreporter.nih.gov/reporter.cfm).

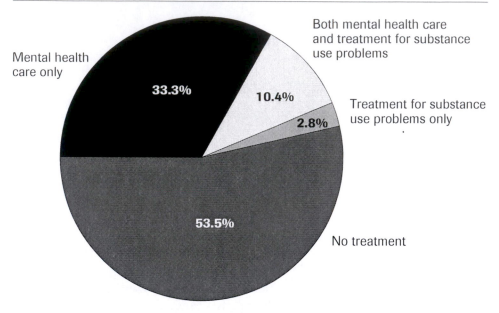

5.4 million adults with co-occurring SPD
and substance use disorder

FIGURE 14.1 Past year mental healthcare among adults aged 18 or older with both
serious psychological distress and a substance use disorder[5]

substance abuse or mental health treatment, 33.3% received only mental healthcare,
2.8% received only specialty substance use treatment, and 10.4% received both
mental healthcare and specialty substance use treatment.[5]

There is abundant evidence that problems associated with mental health–
substance use disorders are typically more severe and chronic than problems
associated with single psychiatric disorders.[7,10] In the general population, persons
with lifetime comorbidity are more likely than those with only one disorder to
experience major impairments with economic domains (e.g. unemployment,
financial problems), social isolation and interpersonal conflicts.[7] The hospitalisation rate among persons experiencing mental health–substance use disorders is
more than 20 times the rate for people experiencing substance use disorder-only
and more than five times the rate for people experiencing mental illness.[11] Mental
health–substance use is highly predictive of other negative treatment outcomes.[12,13]
Among people experiencing mental health problems, particularly persons with
schizophrenia, a substance use disorder has been associated with emergency room
visits, homelessness, involvement with the criminal justice system, suicide attempts,
more severe psychiatric symptoms, and human immunodeficiency virus (HIV)
and hepatitis C virus (HCV) infection.[10,14–17] Among substance abuse patients, the
severity of psychiatric symptoms has also been associated with poorer outcomes[18,19]
although equivalent improvement among substance abuse patients with and without psychiatric problems has also been reported.[20,21]

EFFECTIVENESS OF MUTUAL AID

Mutual aid groups (often termed 'self-help groups') are based on the premise that a group of individuals who share a common problem can collectively support each other and mitigate or eliminate that problem and its personal and social consequences. Members learn about their problem and share their experiences, strengths and hopes for recovery. The group is a setting where individuals' socially stigmatised attributes and behaviours can be discussed in an accepting, trusting environment. Mutual aid groups also provide a source of strategies to cope with the problem and, as a person progresses through the recovery process, the opportunity to become a role model. Thus, the term 'mutual' is an important descriptor since a group member can both give and receive help. The process of giving (sometimes conceptualised as 'helper therapy') is recognised as an important feature of sustaining one's recovery,[22] as illustrated by the Alcoholics Anonymous (AA) slogan, 'You can't keep it unless you give it away'.[23] Many mutual aid groups follow some version of the 12-step model of recovery originally developed by the founders of AA.[24,25]

Mutual aid groups include appealing features that are typically not representative of formal treatment modalities such as no fees, no requirements for appointments, no limit on number of visits, and consumer empowerment.[26] It is noteworthy that one of the early and abiding features of Alcoholics Anonymous (consistent with current theories of addiction) is the recognition that alcoholism is a chronic disorder, that there is no such thing as a cure (since there is always a risk of relapse) and that recovery is a lifelong process. This is evident at most 12-step based meetings where an individual introduces himself/herself with his/her first name and makes the disclosure, 'I am an alcoholic' (or 'addict' or, in the case of dual-focus recovery groups, 'I am dually diagnosed'), regardless of how long one has been abstinent and attending meetings.

A growing body of evidence indicates that 12-step groups are helpful in maintaining abstinence from substances of abuse,[27-29] especially for those who attend regularly or become affiliated (for review, *see* Tonigan[30]). In addition to abstinence, several other outcomes have been found to be associated with 12-step affiliation, such as less severe psychiatric symptoms and higher employment.[31]

There is less research on mutual aid for persons in mental health recovery, but available findings suggest a positive effect.[32] For example, a survey of members of Recovery, Inc., a mutual aid programme for people with mental illness, found a decline in psychiatric symptoms for both peer-leaders and recent members since first joining the programme, although significantly more so for the leaders, who had longer periods of participation.[33]

TRADITIONAL MUTUAL AID AND MENTAL HEALTH–SUBSTANCE USE

Studies have indicated that professionals are less likely to refer persons experiencing mental health–substance use disorders than those with a single diagnosis to mutual aid groups.[34-36] Traditional 12-step groups have substantial limitations for people experiencing mental health–substance use disorders. Identifying and bonding with other members may be difficult if they feel different from other group members. Newcomers to 12-step meetings often find a lack of acceptance and empathy.[37,38] Some members experiencing mental health–substance use disorders report receiving misguided advice about psychiatric illness and the use of medications, which are seen as 'drugs',[35,39] although this is not the official view of AA and NA World Services.[40,41] In many local 12-step chapters, aversion continues against the use of psychoactive medications, where the potential for 'abuse' of these medications has concrete consequences, such as not being allowed to speak (or 'testify') at meetings. This occurs even though the medications may be for treating SUD (e.g. methadone) or mental illness (e.g. antidepressants). A survey of AA leaders revealed their belief that individuals should take their medications as prescribed, but most felt that individuals experiencing mental health–substance use disorders would not fit in their AA group and that *'participation in a group especially* [designed] *for persons with a dual diagnosis would be more desirable than a traditional AA group'.*[42]

Studies have generally indicated that 12-step attendance rates are equal for persons who are and are not experiencing mental health–substance disorders, although attendance rates for substance users with a psychotic disorder are somewhat lower.[43,44] However, even in instances where attendance rates appear to be high, individuals experiencing mental health–substance use disorders report difficulties with traditional 12-step meetings, such as disapproval from other members about taking psychiatric medication and lack of understanding of mental illness.[45,46] Furthermore, although several studies have documented that dually diagnosed patients benefit by participating in traditional 12-step groups,[43,47] other studies have found that these benefits are limited.[45,48]

'DUAL RECOVERY' MUTUAL AID

The recognition of the limitations of traditional 'single focus' 12-step groups for individuals experiencing mental health–substance use disorders has led to the development of several fellowships specifically to address dual-recovery needs. There are AA groups specifically for alcohol-dependent persons who have a co-occurring mental disorder and specialised 12-step fellowships that have emerged to address the recovery needs of people experiencing mental health–substance use disorders: Dual Recovery Anonymous (DRA),[39] Dual Disorders Anonymous (DDA) and Double Trouble in Recovery (DTR).[38] The studies of DTR conducted by the authors of this review appear to be the only research on the effectiveness of dual-focus fellowship participation. Although specialised 12-step facilitation (TSF) models for persons experiencing mental health–substance use disorders have been developed and are useful,[49,50] they are professionally led therapies designed to prepare individuals for peer-led dual-focus 12-step groups. Below we provide an outline of a typical DTR meeting format and describe our continuing research on the outcomes of participating in dual-focus, 12-step mutual aid groups, including improved understanding of the mechanisms of attitudinal and behavioural change in such groups.

FORMAT AND STRUCTURE OF A DUAL RECOVERY MUTUAL AID GROUP

In the 12-step tradition, meetings are led by recovering individuals who are experiencing mental health–substance use disorders. These meetings also typically follow a traditional 12-step format.[1] An outline of this format and structure as described in the DTR Manual[51] is given below.

Each group has a chairperson

Ideally, the chairperson (also known as the facilitator) would have experienced a sustained period of recovery, e.g. at least one year of abstinence from drugs and alcohol and at least one year since having been an inpatient in a psychiatric hospital. If no such person can be found in the core group, the person with the longest history of sobriety and avoidance of psychiatric hospitalisation can be selected as the chair. The chairperson's role is to lead the meetings, maintain adherence to the guidelines (see below), and provide support to other members less advanced in their recoveries. As the group develops, co-chairs (co-facilitators) may also be selected by the members; the co-chairs are members who show particular progress in their recoveries.

The basic features of a DTR meeting are as follows.

Welcoming

Before a meeting formally starts, the DTR group chair welcomes members as they come in. This helps create a climate of warmth and hospitality.

Introduction by chairperson

The chairperson introduces himself/herself as being dually diagnosed ('Hi, my name is Juan, I am dually diagnosed').

Moment of silence

The chair invites everyone to observe a moment of silence for members who are absent, hospitalised or still suffering with addictions and mental disorders and then the group is invited to recite the Serenity Prayer.

Reading of DTR mission

Various members read different parts of the DTR mission as follows:
➤ DTR preamble
➤ DTR – how it works/Twelve Steps of DTR
➤ the Promises
➤ on recovery.

Group member introductions

Group members introduce themselves (first name only) and identify themselves as being dually diagnosed.

Group guidelines

Members are reminded of group guidelines and norms for behaviour. Members are:
➤ required not to bring alcohol or non-prescribed drugs to the meeting
➤ not to share (i.e. relate their experiences with drugs, alcohol and mental illness) during the second half of the meeting if they have used such substances in the past 24 hours
➤ reminded that this is an anonymous programme
➤ asked to limit comments during the sharing time to five minutes
➤ encouraged to express their own experience and feelings in response to others

➤ avoid cross-talk or lecturing
➤ be minded that sharing is voluntary.

Speaker
Fifteen to 20 minutes is provided for a speaker to share his/her experience, strength and hope dealing with and recovering from dual diagnosis. (This could be the chair or co-chair.)

Sharing
Group members are invited to share their experience in response to the speaker.

Closing
Group members are invited to recite the Serenity Prayer.

Pre- and post-meeting activities
Members are asked to accept responsibility for setting up the room for the DTR meeting, straightening and cleaning up the room after the meeting. Pre-meeting activities may involve bringing in and setting out the refreshments, making the hot water and coffee, and placing the chairs as required. Post-meeting activities include sweeping or wiping the table and floor and replacing the furniture in its initial position.

As noted elsewhere, most of the characteristics of DTR are similar to single focus, 12-step groups.[52] However, there also are important differences. Unlike most traditional mutual aid groups, which are held in a variety of community settings, most DTR meetings are typically held in hospitals or other treatment facilities.

Additional differences include:
➤ modifying the first and twelfth steps of AA to include mental health issues, i.e. reference to being powerless over *mental disorders* and substance use (Step 1) and acknowledging the intention to carry the message of recovery to other *dually diagnosed* people (Step 12)
➤ recognition that dually diagnosed people experience the double stigma of mental illness and chemical dependency and that negative attitudes toward the dually diagnosed are prevalent
➤ since many dually diagnosed people are on a prescribed regimen of psychiatric medication, DTR provides an opportunity for individuals to receive peer support for taking prescribed psychiatric medication from other group members.

As noted earlier, although AA and NA World Services accept prescribed psychiatric medication, these addiction-focused fellowships typically are not settings to discuss medication challenges. The relative absence of explicit recognition of mental illness and the opportunity to discuss psychiatric medication in addiction-focused 12-step groups is consistent with the principles of AA and NA. One of the cornerstones of the 12-step programme is 'singleness of purpose'. People come to AA/NA to discuss and overcome addiction, exemplified by the statement frequently made at AA meetings, 'in keeping with AA's singleness of purpose, please limit your sharing to alcohol'.[53]

Observations made by persons familiar with DTR indicate some additional characteristics on how DTR differs from other mutual aid groups.[54,55] During the early period of DTR (1989 through 2002) most groups did not include sponsorship, as typically occurs in AA and other traditional 12-step groups. In 2009, sponsorship does occur at some DTR meetings, although it is less prevalent than found in traditional single-focused groups. One of the challenges in facilitating a DTR meeting is that it can be difficult to get some of the DTR attendees to share at meetings, possibly because of problems associated with severe mental illness (SMI). Reticence to share may be especially prevalent among newcomers who may have a hard time understanding how mutual aid works.

RESEARCH ON MUTUAL AID FOR INDIVIDUALS EXPERIENCING MENTAL HEALTH–SUBSTANCE USE DISORDERS

The DTR model, founded in 1989, has a presence in NYC (more than 40 meetings), expanding nationally throughout the US (an estimated 200 groups nationwide) and has a presence in Toronto, Canada. Since 1997, our research team has described the population, studied outcomes and identified several common therapeutic factors and unique self-help processes that mediate the influence of DTR participation on outcomes for members. The bulk of our past research has been supported by two National Institute on Drug Abuse (NIDA) funded research grants. The first study was conducted from 1997 to 2002. Study participant volunteers were 310 dual-diagnosed persons attending 24 DTR meetings in treatment programmes and community-based organisations in New York City. Participants had been attending DTR for at least one month and were followed up for two years. The second study introduced and sustained DTR groups in a psychiatric outpatient programme serving a large proportion of people experiencing metal health–substance use disorders, and conducted a pre/post analysis, including a historical control, of the effects of DTR participation on members and the clinic. Both studies used $p < 0.05$ as the criterion for statistical significance and employed various multivariate models (e.g. multiple ordinary least squares regression, multiple logistic regression, general estimating equations) to control for and identify covariates when examining correlates of mediating and outcome variables.

Study one

The study methods and many of the findings described below can be found in a comprehensive review and synthesis of DTR.[52]

Characteristics of DTR members

Among the 310 study participants attending 24 DTR groups in NYC, the mean age was 40 years, slightly more than one-quarter (27%) were women, nearly three-quarters were minority (59% black; 13% Hispanic) and only 7% were currently married/common law unions; 60% had never been married. The majority (53%) lived in a community residence. The three most frequent self-reported psychiatric diagnoses were: schizophrenia (39%), major depression (21%) and bipolar disorder (20%); 92% were currently prescribed psychiatric medication. The three most frequent primary substance use problems were: cocaine/crack (39%), alcohol

(35%), and heroin (12%).[56] Most respondents were currently receiving outpatient mental health or substance use treatment, 91% and 77%, respectively. Age for first treatment was 22 years for mental illness and 28 years for substance use. History of hospitalisation was prevalent; 89% had been hospitalised for mental illness and 75% for substance use problems. Five or more mental health hospitalisations were reported by 49% of the sample.[57]

Association between substance abuse and mental illness

The saliency of substance use among this serious mentally ill population is underscored by participants' response to the question, '*Overall what* [substance abuse or mental illness] *caused you the most problems?*' Half (49%) reported both equally, 29% identified drug or alcohol problems, and 17% cited mental health problems. Response to two questions illustrated how psychiatric symptoms and drug/alcohol use are intertwined. More than half (61%) reported that they felt like using when experiencing psychiatric symptoms and 69% said their symptoms got worse when using drugs or alcohol.[57]

Initial and sustained DTR participation

Most members were introduced to DTR through a mental health or dual diagnosis treatment programme (51%), a substance use treatment programme (16%), or a friend (20%). The two most frequent reasons for coming to DTR were: opportunity to be with other dually diagnosed people (33%) and desire to stop using drugs or

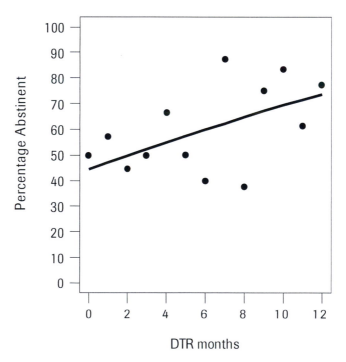

FIGURE 14.2 Percentage abstinent in relation to DTR attendance at one-year follow-up (adapted from Laudet, Magura, Cleland, *et al.*[59])

avoid relapse (32%). One-quarter (25%) said they came because they were referred by their treatment provider. At one-year follow-up, nearly three-quarters (71%) were still attending DTR and attended at least once a week. The main reasons for not continuing to attend were either that there was no meeting to go to or difficulty finding transportation to attend meetings.[58] As shown in Figure 14.2,[59] there was an association between drug/alcohol abstinence and number of months attending DTR during the first year of follow-up. Abstinence rates were sustained from year 1 to year 2 follow-up (72% and 74%, respectively). Other predictors of abstinence at follow-up were drug/alcohol abstinence at study entry, lower psychiatric symptom severity, and not receiving inpatient treatment during the study period.[59]

Medication adherence

Medication adherence is a major public health problem, especially among the mentally ill because lack of adherence has been associated with psychotic relapse, significant impairment in functioning and hospitalisation.[60] Eighty-seven per cent of study participants interviewed one year after enrolling in the study reported that they had taken their medication as prescribed during the previous year. As can be seen in the path diagram (Figure 14.3), medication adherence was associated with DTR attendance plus three baseline variables: living in supported housing, fewer stressful life events, and lower psychiatric symptom severity. In addition, adherence was associated with lower symptom severity at one year and no psychiatric hospitalisation during the follow-up period. Symptom severity at follow-up was also associated with symptom severity at baseline and more stressful life events.[61]

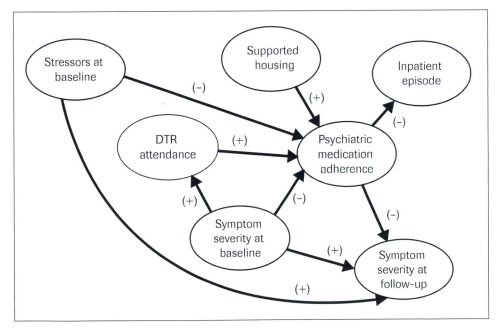

FIGURE 14.3 DTR attendance and psychiatric medication adherence (adapted from Magura, Laudet, Mahmood, *et al.*[61])

An interesting, unexpected finding was an association between elevated psychiatric symptom severity and DTR attendance.

Common and unique 12-step process factors as mediators of outcomes of DTR participation

The study tested the hypotheses that two common process factors (internal locus of control and sociability) and two factors unique to 12-step (spirituality and installation of hope) mediate the effects of DTR group affiliation on drug/alcohol abstinence and a composite measure of health promoting behaviour (medication adherence, medical care and self-care). The degree of DTR group affiliation during the study period was associated with more positive outcomes at follow-up. Internal locus of control and sociability mediated the effects of DTR group affiliation on abstinence and on health-promoting behaviour, whereas spirituality and hope acted as mediators only for health promoting behaviour.[62]

The role of interpersonal self-help processes in achieving abstinence

The study hypothesised that the following three 'active ingredients' characterising mutual aid would mediate the effects of DTR participation on drug/alcohol abstinence outcomes:
1 helper-therapy
2 reciprocal learning
3 peer emotional support processes.

Psychometrically valid measures of each process variable were constructed. To our knowledge, this is the first time that these key theoretical variables have been

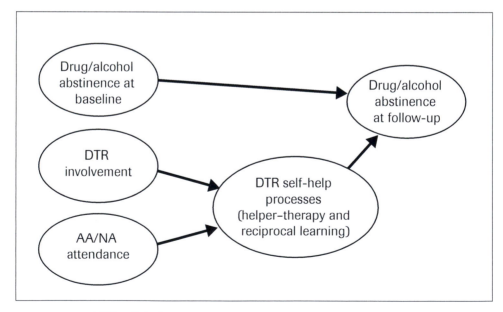

FIGURE 14.4 DTR self-help process and abstinence on one-year follow-up[63] (based on data from Magura, Laudet, Mahmood, *et al.*[63])

examined in research on mutual aid. The study's hypothesis was partially supported; greater DTR involvement at baseline predicted more helper-therapy and reciprocal learning experiences, but not more emotional support during the follow-up period, independent of a range of other factors. Higher levels of self-esteem and recovery self-efficacy and more frequent attendance at traditional 12-step groups also directly predicted interpersonal mutual aid processes. Helper-therapy and reciprocal learning activities were also associated with the better drug/alcohol abstinence outcomes and showed the hypothesised mediation effect. Interestingly, attendance at traditional (e.g. AA/NA) 12-step meetings and a general measure of DTR involvement were also correlated with abstinence at follow-up, but dropped out in the multivariate analysis, indicating that certain therapeutic mechanisms characterising mutual aid, i.e. helper-therapy and reciprocal learning processes, accounted for the sustained and increased abstinence benefits of DTR more so than attendance or involvement alone.[63] The path diagram in Figure 14.4[63] illustrates the mediating role of these two self-help processes (other than drug and alcohol use at baseline, other baseline variables are excluded from this diagram). The non-significant result for emotional support is consistent with members' reports that the most difficult 'recovery challenge' is emotions and feelings.[57]

DTR affiliation, social support, self-efficacy and quality of life

Higher levels of social support and affiliation with DTR (attendance and involvement) in the previous year were significantly associated with lower levels of substance use and mental health distress and higher levels of well-being.[64] DTR affiliation was also found to be significantly associated with self-efficacy for mental health recovery and three quality of life measures:

1 leisure time activities
2 feelings of well-being
3 social relationships.[56]

Self-efficacy fully mediated the effects of DTR affiliation on leisure time and well-being and partially mediated DTR's effect on social relationships. The association of DTR affiliation with self-efficacy is consistent with the social learning processes inherent in mutual aid[65] and suggests the value of facilitating affiliation among persons experiencing mental health–substance use disorders as part of a comprehensive approach to promoting wellness.

Study two

Efficacy of dual-focus mutual aid to reduce substance use and increase health-promoting behaviours

We conducted·a controlled trial using a quasi-experimental design to determine whether adding dual-focus, 12-step self-help groups to regular treatment for dually diagnosed patients can help improve patients' behavioural outcomes.[66] Patient outcomes in a psychiatric day treatment programme were compared for two consecutive admission cohorts characterised by high rates of co-occurring disorders. The first cohort did not have DTR available (termed the Pre-DTR cohort; n = 81) and the second cohort was exposed to DTR after it was established at the

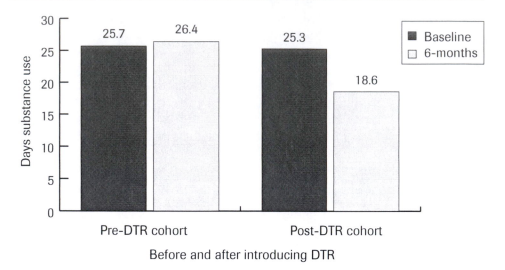

FIGURE 14.5 Days substance use, past 90 days (adapted from Magura, Rosenblum, Villano, *et al.*[66])

programme (termed the Post-DTR cohort; n = 148). Both cohorts were assessed at programme admission and at a six-month follow-up. At follow-up, using intent to treat analysis, the Post-DTR cohort as compared with the Pre-DTR cohort had significantly fewer days of alcohol and drug use (*see* Figure 14.5), more frequent attendance at traditional 12-step groups (AA and NA) outside the treatment programme and higher psychiatric medication adherence.

The feasibility of introducing and sustaining dual-focus 12-step groups in a day treatment programme

DTR was well accepted by patients: two years after we implemented DTR in a psychiatric ambulatory facility, DTR groups were the best-attended groups in the programme. On periodic surveys, DTR members reported a high level of satisfaction with their participation. Professionals at the psychiatric facility, who were initially unfamiliar with the potential of 12-step mutual aid for dually diagnosed patients, later reported that DTR facilitates the recovery process for many patients, and began to encourage patients to attend the groups.[67] Some comments received from staff were: 'The patients love DTR', 'The patients want DTR in this clinic', 'They want more DTR groups'. These findings indicate that dual-focus 12-step groups can be successfully established and sustained in an ambulatory treatment facility. However, based on our experience, sustaining DTR in an institution requires strong professional support and a committed and experienced DTR facilitator. A clinician survey conducted at the programme showed that clinicians who were optimistic about their patients' capacities to show improvement in their mental health or who had personal 12-step experience were more likely to refer their patients to 12-step groups.[36]

Consumer evaluation of DTR

Consistent with findings from our earlier effectiveness study (Study 1), participants who attended DTR groups at the psychiatric programme reported a moderately high level of satisfaction with these groups. Continued attendance in DTR was significantly associated with increased confidence to cope with mental illness (self-efficacy for recovery) and with positive changes in recovery-oriented behaviours such as relationship with counsellor, fewer cravings, less drug use and improved assertiveness. These relationships remained significant even after statistically controlling for time in the psychiatric treatment programme. Perceived DTR usefulness was significantly associated with greater engagement in three specific self-help processes (helper-therapy, reciprocal learning, and emotional support) and increased self-efficacy for recovery. Notably, these associations were independent of consumers' overall satisfaction with the treatment programme. When asked 'What do you get out of coming to DTR – how does it help you (in your own words)?', the two most frequent responses were that DTR was helpful in 'staying clean and sober' (36%) and in providing peer support (25%).[68]

CONCLUSION

Implications for clinical practice

Collectively, both studies indicate that participation in a mutual aid group for the individual experiencing mental health–substance use disorders is associated with reductions in substance 'abuse' and other health promoting behaviours, and positive experiences such as medication adherence, increased attendance at traditional 12-step groups and quality of life. The studies have also identified common and unique process factors that are associated with mutual aid affiliation and that serve as mediators between mutual aid affiliation and outcomes. The importance of affiliation with other individuals experiencing mental health–substance use disorders in a supportive environment is underscored by:

➤ reports from DTR participants that affiliating with others was the first (Study 1) or second (Study 2) most-cited reason for attending DTR groups
➤ identification of helper-therapy and reciprocal learning (activities requiring some level of affiliation) as factors that mediate between DTR participation and substance use outcomes (Study 1)
➤ the finding that DTR groups at an outpatient psychiatric programme were the best-attended groups (Study 2).

Specialised self-help groups for persons experiencing substance use disorders and SMI have a unique advantage of offering a safe and comfortable environment where often-stigmatised topics – mental health symptoms and the use of medication – can be openly discussed. When dual-focus groups are available, professionals should encourage the individual to attend. Because most dual-focus groups are held in hospitals or other treatment facilities, professionals should seek information about such groups and support the individual initiative to start such meetings. In view of the restricted availability of dual-focus groups and the strong need for peer support among people experiencing mental health–substance use disorders in recovery, affiliation with traditional 12-step groups should also be encouraged, although obstacles to participation should be identified and addressed. Our finding that DTR attendance is associated with subsequent attendance at traditional 12-step groups underscores the acceptability of single-focused 12-step for some people experiencing mental health–substance use disorders. This finding also suggests that dual-focus mutual aid may strengthen self-efficacy and help increase comfort levels in participating in single-focused mutual aid groups.

REFERENCES

1 Center for Substance Abuse Treatment. *Substance Abuse Treatment for Persons with Co-Occurring Disorders.* Treatment Improvement Protocol (TIP) Series 42. DHHS Publication No. SMA 05–3922. Rockville, MD: Substance Abuse and Mental Health Services Administration; 2005. Available at: www.ncbi.nlm.nih.gov/book/NBK14528 (accessed 13 August 2010).

2 Clark HW, Power AK, Le Fauve CE, *et al.* Policy and practice implications of epidemiological surveys on co-occurring mental and substance use disorders. *Journal of Substance Abuse Treatment.* 2008; **34**: 3–13.

3 NIAAA. Alcohol use and alcohol use disorders in the United States. Main findings from the 2001–2002 National Epidemiologic Survey on Alcohol and Related Conditions (NESARC). *US Alcohol Epidemiologic Data Reference Manual*, Vol. 8(1). Bethesda, MD: National Institutes of Health; 2006. Available at: http://pubs.niaaa.nih.gov/publications/NESARC_DRM/NESARCDRM.htm (accessed 26 August 2010).

4 National Comorbidity Survey (NCS) and National Comorbidity Survey Replication (NCS-R). Available at: www.hcp.med.harvard.edu/ncs/index.php (accessed 13 August 2010).

5 Substance Abuse and Mental Health Services Administration. *Results from the 2007 National Survey on Drug Use and Health: national findings.* NSDUH Series H-30, DHHS Publication No. SMA 06–4194. Rockville, MD: Substance Abuse and Mental Health Services Administration; 2008. Available at: www.oas.samhsa.gov/NSDUH/2k7NSDUH/2k7results.cfm#8.1.4 (accessed 13 August 2010).

6 Regier DA, Farmer ME, Rae DS, *et al.* Comorbidity of mental disorders with alcohol and other drug abuse: results from the Epidemiologic Catchment Area (ECA) study. *Journal of the American Medical Association.* 1990; **264**: 2511–18.

7 Kessler RC. The national comorbidity survey: preliminary results and future directions. *International Journal of Methods in Psychiatric Research.* 1995; **5**: 139–51.

8 Sacks S, Sacks J, De Leon G, *et al.* Modified therapeutic community for mentally ill chemical abusers: background; influences; program description; preliminary findings. *Substance Use and Misuse.* 1997; **32**: 1217–59.

9 Carrà G, Johnson S. Variations in rates of comorbid substance use in psychosis between mental health settings and geographical areas in the UK. A systematic review. *Society of Psychiatry and Psychiatric Epidemiology.* 2009; **44**: 429–47.

10 Drake RE, Brunette MF. Complications of severe mental illness related to alcohol and drug use disorders. *Recent Developments in Alcoholism.* 1998; **14**: 285–99.

11 Coffey R, Graver L, Schroeder D, *et al. Mental Health and Substance Abuse Treatment: results from a study integrating data from state mental health, substance abuse, and medicaid agencies.* DHHS Publication No. SMA 01–3528. Rockville, MD: Substance Abuse and Mental Health Services Administration; 2001. Available at: http://csat.samhsa.gov/IDBSE/idb/reports/FinalReportv9.pdf (accessed 13 August 2010).

12 Gonzalez G, Rosenheck R. Outcome and service use among homeless persons with serious mental illness and substance abuse. *Psychiatric Services.* 2002; **53**: 437–46.

13 Donat DC, Haverkamp J. Treatment of psychiatric impairment complicated by co-occurring substance use: impact of rehospitalization. *Psychiatric Rehabilitation Journal.* 2004; **28**: 78–82.

14 Curran GM, Sullivan G, Williams K, *et al.* The association of psychiatric comorbidity and use of the emergency department among persons with substance use disorders: an observational cohort study. *BMC Emergency Medicine.* 2008; **3**: 17.

15 Dixon L. Dual diagnosis of substance abuse in schizophrenia: prevalence and impact on outcomes. *Schizophrenia Research.* 1999; **35**(Suppl. 1): S93–100.

16 Rosenberg SD, Drake RE, Brunette MF, *et al.* Hepatitis C virus and HIV co-infection in people with severe mental illness and substance use disorders. *AIDS.* 2005; **19**(Suppl. 3): S26–33.

17 Osher FC, Drake RE, Noordsy DL. Correlates and outcomes of alcohol use disorder among rural outpatients with schizophrenia. *Journal of Clinical Psychiatry.* 1994; **55**: 109–13.

18 McLellan AT, Luborsky L, Woody GE, *et al.* Predicting response to alcohol and drug abuse treatments: role of psychiatric severity. *Archives of General Psychiatry.* 1983; **40**: 620–5.

19 Rounsaville BJ, Kosten TR, Weissman MM, *et al.* Prognostic significance of psychopathology in treated opiate addicts. *Archives of General Psychiatry.* 1986; **43**: 739–45.

20 Cacciola JS, Alterman AI, Rutherford MJ, *et al.* The relationship of psychiatric comorbidity to treatment outcomes in methadone maintained patients. *Drug Alcohol Dependence.* 2001; **61**: 271–80.

21 Saxon AJ, Calsyn DA. Effects of psychiatric care for dual diagnosis patients treated in a drug dependence clinic. *American Journal of Drug and Alcohol Abuse.* 1995; **21**: 303–13.

22 Zemore SE, Pagano ME. Kickbacks from helping others: health and recovery. *Recent Developments in Alcoholism.* 2008; **18**: 141–66.

23 Narcotics Anonymous World Services. *Narcotics Anonymous.* 6th ed. Chatsworth, CA: Narcotics Anonymous World Services; 2008. Available at: www.na.org/admin/include/spaw2/uploads/pdf/BT6E_Webposting.pdf (accessed 24 August 2010).

24 Alcoholics Anonymous. *Alcoholics Anonymous: the story of how many thousands of men and women have recovered from alcoholism.* 3rd ed. New York: Alcoholics Anonymous World Services; 1939/1976.

25 Alcoholics Anonymous. *Twelve Steps and Twelve Traditions.* New York: Alcoholics Anonymous World Services; 1952.

26 Humphreys K, Mavis BE, Stöffelmayr BE. Are twelve-step programs appropriate for disenfranchised groups? Evidence from a study of posttreatment mutual help group involvement. *Prevention in Human Services.* 1994; **11**: 165–80.

27 Timko C, Debenedetti A, Billow R. Intensive referral to 12 step self-help groups and 6-month substance use disorder outcomes. *Addiction.* 2006; **101**: 678–88.

28 Kelly JF, Stout R, Zywiak W, *et al.* A 3-year study of addiction mutual-help group participation following intensive outpatient treatment. *Alcohol and Clinical Experimental Research.* 2006; **30**: 1381–92.

29 Humphreys K, Moos RH. Encouraging post-treatment self-help group involvement to reduce demand for continuing care services: two-year clinical and utilization outcomes. *Alcohol and Clinical Experimental Research.* 2007; **31**: 64–8.

30 Tonigan JS. Alcoholics anonymous outcomes and benefits. *Recent Developments in Alcoholism.* 2008; **18**: 357–72.

31 Moos R, Finney J, Ouimette PC, *et al.* A comparative evaluation of substance abuse

treatment: I. Treatment orientation, amount of care, and 1-year outcomes. *Alcoholism Clinical and Experimental Research.* 1999; **23**: 529–36.

32 Kyrouz EM, Humphreys K, Loomis C. A review on research on the effectiveness of self-help mutual aid groups. In: White BJ, Madara EJ, editor. *American Self-Help Clearinghouse Self-Help Group Sourcebook.* 7th ed. Denville, NJ: American Self-Help Clearinghouse Self-Help Group Sourcebook; 2002. Available at: http://facesandvoicesofrecovery.org/pdf/kyrouz%20 humphreys%20loomis%202002.pdf (accessed 23 August 2010).

33 Galanter M. Zealous self-help groups as adjuncts to psychiatric treatment: a study of Recovery, Inc. *American Journal of Psychiatry.* 1988; **145**: 1248–53.

34 Humphreys K. Clinicians' referral and matching of substance abuse patients to self-help groups after treatment. *Psychiatric Services.* 1997; **48**: 1445–9.

35 Laudet AB. Substance abuse treatment providers' referral to self-help: review and future empirical directions. *International Journal of Self Help and Self Care.* 2000; **1**: 195–207.

36 Villano CL, Rosenblum A, Magura S, *et al.* Mental health clinicians' 12-step referral practices with dually diagnosed clients. *International Journal of Self Help and Self Care.* 2005; **3**: 63–71.

37 Noordsy DL, Schwab B, Fox L, *et al.* The role of self-help programs in the rehabilitation of persons with severe mental illness and substance use disorders. *Community Mental Health Journal.* 1996; **32**: 71–81.

38 Vogel HS, Knight E, Laudet, AB, *et al.* Double Trouble in Recovery: self-help for the dually diagnosed. *Psychiatric Rehabilitation Journal.* 1988; **21**: 356–64.

39 Hazelden Foundation. *The Dual Diagnosis Recovery Book.* Center City, MN: Hazelden; 1993.

40 Alcoholics Anonymous. *The AA Member-Medications and other Drugs.* New York: Alcoholics Anonymous World Services; 1984.

41 Narcotics Anonymous (NA). *Facts About NA.* Van Nuys, CA: Narcotics Anonymous World Services; 2008. Available at: www.na/org (accessed 13 August 2010).

42 Meissen G, Powell TJ, Wituk SA, *et al.* Attitudes of AA contact persons toward group participation by persons with a mental illness. *Psychiatric Services.* 1999; **50**: 1079–81.

43 Bogenschutz MP. 12-step approaches for the dually diagnosed: mechanisms of change. *Alcoholism: clinical and experimental research.* 2007; **31**(Suppl. 3): S64–6.

44 Jordan LC, Davidson WS, Herman SE, *et al.* Involvement in 12 step programs among persons with dual diagnosis. *Psychiatric Services.* 2002; **53**: 894–6.

45 DiNitto DM, Webb DK, Rubin A, *et al.* Self-help group meeting attendance among clients with dual diagnosis. *Journal of Psychoactive Drugs.* 2001; **33**: 263–72.

46 Bogenschutz M, Akin S. 12-Step participation and attitudes towards 12-step meetings in dual diagnosis patients. *Alcoholism Treatment Quarterly.* 2000; **18**: 31–45.

47 Moggi F, Ouimette PC, Moos RH, *et al.* Dual diagnosis patients in substance abuse treatment: relationship of general coping and substance-specific coping to 1-year outcomes. *Addiction.* 1999; **94**: 1805–16.

48 Ritsher JB, McKellar JD, Finney JW, *et al.* Psychiatric comorbidity, continuing care and mutual help as predictors of five-year remission from substance use disorders. *Journal of Studies on Alcohol.* 2002; **63**: 709–15.

49 Brooks AJ, Penn PE. Comparing treatments for dual diagnosis: twelve-step and self-management and recovery training. *American Journal of Drug Alcohol Abuse.* 2003; **29**: 359–83.

50 Bogenschutz MP. Specialized 12-Step programs and 12-Step facilitation for the dually-diagnosed. *Community Mental Health Journal.* 2005; **41**: 7–19.

51 Vogel H. *How to Start a Double Trouble in Recovery Group: a guide for professionals.* Center City, MN: Hazelden; 2010.

52 Magura S. Effectiveness of dual focus mutual aid for co-occurring substance use and mental health disorders: a review and synthesis of the 'Double Trouble' in Recovery evaluation. *Journal of Substance Use and Misuse.* 2008; **43**: 1904–26.

53 Magura S, Cleland C, Vogel HS, *et al.* Effects of 'dual focus' mutual aid on self-efficacy for recovery and quality of life. *Administration and Policy in Mental Health and Mental Health Services Research.* 2007; **34**: 1–12.

54 Laudet AB. The impact of alcoholics anonymous on other substance abuse-related twelve-step programs. *Recent Developments in Alcoholism.* 2008; **18**: 71–89.

55 Vogel H. Executive Director of DTR. Personal communication; 29 October 2009.

56 Reggie W. Personal communication; 29 October 2009.

57 Laudet AB, Magura S, Vogel HS, *et al.* Recovery challenges among dually diagnosed individuals. *Journal of Substance Abuse Treatment.* 2000; **18**: 321–9.

58 Laudet AB, Magura S, Cleland CM, *et al.* Predictors of retention in dual-focus self-help groups. *Community Mental Health Journal.* 2003; **39**: 281–97.

59 Laudet AB, Magura S, Cleland CM, *et al.* The effect of 12-step based fellowship participation on abstinence among dually diagnosed persons: a two-year longitudinal study. *Journal of Psychoactive Drugs.* 2004; **36**: 207–16.

60 Velligan DI, Weiden PJ, Sajatovic M, *et al.* Expert Consensus Panel on Adherence Problems in Serious and Persistent Mental Illness. The expert consensus guideline series: adherence problems in patients with serious and persistent mental illness. *Journal of Clinical Psychiatry.* 2009; **70**: 1–46.

61 Magura S, Laudet AB, Mahmood D, *et al.* Adherence to medication regimens and participation in dual-focus self-help groups. *Psychiatric Services.* 2002; **53**: 310–16.

62 Magura S, Knight EL, Vogel HS, *et al.* Mediators of effectiveness in dual-focus self-help groups. *American Journal of Drug Alcohol Abuse.* 2003; **29**: 301–22.

63 Magura S, Laudet AB, Mahmood D, *et al.* Role of self-help processes in achieving abstinence among dually diagnosed persons. *Addictive Behaviours.* 2003; **28**: 399–413.

64 Laudet AB, Magura S, Vogel HS, *et al.* Support, mutual aid and recovery from dual diagnosis. *Community Mental Health Journal.* 2000; **36**: 457–76.

65 Moos RH. How and why twelve-step self-help groups are effective. *Recent Developments in Alcoholism.* 2008; **18**: 393–412.

66 Magura S, Rosenblum A, Villano CL, *et al.* Dual-focus mutual aid for co-occurring disorders: a quasi-experimental evaluation study. *American Journal of Drug and Alcohol Abuse.* 2008; **34**: 61–74.

67 Villano CL, Rosenblum A, Magura S, *et al.* Challenges to implementing a 12-step group for dually diagnosed consumers. Oral presentation at the 113th Convention of the American Psychological Association (APA); 18–23 Aug 2005; Washington, DC.

68 Magura S, Villano CL, Rosenblum A, *et al.* Consumer evaluation of dual focus mutual aid. *Journal of Dual Diagnosis.* 2008; **4**: 170–85.

TO LEARN MORE

- Vogel H. Double Trouble. In: *Recovery: basic guide.* Center City, MN: Hazelden; 2010.
- Vogel H. *How to Start a Double Trouble in Recovery Group: a guide for professionals.* Center City, MN: Hazelden; 2010.
- Most of the peer-reviewed journal articles on Double Trouble in Recovery are cited on

Pubmed.gov. A list of these articles (which links to the abstract and, in most cases, to the full text article) are available at: http://doubletroubleinrecovery.org/research.htm

- A review of Double Trouble in Recovery can be found on the website of the National Registry of Evidence-Based Programs (NREPP). Available at: www.nrepp.samhsa.gov/ViewIntervention. aspx?id=13

    NREPP is a searchable online registry of more than 160 interventions supporting mental health promotion, substance abuse prevention, and mental health and substance abuse treatment. NREPP connects members of the public to intervention developers so they can learn how to implement these approaches in their communities.

ACKNOWLEDGEMENT

This literature review was supported by the grant: Efficacy of 'Dual Focus' Mutual Aid for Persons with Co-Occurring Disorders (R01 DA023119, S. Magura, Principal Investigator).

CHAPTER 15

Empowering life choices

Catherine Dixon

INTRODUCTION

The Empower Your Life programme was written to complement existing aftercare services. Maintaining abstinence from alcohol successfully post-rehabilitation depends on the individual developing a reliable interpersonal support network, powerful coping mechanisms and a personal commitment to abstinence.

Much of what is currently available to the individual in recovery involves relapse prevention groups or Alcoholics Anonymous. This programme focuses on what the individual is going to do with his/her life now the person is no longer dependent on alcohol or other substances – this aftercare treatment focuses on relapse prevention. There is a need for practical life skills that increase confidence by setting goals and asking the individual to commit to the goals. This is the first programme that has addressed these issues in a group setting and takes the individual through those steps.

The idea of putting together a programme such as this came from asking the individual about how they filled their time now they did not drink. This included an enquiry on how people put their lives together after major trauma. In almost all the cases of success there was an imperative to change, to re-examine assumptions about life and to start taking personal responsibility for outcomes, i.e. understanding that the decision not to drink was theirs and their alone. It was clear that those who had successfully created a new life had created inspiring goals and had a powerful internal motivation to fulfil those goals. The individual also builds up self-empowerment skills (self-reliance, confidence, accountability, awareness, ability to set and commit to goals, ability to learn new skills and adapt and change to different circumstances). Most of all they learn now to motivate themselves.

The interventions most needed were ones of support and guidance and providing the individual with powerful tools so she/he could learn to apply them in their lives.

The authors work in the private sector was almost exclusively on goal-setting and providing a coaching and mentoring facility to the individual. It seemed that when the individual committed to goals they got better quicker, and that what she/he needed was a space to formulate the goals and a process of accountability offered in the group setting. It appears that this innovative programme may be the first of its kind.

Consistent anecdotal feedback from several hundred individuals over three years of practice in well-being groups suggested that there is an imperative for the individuals to feel better about the present, and to believe that the future can be different. Without the support of alcohol, individuals are left with either a complete void or a mass of uncomfortable feelings and emotions to manage, and an uncertainty and pessimism about the future. Feeling good about oneself requires emotional, physical and psychological stability and an empowered sense of identity. This requires a change in mindset, attitudes and beliefs as well as a different perspective on how to relate to the idea of the future. Change is always problematic when the means of obtaining that change are unknown and the benefits of undergoing such a change process uncertain.

Empower Your Life is not therapy or counselling. It is an educational programme that delivers a methodology for change and transformation. The individuals are informed that the programme is not therapy and that it has an educational focus. The individual is requested to sign a confidentiality agreement with terms of engagement that need to be respected if she/he chooses to participate in the programme. The individual needs to be assessed by the key-worker to establish whether he/she has reached a suitable level of sustained recovery for this to be of benefit. If the individual is not ready, embarking on Empowering Your Life could be destabilising.

Empower Your Life is a challenging programme – it is a call to action. The problem with setting goals and not fulfilling them is that it can reinforce a negative programming that 'nothing works for me' that damages self-esteem and develops an attitude of learned helplessness, which is counterproductive to successful learning and successful outcomes. It is better to wait until the individual is ready to do this programme than to introduce it to them too early.

Learning from practice experience, and in order to address these needs, the author wrote a complementary foundation programme called Empower Your Health. This is a step-by-step approach through following practical advice and processes to commit to daily actions that start to lay down some good habits that are essential to acquire stability. This is proving very popular because it provides the individual with practical tools to embed good habits or self-care into their lives, and a stepping stone and preparation towards the Empower Your Life Goal Setting Programme.

OBJECTIVES

The programme objective is to help the individual develop self-reliance and independence in maintaining and sustaining abstinence/safe drinking patterns. Other objectives include:

➤ to present an empowering framework that supports the desire to remain abstinent
➤ to enable the individual to identify her/his motivating life goals
➤ to equip the individual with information, resources and tools enabling him/her to achieve the desired goal
➤ to increase confidence in independent coping mechanisms
➤ to establish a daily personal practice and develop a self-care routine

> to create a peer support system and feedback loop during the programme, and maintain this support system after the programme, through monthly meetings
> evaluate feedback pre- and post-programme.

BENEFITS OF PROGRAMME

Benefits of the Empower Your Life programme are:
> It complies with the drive for aftercare programmes to include the individual.
> The strategies place the responsibility of recovery on the individual rather than on an external authority, thereby instilling a sense of personal responsibility.
> Group dynamics focus on creating a mutually supportive environment with less focus on individuals and analysis of personal stories.
> It is highly solution focused.
> The programme runs within a set time frame so it can be accessed by a greater number of individuals throughout the year.
> It complements other treatment interventions, such as counselling, key-worker sessions, meditation and well-being groups.
> Pre- and post-evaluation and weekly feedback continually assesses progress from the individual's perspective.
> Monthly peer supervision groups monitor progress and provide the individuals with further support.
> It introduces empowering concepts, such as mindfulness, creating positive intention, developing individual awareness, value-centred goal-setting and embodiment.

DELIVERY

Delivery of the programme includes:
> weekly modular handouts
> presentation of material
> group discussion
> pair work and group work
> visualisation and consolidation
> task-setting between modules to be completed during the week.

THEORY AND CONTENT

The theory underpinning the concepts and contents presented in the programme are adapted from the fields of:
> positive psychology
> neurolinguistic programming
> cognitive behavioural therapy
> performance coaching
> hypnotherapy
> energy therapies (Chi Kung Emotional Freedom Technique[1]) and phenomenology.

They are included because of efficacy, feedback and successful involvement by the individual. The major themes are:

➤ presenting information that supports the mind/body connection and the link between physical, mental and emotional health
➤ developing a robust sense of personal acceptance, awareness and commitment to personal growth
➤ identification of values and beliefs and individual needs
➤ introduction of the value-driven decision and goal-setting process
➤ setting life goals linked to specific measurable outcomes
➤ creating mental stability with mindfulness, meditation and visualisation.

This material is presented and practised during the programme to encourage the individual to develop a daily personal practice that integrates exercise, healthy eating and lifestyle and rituals. This helps maintain a positive outlook and emotional stability until well-being becomes a reinforced habit and the preferred way of relating to themselves and others.

Module one

Module one presents a theoretical model of how negative thinking impacts emotions and well-being. This model draws on cognitive behavioural therapy which maintains that feelings, whether good or bad, are the direct product of good or bad thoughts, and consequently produce an emotional response.

Module one presents core research from the field of positive psychology[2] and the factors that contribute to feelings of happiness, such as the need to identify personal strengths and a supportive personal value system. The individual is presented with the information regarding the mind–body link and phenomenology – namely that our energy levels directly correlate to our mental, emotional and physical health, and that improving levels of energy has a positive impact in all areas of our well-being. Therefore the concept of positive thinking is not to deny uncomfortable feelings or personal difficulties but to raise the energy system of the individual, thereby improving her/his ability to cope with stressful conditions.

Module two

Module two builds awareness of core strengths and attributes – the recognition of which is important in building self-esteem and self-awareness. This module also encourages the individual to identify vulnerabilities and the internal and external factors that both contribute to and drain his/her personal strengths. Individuals start to gain insight and awareness of patterns that need strengthening and unhelpful patterns that do not contribute to well-being. This module also invites the individual to examine core values and beliefs that support those values.

Module three

Module three takes the individual though an envisioning process that combines values with desires – what they most wish for in their life and how to create overall well-being. This builds awareness of a higher level of existence and demonstrates how what the individual wishes to create in his/her life – whether positive or negative – manifests at some level. The individual articulates this vision in positive and affirmative language which reinforces a positive sense of identity. These wishes are also mapped out against the GROW model:[3]

➤ **G**oal
➤ **R**eality
➤ **O**ptions
➤ **W**ill

. . . wheel of life which identifies the core areas of life that affect human stability and growth.

Module four

Module four enables the individual to translate her/his vision into goal-setting. The individual is presented with best practice models of goal-setting adapted from neurolinguistic programming's outcome setting, SMART goals:[4]

➤ **S**trategic and **S**pecific – the goal should identify a specific action or event that will take place. Answers the questions: Who? and What?
➤ **M**easurable – include in the specific goal statement the measurements to be used to determine that the results or outcomes expected have been achieved. It answers the question: How?
➤ **A**ttainable – goals should challenge people to do their best, but they need also be achievable.
➤ **R**elevant/**R**igorous – goals need to pertain directly to the performance challenge being managed.
➤ **T**ime bound – enough time to achieve the goal, and not too much time, which can affect project performance. It answers the question: When?[4]

The individual is also presented with PRINCE2 project management guidelines.[5] The key features of PRINCE2 are:

➤ its focus on business justification
➤ a defined organisation structure for the project management team
➤ its product-based planning approach
➤ its emphasis on dividing the project into manageable and controllable stages
➤ its flexibility to be applied at a level appropriate to the project.[5]

The individual writes up her/his goals, which have a six-month time frame, and is encouraged to identify all the variables associated with the goals including deliverables, milestones, stakeholders and contingencies.

Module five

Module five introduces the individual to transformational tools that break through the resistance to the goal being fulfilled, namely lack of planning, insufficient motivation or lack of belief that the outcome can be achieved. Individuals are taught how to deeply relax their conscious mind to bypass critical thought so they can visualise themselves succeeding and achieving their goal. This reinforces the outcome in the subconscious mind. Emotional Freedom Technique[6] is introduced to deal with resistance in the form or sabotaging thoughts and negative beliefs.

Modules six and seven

Modules six and seven provide the individual with a range of techniques that help maintain a positive outlook and high levels of motivation. They include:
➤ planning days that do not overwhelm
➤ commitment strategies
➤ affirmations of positive intentions
➤ visual reminders of their goal
➤ listing and recognising achievements
➤ written statement of gratitude
➤ recognition of the progress made to date.

The deliberate cataloguing of this information keeps the mind attuned to what the individual is creating rather than past failures. Individuals learn that daily self-care strategies, rituals and habits enable them to sustain positive, gradual change.

FEEDBACK
January–March 2009: Empower Your Life 1

This feedback has been reproduced from the feedback sheets that were handed out on the final day of the first programme. Names are not included on the feedback form for reasons of confidentiality. The comments indicated that the group setting was very well received and that individuals appreciated the level of support, the techniques learnt, and what he/she learnt about themselves. Feedback questions included:
➤ Has this course met your expectations? Yes/No. Please provide a full explanation to either answer
➤ Did you find this course useful? Yes/No
➤ What aspects did you find the most useful?
➤ Will any of the material enable you to live your life differently? If yes, please specify which parts.
➤ Did you enjoy the programme? Yes/No
➤ Please provide any additional feedback you have concerning course contents, delivery, structure or anything else you would like to tell us.

There were between four and six participants in each group. Written feedback was taken after each session. Empowerment is a process rather than a measurement so the comments were more significant than anything else was. The comments reflected that the individual appreciated the content of the information and the practicality of the exercises that they could apply into their lives. The comments reflected that the need to provide practical tools and exercises to reinforce the skills needed to acquire empowerment and this was the aspect of the course that was most appreciated by participants.

One individual commented that the programme actually delivered what had been described. Another said that all the elements of the programme helped create a personal practice and commitment to stability. Attendance was very good, as was timekeeping and punctuality. Commitment to the process was one of the embedded skills learnt as a result of attending this programme.

All members completed tasks set as homework, including a keeping a weekly journal. All individuals remained stable/abstinent during the programme and stated it was their intention to remain stable/abstinent.

All mentioned that the Empower Your Life programme complemented the treatment they had received in the well-being acupuncture group (one provides intervention and treatment and the other a framework for self-development).

RECOMMENDATIONS

The evaluation produced several recommendations for future development of this service provision.

1 Ensure that the well-being group and the Empower Your Life programme is a core component of aftercare services.
2 Publish the resource booklet of the self-care strategies and health information and distribute out to *all* individuals accessing the aftercare services.
3 Write an additional section containing up-to-date information about where the individual can access further low-cost or free services in various districts and boroughs, such as yoga, meditation, etc. This would be extremely useful and can be developed with the individuals' participation.
4 Provide the individual with audio materials so that he/she can listen to the material presented as this reinforces core concepts of transformational thinking.
5 Provide individuals with a video of the Chi Kung exercises as part of the self-care plan.
6 Provide monthly follow-up meetings for all individuals to discuss progress.

CONCLUSION

The efficacy of the Empower Your Life approach to aftercare is still being developed and redefined. However, the feedback is encouraging and appears to support that this approach can open up the mind to a different way of thinking, which in turn leads to different habits and different choices.

The tools on this programme are life skills, coping mechanisms, and a way of structuring goals so the individual can identify potential hazards and deal with them effectively. The Empower Your Life programme could be adapted to most existing aftercare services such as well-being groups, complementary therapies, one-to-one support, life skills and relapse prevention.

There is a need to undertake a full-scale evaluation of the programme, but it is hoped that this will introduce the approach to those able to undertake appropriately funded research. It is recognised that this approach will not suit all. However, it may be an important tool for individuals experiencing mental health–substance use concerns and dilemmas.

REFERENCES

1 Dixon C. *Versatility of EFT Applications.* Available at: www.energyroots.co.uk/articles/Versatility%20of%20EFT%20Applications%20Article.pdf (accessed 14 August 2010).
2 Positive Psychology Center, University of Pennsylvania. Available at: www.ppc.sas.upenn.edu (accessed 29 December 2010).

3 Mind Tools. The GROW model. Available at: www.mindtools.com/pages/article/newLDR_89.htm (accessed 14 August 2010).

4 SMART goals. Available at: www.smart-goals.org (accessed 14 August 2010).

5 PRINCE2: Projects in Controlled Environments. Available at: www.prince2.com/what-is-prince2.asp

6 Emotional Freedom Techniques. Available at: www.eftuniverse.com (accessed 14 August 2010).

TO LEARN MORE

- For more information please contact Catherine Dixon – Tel: 020 8998 8556. Email: info@energyroots.co.uk

Useful chapters

The *Mental Health–Substance Use* series comprises six books. To develop knowledge and understanding, chapters are interlinked, building and exploring specific areas. It is hoped the following will help readers locate relevant chapters easily.

BOOK 1: INTRODUCTION TO MENTAL HEALTH–SUBSTANCE USE

BOOK 2: DEVELOPING SERVICES IN MENTAL HEALTH–SUBSTANCE USE

Useful contacts

Collated by Jo Cooper

Addiction Arena – www.addictionarena.com
Addiction Medicine – http://listserv.icors.org/SCRIPTS/WA-ICORS.
   EXE?A0=ADD_MED
The Addiction Project – www.theaddictionproject.com
Addiction Rehabilitation Facilities – www.arf.org/isd/bib/mental.html
Addiction Technology Transfer Center (ATTC) Network– www.attcnetwork.org
Addiction Today – www.addictiontoday.org
ADDICT-L List – http://listserv.kent.edu/archives/addict-l.html
Alcohol and Alcohol Problems Science Database – http://etoh.niaaa.nih.gov
Alcohol and Drug History Society – http://historyofalcoholanddrugs.typepad.com
Alcohol Concern (64 Leman Street, London E1 8EU, UK; Tel: 020 7264 0510;
   Fax: 020 7488 9213; Email: contact@alcoholconcern.org.uk) – www.alcoholconcern.
   org.uk/servlets/home
Alcohol Drugs and Development – www.add-resources.org
Alcohol Focus Scotland – www.alcohol-focus-scotland.org.uk
Alcohol Misuse (Department of Health) – www.dh.gov.uk/en/Publichealth/
   Healthimprovement/Alcoholmisuse/index.htm
Alcohol Misuse List – www.jiscmail.ac.uk/lists/ALCOHOL- MISUSE.html
Alcohol, other Drugs and Health: current evidence – www.bu.edu/
   aodhealth/index.html
Alcohol Policy Network – www.apolnet.ca
Alcohol Reports – www.alcoholreports.blogspot.com
Alcoholics Anonymous – www.aa.org
Alcoholism and Substance Abuse Providers – www.asapnys.org
American Association of Colleges of Nursing. *Tool Kit for Cultural Competent*
   Baccalaureate Nurses; 2008. (This site will soon have a toolkit for graduate education
   as well.) – www.aacn.nche.edu/Education/pdf/toolkit.pdf
American Psychiatric Association – www.psych.org
American Society of Addiction Medicine – www.asam.org/CMEonline.html
Australasian Professional Society on Alcohol and other Drugs – www.apsad.org.au
Australian Drug Foundation – www.adf.org.au
Australian Drug Information Network – www.adin.com.au

Australian Government Department of Health and Ageing:
> Alcohol – www.alcohol.gov.au
> Illicit drugs – www.health.gov.au/internet/main/publishing.nsf/content/healthpubhlth-strateg-drugs-illicit-index.htm
> Mental health publications – www.health.gov.au/internet/main/publishing.nsf/Content/mental-pubs

Berman Institute of Bioethics – www.bioethicsinstitute.org

Best Practice Portal – www.emcdda.europa.eu/best-practice

BioMed Central – www.biomedcentral.com

Brain Injury Australia – www.bia.net.au

Brain Trauma Foundation – www.braintrauma.org

Brief Addiction Science Information Source (BASIS) – www.basisonline.org

Campaign for Effective Prevention and Treatment of Addiction – www.solutionstodrugs.com

CASA: The National Centre on Addiction and Substance Abuse – www.casacolumbia.org

Centre for Addiction and Mental Health – www.camh.net

Centre for Clinical and Academic Workforce Innovation (Tel: 01623 819140; Email: ccawi@lincoln.ac.uk) – www.lincoln.ac.uk/ccawi

Centre for Evidence-based Mental Health (CEBMH) – www.cebmh.com

Centre for HIV and Sexual Health, Sheffield Primary Care NHS Trust – www.sexualhealthsheffield.nhs.uk

Centre for Independent Thought – www.centerforindependentthought.org

Centre for Mental Health – www.centreformentalhealth.org.uk

Clan Unity – www.clan-unity.co.uk

Clifford Beers Foundation. *Promotion of Mental Health*, vol. 1 (1992) – www.cliffordbeersfoundation.co.uk/jcont91.htm

Committee on Publication Ethics – http://publicationethics.org

Communities of Practice for Local Government – www.communities.idea.gov.uk

Community Nursing Network – www.communitynursingnetwork.org

Co-morbid Mental Health and Substance Misuse in Scotland – www.scotland.gov.uk/Publications/2006/06/05104841/0

Co-occurring Centre for Excellence (US) – www.coce.samhsa.gov

Co-occurring Mental and Substance Abuse Disorders: a guide for mental health planning and advisory councils (2003) – www.namhpac.org/PDFs/CO.pdf

Creative Commons – http://creativecommons.org

Cultural Competency in Health: a guide for policy, partnership and participation (2005) – www.nhmrc.gov.au/publications/synopses/hp25syn.htm

Daily Dose: drug and alcohol news from around the world. (This website is no longer in continuous service, but the archives are still available.) – http://dailydose.net

Dartmouth Psychiatric Research Centre – http://dms.dartmouth.edu/~prc

Department of Health – www.dh.gov.uk

Department of Primary Health Care – www.primarycare.ox.ac.uk/research/dipex

Doctors.net.uk – www.doctors.net.uk

Double Trouble in Recovery: http://doubletroubleinrecovery.org
> A list of peer-reviewed journal articles on Double Trouble in Recovery: http://doubletroubleinrecovery.org/research.html

Citations for biomedical literature published in peer- reviewed journals. Most citations resulting from a search for Double Trouble in Recovery link to the full text article: www.ncbi.nlm.nih.gov/pubmed

Drink and Drugs News – www.drinkanddrugs.net

Drinks Media Wire – www.drinksmediawire.com

Drug and Alcohol Findings – http://findings.org.uk

Drug and Alcohol Nurses of Australia – www.danaonline.org

Drug and Alcohol Services South Australia – www.dassa.sa.gov.au

Drug Day Programmes list – http://health.groups.yahoo.com/group/drug_day_programmes

DrugInfo Clearinghouse – http://druginfo.adf.org.au

Drug Misuse Information Scotland – www.drugmisuse.isdscotland.org

Drug Misuse Research list – www.jiscmail.ac.uk/lists/DRUG- MISUSE-RESEARCH.html

Drugs and Mental Health –www.thesite.org/drinkanddrugs/drugsafety/drugsandyourbody/drugsandmentalhealth

Drug Talk list – http://lists.sublimeip.com/mailman/listinfo/drugtalk

Drugtext Internet Library – www.drugtext.org

Dual Diagnosis – www.hoseahouse.org/infirmary/dualdx.html

Dual Diagnosis: Australia and New Zealand – www.dualdiagnosis.org.au

Dual Diagnosis Toolkit – www.rethink.org/dualdiagnosis/toolkit.html

Dual Diagnosis Website – http://users.erols.com/ksciacca

Enter Mental Health: www.entermentalhealth.net

European Alcohol Policy Alliance – www.eurocare.org

European Association for the Treatment of Addiction – www.eata.org.uk

European Federation of Nurses Associations – www.efnweb.org

European Monitoring Centre for Drugs and Drug Addiction – www.emcdda.europa.eu

European Working Group on Drugs Oriented Research – www.dass.stir.ac.uk/old-site/sections/scot-ad/ewodor.htm

Evidence-based Practice websites – http://davisplus.fadavis.com/purnell/evidence_based_weblinks.cfm

Eye Movement Desensitisation and Reprocessing Training Workshops – www.emdrworkshops.com

Faces and Voices of Recovery – www.facesandvoicesofrecovery.org

Federation of Drug and Alcohol Professionals – www.fdap.org.uk/certification/dap.html

Gambling International list – http://health.groups.yahoo.com/group/GamblingIssuesInternational/join?

Global Alcohol Harm Reduction Network – http://groups.google.com/group/gahrnet

Global Health Council – www.globalhealth.org

Guardian UK: The most useful websites on dual diagnosis – http://society.guardian.co.uk/mentalhealth/page/0,8149,688817,00.html

Headway – www.headway.org.uk

Health and Safety Executive (HSE) – www.hse.gov.uk/stress

HIT – www.hit.org.uk

Horatio: European Psychiatric Nurses – www.horatio-web.eu

Hub of Commissioned Alcohol Projects and Policies (HubCAPP) (This is an online resource of local alcohol initiatives throughout England and Wales.) – www.hubcapp.org.uk

Inexcess: in search of recovery – www.inexcess.tv

International Brain Injury Association – www.internationalbrain.org
International Centre for Alcohol Policies – www.icap.org
International Council of Nurses – www.icn.ch
International Council on Alcohol and Addictions – www.icaa.ch
International Drug Policy Consortium – www.idpc.net
International Harm Reduction Association – www.ihra.net
International Network on Brief Interventions for Alcohol Problems (INEBRIA) –
    www.inebria.net
International Nurses Society on Addictions – www.intnsa.org
International Society for the Study of Drug Policy – www.issdp.org
International Society of Addiction Journal Editors – www.parint.org/isajewebsite/
Intervoice: the International Community for Hearing Voices – www.intervoiceonline.org
IVO: scientific institute in lifestyle, addiction and related social developments –
    www.ivo.nl
James Lind Alliance Guidebook – www.jlaguidebook.org
James Lind Library – www.jameslindlibrary.org
Join Together: advancing effective alcohol and drug policy, prevention and treatment –
    www.jointogether.org
Madness and Literature Network – www.madnessandliterature.org
Medical Council on Alcohol – www.m-c-a.org.uk
Medline Plus – www.nlm.nih.gov/medlineplus/dualdiagnosis.html
Mental Health (About.com) – http://mentalhealth.about.com
Mental Health and Addiction 101 (Centre for Addiction and Mental Health, Canada) –
    www.camh.net/MHA101/
Mental Health Europe – www.mhe-sme.org/en.html
Mental Health First Aid: Australia – www.mhfa.com.au
Mental Health First Aid: Canada – www.mentalhealthfirstaid.ca
Mental Health First Aid: England – www.mhfaengland.org.uk
Mental Health First Aid: Hong Kong – www.mhfa.org.hk
Mental Health First Aid: Scotland – www.smhfa.com
Mental Health First Aid: Singapore – www.mhfa.sg
Mental Health First Aid: South Africa – www.mhfasa.co.za
Mental Health First Aid: USA – www.thenationalcouncil.org/cs/program_overview
Mental Health First Aid: Wales – www.mhfa-wales.org.uk
Mental Health Forum – www.mentalhealthforum.net/forum
Mental Health Foundation – www.mentalhealth.org.uk
Mental Health in Higher Education – www.mhhe.heacademy.ac.uk/sitepages/
    educators/?edid=239
Mental Health Information for All (RCPSYCH) – www.rcpsych.ac.uk/
    mentalhealthinfoforall.aspx
*Mental Health Policy Implementation Guide: dual diagnosis good practice
    guide* (2002) – www.dh.gov.uk/en/Publicationsandstatistics/Publications/
    PublicationsPolicyAndGuidance/DH_4009058
Mental Health Research Network – http://homepages.ed.ac.uk/mhrn
The Mentor Foundation – www.mentorfoundation.org
The Methadone Alliance Forum – www.m-alliance.org.uk/forum.html
Middlesex University Dual Diagnosis Courses – www.mdx.ac.uk/courses/postgraduate/
    nursing_midwifery_health/index/aspx

MIND: for better mental health – www.mind.org.uk

Ministry of Justice: National Offender Management Service – www.justice.gov.uk/about/noms.htm

Mood Disorders Association of Canada – www.mooddisorderscanada.ca

Motivational Interventions for Drugs and Alcohol Misuse in Schizophrenia – www.midastrial.ac.uk

Motivational Interviewing – www.motivationalinterview.org

National Alliance on Mental Illness (US) – www.nami.org

National Centre for Education and Training on Addiction Australia – www.nceta.flinders.edu.au

National Comorbidity Initiative Australia – www.health.gov.au/internet/main/publishing.nsf/Content/health-pubhlth-publicat-document-metadata-comorbidity.htm

National Consortium of Consultant Nurses in Dual Diagnosis and Substance Use – www.dualdiagnosis.co.uk

National Drug and Alcohol Research Centre – http://ndarc.med.unsw.edu.au

National Drug Research Institute – http://ndri.curtin.edu.au

National Health Service – www.nhs.uk

National Health Service Litigation Authority – www.nhsla.com

National Institute for Health and Clinical Excellence (Midcity Place, 71 High Holborn, London, WC1V 6NA, UK; Tel: 0845 003 7780; Fax: 0845 003 7784; Email: nice@nice.org.uk) – www.nice.org.uk

National Institute of Mental Health – www.nimh.nih.gov

National Institute on Alcohol Abuse and Alcoholism (NIAAA) (5635 Fishers Lane, MSC 9304, Bethesda, MD 20892-9304, USA; Tel: 301-443-3860; Email: www.niaaa.nih.gov/ContactUs.htm) – www.niaaa.nih.gov

National Institute on Drug Abuse, National Institutes of Health (6001 Executive Boulevard, Room 5213, Bethesda, MD 20892-9561, USA; Tel: 301-443-1124; Email: information@nida.nih.gov) – www.nida.nih.gov

National Treatment Agency for Substance Misuse – www.nta.nhs.uk

New Directions in the Study of Alcohol – www.newdirections.org.uk

New South Wales Health Dual Disorders resources – www.druginfo.nsw.gov.au/illicit_drugs

NHS Institute for Innovation and Improvement – www.institute.nhs.uk

Nordic Council for Alcohol and Drug Research (NAD) – www.norden.org/en/areas-of-co-operation/alcohol-and-drugs

O'Grady CP, Skinner WJ. *A Family Guide to Concurrent Disorders* (2007) – www.camh.net/Publications/Resources_for_Professionals/Partnering_with_families/partnering_families_famguide.pdf

Ontario Mental Health and Addictions Knowledge Exchange Network – www.ehealthontario.ca/portal/server.pt?open=512&objID=1398&PageID=0&mode=2

Oxford Centre for Neuroethics – www.neuroethics.ox.ac.uk

Partnership in Coping – www.pinc-recovery.com

Progress: National Consortium of Consultant Nurses in Dual Diagnosis and Substance Use – www.dualdiagnosis.co.uk

Promoting Adult Learning – www.niace.org.uk/current-work/area/mental-health

Psychiatric Nursing – www.citypsych.com/index.html

Psychminded – www.psychminded.co.uk

Public Access (National Institutes of Health) – http://publicaccess.nih.gov/index.htm

Recovery Workshop – www.recoveryworkshop.com

Rethink (UK) – www.rethink.org/dualdiagnosis

Royal College of General Practitioners – www.rcgp.org.uk

Royal College of Psychiatrists – www.rcpsych.ac.uk

Royal College of Psychiatrists. *Changing Minds Campaign* – www.rcpsych.ac.uk/
campaigns/previouscampaigns/changingminds.aspx

Royal Society for the encouragement of Arts, Manufactures and Commerce (RSA) –
www.thersa.org

Sacred Space Foundation – www.sacredspace.org.uk

SANE Australia – www.sane.org

Schizophrenia Society of Canada – www.schizophrenia.ca

Scholarship Society – www.scholarshipsociety.org

Scottish Addiction Studies – www.dass.stir.ac.uk/sections/showsection.php?id=4

Scottish Addiction Studies Library – www.drugslibrary.stir.ac.uk

Social Care Institute for Excellence – www.scie.org.uk

Social Care Online – www.scie-socialcareonline.org.uk

Society for the Study of Addiction – www.addiction-ssa.org

Spanish Peaks Mental Health Centre – www.spmhc.org

Stigma in Mental Health and Addiction – www.cmhanl.ca/pdf/Stigma.pdf

Substance Abuse and Mental Health Center toolkit for integrated treatment for
co-occurring disorders – http://mentalhealth.samhsa.gov/cmhs/CommunitySupport/
toolkits/cooccurring

Substance Abuse and Mental Health Data Archive – www.icpsr.umich.edu/SAMHDA

Substance Abuse and Mental Health Services Administration – www.samhsa.gov

Substance Misuse Management in General Practice – www.smmgp.org.uk

The International Network of Nurses (TINN) – www.tinnurses.org

The Management Standards Consultancy – www.themsc.org

Therapeutic Communities list – www.jiscmail.ac.uk/lists/
THERAPEUTICCOMMUNITIES.html

Think Cultural Health: bridging the healthcare gap through cultural competence
continuing education. (This site, developed by the US Department of Minority
Health, has continuing education modules for physicians, nurses and other healthcare
providers, and the Health Care Languages Implementation Guide.) – www.
thinkculturalhealth.org and https://hclsig.thinkculturalhealth.hhs.gov

Tidal Model – www.tidal-model.com

Tilburg University, Department of Tranzo – www.uvt.nl/tranzo

Toc H – www.toch-uk.org.uk

Treatment Improvement Exchange – www.treatment.org

Trimbos Institute: Netherlands Institute on Mental Health and Addiction –
www.trimbos.org

Turning Point – www.turning-point.co.uk

Tx Director – www.txdirector.com

UK Database of Uncertainties about the Effects of Treatment – www.library.nhs.uk/
DUETs/Default.aspx

UK Drug Policy Commission – www.ukdpc.org.uk

UNGASS: United Nations General Assembly Special Session on the World Drug Problem
– www.ungassondrugs.org

United Nations Office on Drugs and Crime – www.unodc.org

University of Toronto Joint Centre for Bioethics Centre for Addiction and Mental Health Bioethics Service – www.jointcentreforbioethics.ca/partners/camh.shtml

Update: an alcohol and other drugs information bulletin board –http://lists.sublimeip.com/mailman/listinfo/update

US Department of Health and Human Services. *Co-occurring Mental and Substance Abuse Disorders: a guide for mental health planning and advisory councils* (2003) – www.namhpac.org/PDFs/CO.pdf

Victorian Alcohol and Drug Association – www.vaada.org.au

Web of Addictions: links to other websites related to addiction – www.well.com/user/woa/aodsites.htm

Wired In to Recovery: empowering people to tackle substance use problems – http://wiredin.org.uk

World Health Organization: Climate change and human health – www.who.int/globalchange/en

World Health Organization: Management of substance abuse – www.who.int/substanceabuse/en

World Health Organization: Mental health – www.who.int/mental_health/policy/en

World Medical Association – www.wma.net/en/10home/index.html

Youth Drug Support, Australia – www.yds.org.au

Youth Health Talk – www.youthtalkonline.com

Index